The Jossey-Bass Health Care Series brings together the most current information and ideas in health care from the leaders in the field. Titles from the Jossey-Bass Health Care Series include these essential health care resources:

GLOBAL
HEALTH CARE MARKETS

GLOBAL
HEALTH CARE
MARKETS

A Comprehensive Guide to Regions, Trends, and Opportunities Shaping the International Health Arena

Walter W. Wieners, Editor

Foreword by Marion J. Ball

Sponsored by the
Academy for International Health Studies

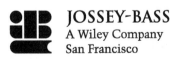

JOSSEY-BASS
A Wiley Company
San Francisco

Jossey-Bass books and products are available through most bookstores. To contact Jossey-Bass
directly, call (888) 378-2537, fax to (800) 605-2665, or visit our website at www.josseybass.com.

Substantial discounts on bulk quantities of Jossey-Bass books are available to corporations,
professional associations, and other organizations. For details and discount information, contact
the special sales department at Jossey-Bass.

Library of Congress Cataloging-in-Publication Data

Global health care markets: a comprehensive guide to regions, trends, and opportunities
shaping the international health arena/Walter W. Wieners, editor; foreword by Marion
J. Ball.
     p. cm—(The Jossey-Bass health series)
    Includes bibliographical references and index.
     ISBN 978-0-7879-5307-2   ISBN 0-7879-5307-5 (alk. paper)
     1. Medical care—Marketing. 2. Medical policy. 3. Medical economics. I. Wieners,
Walter W. II. Series.

RA410.56.G59 2000
362.1—dc21   00-060179

FIRST EDITION
       10 9 8 7 6 5 4 3 2 1

CONTENTS

FIGURES AND TABLES

Figures

Tables

FOREWORD

As we begin the new century, we are accumulating more and more evidence that the world is no longer regional. We have evolved into one world with a global economy—a world in which individual citizens have unprecedented means to traverse cities, nations, and continents. Health care has felt the effects of this shift. As population mobility increases, our countries' borders are becoming largely invisible, bringing the health status of the world under one umbrella. Along with this mega-change comes the opportunity to learn from the policy and managerial changes that are occurring and understand how businesses and the public sector can work together to improve health care delivery.

This book encompasses a broad cross-section of health care systems around the world, examining such timely topics as policy reforms and factors affecting health care in the new century. Each contributor has described a system's organizational and financial issues, some of which address the legislation and regulatory issues dominating different parts of the world. Even though the countries and regions differ in some ways, a striking number of similarities come to light.

Additional chapters cover such topics as (1) comparing global health care systems, (2) exporting a brand of private health care insurance, (3) using e-commerce to improve administration and delivery of care, (4) accreditation, (5) benefiting from an insurance case study, and (6) understanding trade regulations.

Contributors to this book have also worked to address the globalization of health care and its implications. They highlight the importance of using the enabling technologies developed during the second half of the twentieth century to change health care in the twenty-first century. Finally, they demonstrate how the "business" of health care delivery will be transformed, just as the day-to-day professional activities of other industries have been transformed by technological advancement.

The book's title, *Global Health Care Markets: A Comprehensive Guide to Regions, Trends, and Opportunities Shaping the International Health Arena,* skillfully captures its thrust. As a meaningful primer of global issues in health care, this work is a must-read for educators, business readers, and health care professionals involved in all levels of the new global health market. This volume not only addresses such crucial issues as improving health care delivery and seizing the business opportunities to do so, it also underscores what organizations must do to bring about the changes that will transform health care in the twenty-first century.

Special congratulations and thanks go to all the contributors for bringing so much thoughtful knowledge to the readers fortunate enough to study its contents. As the health care industry takes on monumental changes in the next few years, let us all do our part to provide access to the best care possible, thus improving the health status of all citizens of the world.

August 2000

Marion J. Ball
Baltimore, Maryland

PREFACE

The revolution in communications technologies has raised our hopes that earth's current patchwork of regions, nations, and states may yet become a true global community. The growing globalization of businesses and enterprises, facilitated by the communications revolution, leads us to conclude that the journey to a cooperative global community has already begun.

One sphere that stands most to benefit from globalization is health care. This book outlines the opportunities and pitfalls in global health and is intended to inform and enable individuals and organizations in health care who are searching for opportunity in the global arena.

Specifically, this book covers subjects that are essential to understanding the dynamics of global health systems: policy, financing, organization, leadership, and management. Regardless of the country, the health sector responds to the same political and financial pressures as other industries. The chapters that follow reveal differences in history and context that will give the reader insight into many different perspectives. This volume presents many of the factors that account for the diversity in health care systems and the resulting barriers to a global model for health care financing and delivery.

Purpose of the Book

Global Health Care Markets is a single-volume, geographically comprehensive guide to national health care policies and to the financing and delivery of health care in those nations. The book presents a practical business guide or tool for analyzing diverse systems and furthering discussions of the major trends affecting global health care. The reader can find information that will help private and public sector health care leaders learn from each others' experiences.

Readers can use this book in several ways. It can be a guide for businesses seeking to expand into the health care industry or entering new markets, as well as an educator's resource for learning, teaching, and conducting academic research.

The introduction to each section of *Global Health Care Markets* summarizes the relevant content and importance of the chapters within that section. The first section provides concrete analyses and perspective regarding such issues as these:

- Understanding diverse health care systems
- The fundamental health care economics of leading industrial nations
- The effects of the increasing role of private insurance and a related case study
- The effects of key trends (information technology and accreditation, for example) on many countries
- The impact of communications and information system technology
- Understanding regulatory environments and trade regulations

Following the first section, chapters provide comprehensive analyses of national health care systems throughout the world. Each chapter in Parts Two through Six focuses on a single country; each is written to help readers understand the following aspects of that country:

- The nation's health policy and health care financing and delivery systems
- Key historical events that shaped its health care sector as it is today
- Policy decisions expected to affect its health care sector in the future
- Market conditions and opportunities to provide products and services that would expand or enhance health care access and quality in that country

Each contributor was asked to conclude the chapter by expressing an opinion on future developments in the country.

Acknowledgments

Although, as editor, my name is the only one on the cover of the book, the final product is the result of a collegial and diligent peer review process and many long hours invested by members of the editorial board. The board's feedback was instrumental in our editorial process from the book's conception. Reviewers assumed considerable responsibility for content and had authority to veto any proposed chapter.

Each board member assumed a lead responsibility for one section of the book, reviewed and edited chapters from other sections, and participated in regular board meetings. I extend my deepest professional respect and gratitude to Paul Basch (Part One), Donald Duffy (Part Two), Paul Doulton (Part Three), Denise Runde (Part Four), and Neelam Sekhri (Part Five) for contributing and for working with me very closely. The entire board collaborated on Part Six.

One additional board member whose organization cosponsored this book and who provided important overall direction is Jonathan Lewis, president of the Academy for International Health Studies, Davis, California.

Andy Pasternack, senior editor for the Health Series at Jossey-Bass, first proposed this book to me. Throughout the process of developing the manuscript, he provided invaluable editorial and publishing direction. Without Andy and the rest of the Health Team at Jossey-Bass, this book could not have achieved its present level of overall quality.

Barbara Fuller provided valuable editorial assistance in the final months by editing chapters for consistency in terminology, contributing to chapter organization, and readily adapting diverse formats to the uniform digital medium used in the book development process.

Finally, I thank many colleagues who shared their knowledge and perspectives of the health industry, cross-checked information, held discussions with authors, and debated endless issues, topics, and perspectives. I have tried to acknowledge these new friends at the ends of chapters and regret any inadvertent omissions.

As the editor, I invite readers to contact me regarding this book via e-mail at wwieners@w-three.com or by telephone at (415) 331-7832.

August 2000   Walter W. Wieners
                                                                                      Sausalito, California

THE EDITOR

Walter W. Wieners is principal of Walter Wieners & Associates, a globally oriented health care management consulting practice focused on Internet technology. He has more than twenty years of experience in the health care industry in the United States and abroad. A graduate of the Johns Hopkins University with a B.S. in industrial engineering, Wieners holds an M.A. from the University of Chicago, where he specialized in health management.

Wieners has consulted abroad extensively and held senior-level positions with two of the major health care information technology consulting firms: First Consulting Group and Superior Consultant Company. Previously, he served as an executive with information system vendors and with a leading insurance company.

Wieners is a fellow of the Healthcare Information and Management Systems Society, and is a member of the American Medical Informatics Association, the International Federation of Health Funds, and the Friends of the Library of Medicine.

Wieners is a frequent speaker on health information technology and global health care markets. Readers are invited to contact him at (415) 331-7832 or at wwieners@w-three.com. Additional information about the book and the editor can be found at www.w-three.com.

THE EDITORIAL ADVISORY BOARD
AND SPONSORING ORGANIZATION

Paul F. Basch is professor emeritus of health research and policy at the Stanford University School of Medicine. Prior to his appointment at Stanford in 1970, he served for eight years as research parasitologist at the University of California, San Francisco School of Medicine. He has served as a consultant for the U.S. Agency for International Development, the World Health Organization, and other national and international agencies in Ecuador, Egypt, India, Indonesia, Malaysia, Mexico, Pakistan, Singapore, Vietnam, and Zimbabwe. He has published the *Textbook of International Health,* the second edition of which appeared in July 1999.

Paul Doulton is a health care industry consultant. He is the author of *Latin America: Building Business in Pharmaceuticals and Healthcare,* published by Financial Times Healthcare Management Reports. He formerly was chief executive officer of Wellcome Operations in Mexico City, Mexico. He is a visiting speaker for a number of postgraduate institutions.

Donald A. Duffy is a health care consultant and author of *The Compass Report: The Direction and Alignment of Global Health Systems* (Volumes 1 and 2) and *The World Summit Report on Global Healthcare Systems* (Volume 1). His practice is based in Washington, D.C.

Jonathan C. Lewis is president of the Academy for International Health Studies, Inc., in Davis, California. The academy was founded in 1993 to serve senior health care executives from multinational health industries, including health plans, providers, medical device manufacturers, pharmaceutical companies, and information technology vendors. The academy stages the annual International Summit on the Private Health Sector. Lewis formerly was executive officer of the California Association of Health Plans in Sacramento.

Denise M. Runde is the former director of health care at the Institute for the Future in Menlo Park, California. She is now an executive in the Internet health industry, with a start-up company headquartered in Sunnyvale, California.

Neelam Sekhri is the chief executive officer of Healthcare Redesign Group, Inc. and a founding partner of Healthcare Redesign International, Oakland, California. Her organization's clients include Kaiser Permanente, Blue Shield of California, Children's Hospitals of America, and Health Net of California.

The *Academy for International Health Studies, Inc.,* in Davis, California, is an educational and networking business organization. Founded in 1993, the Academy serves senior health care executives from multinational health industries: health plans, health care providers, medical device manufacturers, pharmaceutical companies, and information technology vendors. To promote cost-effective, high-quality health care, the Academy arranges trade and study missions for chief executive officers of American health care companies and presents the annual International Summit on the Private Health Sector. The Academy's Web address is www.aihs.com.

THE CONTRIBUTORS

Gerard F. Anderson is director and professor at the Center for Hospital Finance and Management, Johns Hopkins School of Public Health, Baltimore, Maryland. He is also professor of medicine at the Johns Hopkins University School of Medicine, associate chair for health services research in the Department of Health Policy and Management, director of the Johns Hopkins Washington program in health policy, and codirector of the Johns Hopkins Program for Medical Technology and Practice Assessment.

Marion J. Ball is vice president of the First Consulting Group and adjunct professor at Johns Hopkins University. She is the former president of the International Medical Informatics Association in Baltimore, Maryland.

Keith F. Batchelder is the chief technical officer of World Care International in Cambridge, Massachusetts. Previously, he was chief information officer at Harvard Salud Integral, Mexico City, and held a position at Massachusetts General Hospital's Center for Imaging and Pharmaceutical Research.

Mary-Anne Boyd is a consultant focusing on the development of strategic health partnerships in Auckland, New Zealand. She has served on several ministerial advisory groups and boards of directors.

Renata Bushko is founder and chair of the Future of Health Technology Institute in Hopkinson, Massachusetts. She has served on the boards of many national American health care organizations and for fifteen years was an executive in the computer industry.

Reinhard Busse is a senior research fellow at the European Observatory on Health Care Systems. He is also head of Madrid Hub at Escuela Nacional de Sanidad, Madrid, Spain, and the Department of Epidemiology, Social Medicine, and Health System Research, Medizinische Hochschule, Hannover, Germany.

Bianca Camac is an analyst at National Economic Research, International Health Practice Associates in London, United Kingdom, where she focuses exclusively on Latin America.

Yanek S. Y. Chiu is a founding partner of Healthcare Redesign International, Oakland, California. He is a native of Hong Kong and a leading surgeon.

K. Tina Donahue is the former president of Joint Commission Resources, Inc., Joint Commission Worldwide Consulting, and Joint Commission International Accreditation, Oakbrook Terrace, Illinois. She was previously vice president of education for the Joint Commission on Accreditation of Healthcare Organizations.

Paul Doulton is a health care consultant and former chief executive officer of Wellcome Operations in Mexico City, Mexico. He has spent more than thirty years working in Latin America and has written numerous books on the region.

Donald A. Duffy is a health care consultant based in Washington, D.C. He is a former executive of a large U.S. managed care health plan and author of three reports on global trends.

Pedro Gallo is an official of the Catalan Agency for Health Technology Assessment, Barcelona, Spain. He is also an economist and lecturer in the Department of Sociology and Analysis of Organizations at the University of Barcelona.

Brian S. Gould is the former chief executive officer of United HealthCare Global Services in Minneapolis, Minnesota. He was also a venture partner with the investment firm Accel Partners.

Alicia Granados is director of the Catalan Agency for Health Technology Assessment, Barcelona, Spain. She is vice president of the board of directors of the International Society for Technology Assessment in Health Care and a member of the editorial board of the *International Journal of Technology Assessment in Health Care.*

Peter Sotir Hussey is a research assistant in the Center for Hospital Finance and Management, Johns Hopkins School of Public Health, Baltimore, Maryland. His research specializes in comparisons of population aging and its effects on health and social support systems.

Howard A. Kahn is a senior vice president of Cigna International and former vice president of Global Health Business, Aetna International, Inc. He previously had national responsibility for all government-managed health programs, including disease management and Informed Health.

Pierre-Jean Lancry is director of the Department of Pharmaceuticals and Medical Devices, Caisse Nationale d'Assurance Maladie des Travailleurs Salariés, Paris, France. He was formerly in charge of information, research, and quality assurance at the Paris Hospital Administration, associate professor of economics at the University of Paris, and director of the Centre de Recherche d'Étude et de Documentation en Économie de la Santé (CREDES), the leading French research center on health economics.

Youri Lavinski is chairman and chief executive officer of Global Health Systems, Inc., in Aliso Viejo, California. He founded Russia's first private medical group in St. Petersburg and served as its chief executive officer and chairman of the board.

Albert Lowey-Ball is president of Albert Lowey-Ball Associates, Inc., Sacramento, California, and is adjunct associate professor of health policy and economics at the University of San Francisco. Lowey-Ball, a native of the Netherlands, specializes in technical services to hospital and health systems, provider groups, and public agencies.

Theodore R. Marmor is professor of political science and professor of public policy and management in the Yale University School of Management in New Haven, Connecticut. He is director of the Robert Wood Johnson Foundation's postdoctoral program in social science and health policy and a founding board member of the National Academy of Social Insurance.

Laurence Dene McGriff is an international consultant based in Sacramento, California. Previously, he held positions with United HealthCare, AIG, and Travelers and consulted for William M. Mercer, Inc.

Alexandre Alois Mencik is counselor at law with Squire Sanders & Dempsey in Brussels, Belgium. He has held prior positions with Keller and Heckman in Brussels and served as a legal adviser to the Commission of the European Communities.

Jan E. Murray is counselor at law with Squire Sanders & Dempsey in Cleveland, Ohio. She currently serves as vice chair of the committee for teaching hospitals and academic medical centers of the American Health Lawyers Association.

Leslie V. Norwalk is attorney at law with Epstein Becker & Green, Washington, D.C. Prior to joining the firm, she served in the Bush administration in the White House Office of Presidential Personnel and as an assistant to the deputy U.S. trade representative.

T. W. Noseworthy chairs and teaches in the Faculty of Medicine and Dentistry at the University of Alberta in Edmonton, Canada. He served as a member of the Prime Minister's National Forum on Health from 1994 to 1997. He is an internist and physician and holds specialty certification in the Royal College of Physicians and Surgeons of Canada, the American College of Physicians, the American College of Chest Physicians, and the American College of Critical Care Medicine.

Kieke G. H. Okma is senior policy adviser for the Ministry of Health, Welfare, and Sport in The Hague, Netherlands. She is also associate professor in the School of Public Policy Studies of Queen's University, Kingston, Canada.

Benito R. Reverente Jr. is senior adviser and former president and chief executive officer of Philam Care Health Systems, Inc., in Manila, Philippines. He serves as chairman of the Association of HMOs of the Philippines, Inc., and senior consultant to the Secretary of Health and the Philippine Health Insurance Corporation.

Jane Sarasohn-Kahn is a management consultant and health economist with the Kahn Group in Philadelphia, Pennsylvania. She has worked with organizations in the United States, Europe, and Asia for fifteen years and is a research affiliate with the Institute for the Future in Menlo Park, California.

Simone Sandier is research director, Arguments Socio-Économiques pour la Santé, Caisse Nationale d'Assurance Maladie des Travailleurs Salariés, Paris, France. She is honorary president of the French Health Economist College and is a foreign member of the Institute of Medicine of the National Academy of Science (USA).

Franz Schenkel is director and chief executive officer of Salumax S.A. in Santiago, Chile. He is a founder of Salumax and was previously regional director for Sanofi and was responsible for pharmaceutical operations in Chile, Peru, Uruguay, Bolivia, and Paraguay.

Russell J. Schneider is chief executive officer of Australian Health Insurance Association, Deakin, Australia. He has worked as an adviser to federal governments and opposition governments and has worked closely with ministers, shadow ministers, backbench members of Parliament, and senior public servants.

Richard G. Schulze is the business manager of Global Healthcare, Rabobank International, Utrecht, Netherlands. He started Rabobank's health care effort in the United States, and he has worked in Germany, the United Kingdom, France, Saudi Arabia, Egypt, Argentina, Brazil, Mexico, Singapore, and Hong Kong.

Neelam Sekhri is a founding partner of Healthcare Redesign International in Oakland, California. She has provided technical assistance internationally and has worked in countries such as India, Mexico, Singapore, and Ecuador. She has spoken internationally on new models for health care delivery.

Nicolette Sheridan is a health research consultant and senior lecturer at the University of Auckland in Auckland, New Zealand. She is an adviser to Auckland Healthcare, which is New Zealand's largest state-owned hospital and health service.

Lynn Shapiro Snyder is an attorney with Epstein Becker & Green in Washington, D.C. She is currently a member of the Reforming the Fee-for-Service Medicare Program study panel, sponsored by the National Academy of Social Insurance. She is on the advisory boards of the Bureau of National Affairs' Managed Care Reporter, the Academy for International Health Studies, and the Washington Institute for Israel Health Policy Research.

Tan Sri Dato' Dr. Abu Bakar Suleiman is the director general of health, Ministry of Health, in Kuala Lumpur, Malaysia. He holds positions on numerous committees at national and international levels and represents Malaysia at the World Health Assembly. He also continues to practice as a nephrologist.

Steven Vasilev is president and medical director of Global Health Systems, Inc., in Aliso Viejo, California. He holds a faculty appointment as clinical professor at the University of Southern California and previously was the director of gynecologic oncology at the Los Angeles Medical Center with the Southern California Permanente Medical Group.

Pat Vitacolonna is chairman of Salumax S.A., Santiago, Chile. He is the former president and chief operating officer of MetLife Health Care and the former chief operating officer and executive vice president of FHP, Inc. He serves on numerous boards and consults in Latin America and the United States.

Margaret Ware is assistant vice president of Global Health Business, Aetna International, Inc., in Hartford, Connecticut. She directs market development and strategy projects in expansion markets and supports local managers in Mexico, South America, Southeast Asia, India, and Europe.

Daniel Whitaker is associate director of National Economic Research, International Health Practice Associates, London, United Kingdom. He spent five years based in Madrid and has worked for a wide range of public and private sector clients across Latin America and Europe.

Rohaizat bin Yon is principal assistant director of planning and development for the Ministry of Health in Kuala Lumpur, Malaysia.

Aki Yoshikawa is a health economist with the National Bureau of Economic Research in Menlo Park, California. He is chairman of the board of the Global Health Foundation and founded the Comparative Health Care Policy Research Program at Stanford University. He serves as a senior adviser to the CSC Healthcare Group.

GLOBAL
HEALTH CARE MARKETS

PART ONE

UNDERSTANDING GLOBAL HEALTH MARKETS AND THE FORCES THAT SHAPE THEM

This opening section provides a foundation for understanding global health markets, examines extensively the growth of private insurance, and addresses significant issues affecting many nations. Critical global issues we have included are information technology, accreditation, emerging markets, and trade regulations. The purpose of this group of chapters is to provide an overview of the lessons to be learned from comparing global health systems and projecting future developments across borders.

Understanding Global Health Systems

In Chapter One, Theodore R. (Ted) Marmor compares global health care systems and discusses why (or whether) we benefit from doing so. Marmor addresses and refutes two commonly held beliefs: (1) that a "best model" of health care to be found somewhere in the world could be transplanted and work well elsewhere and (2) that because nations always differ in some respects, one cannot learn from the policies of another. The truth, Marmor argues, lies somewhere between.

In Chapter Two, Gerard F. Anderson and Peter Sotir Hussey compare levels and trends in health spending in twenty-nine industrialized nations and reveal the consistent increase in expenditures since 1960. The contributors discuss the impact of aging and per capita income and the position of the United States as outlier. After evaluating insurance coverage, they analyze the share of health resources allocated to hospital services, physician services, and pharmaceuticals; they conclude with a comparison of available health outcome measures.

The Growing Role of Private Insurance

Evaluating and assessing international markets and environments is the focus of Chapter Three. Howard A. Kahn and Margaret Ware find that analyzing an environment first—and not simply from a U.S. perspective—is a critical step when introducing new approaches into a health care system. The top five items in this assessment are (1) the government's role and plans for reform, (2) health care funding sources and uses, (3) consumer expectations and preferences, (4) the local medical provider infrastructure, (5) the health information structure, and (6) the local culture.

We should be prepared to look in depth at actual cases, and this opportunity is provided in Chapter Four. Brian S. Gould presents a case study of his company's effort to introduce managed care in South Africa. Although United HealthCare Global Services decisions were based on seemingly sound criteria and involved successfully recruiting local business partners, the project failed. Reasons for the failure and the lessons learned from it form the analyses presented in this chapter.

Lynn Shapiro Snyder and Leslie V. Norwalk, authors of Chapter Five, look at how regulation abroad has affected attempts to export managed health care. They observe that managed care is evolving throughout the world and encounters similar regulatory activity on the part of governments.

Emerging Developments

In Chapter Six, K. Tina Donahue provides analyses of the evolving international landscape for quality and accreditation issues. She briefly recaps the history of accreditation globally and describes recent and projected changes in accreditation policy.

Another important element in global health markets is information and communications technology, as discussed in Chapter Seven. Although U.S. executives may assume that these are essential to expanding abroad, Jane Sarasohn-Kahn notes important caveats for hardware and software companies wanting to go global.

Finally, Chapter Eight addresses trade regulations that influence the introduction of new drugs and medical devices in Europe, in particular the European Union-home to more than 370 million people. Jan E. Murray and Alexandre Alois Mencik discuss rules that have been developed to govern entry to the European market and what manufacturers should do to keep close tabs on important developments.

UNDERSTANDING GLOBAL
HEALTH SYSTEMS

CHAPTER ONE

COMPARING GLOBAL HEALTH SYSTEMS

Lessons and Caveats

Theodore R. Marmor

The subject of this chapter, although seemingly obvious, is actually far from straightforward. There has been considerable growth in the numbers of comparative studies of health care during the last decade—but growth of many different kinds.[1] Some studies have been statistical in nature and have described the particular features of national health arrangements in many countries. The work of the Organization for Economic Cooperation and Development (OECD) is typical in this regard, as are the numerical portraits regularly distributed by institutions like the World Health Organization and the World Bank.

Other studies have focused on a limited number of nations, with the researchers pursuing selected analytical themes. Topics have varied widely, from cost control to competitive or regulatory policies. But such studies emphasize explanation, evaluation, and prescription more than descriptive statistical portraits. Carolyn Tuohy's recent book *Accidental Logics* (1999), which is an account of stability and change in British, Canadian, and American health care policies, is a good illustration of this type of work.

Finally, some analyses are called comparative but in fact are not. Many books and symposia simply collect national commentaries as chapters. Such works constitute parallel portraits; they do not provide intellecual support for either finding explanations or drawing lessons but are, unfortunately, a quite common form.

This chapter sets out to discuss the forms that cross-national claims about medical care can take. Here I sharply distinguish between "learning about" different health systems and "learning from" comparative studies. Accurate description is the obvious precondition for any learning. Moreover, learning about other national experiences often prompts efforts to understand why those systems have developed as they have. But neither description nor explanation is enough for drawing policy lessons—a task with its own set of opportunities and constraints.

Using that distinction, the chapter first characterizes the growth in numbers of claims to the "comparative" category in the contemporary medical literature. Second, it discusses the variety of approaches taken in comparative commentary, including characterizing the range of possible analytical positions and attempting to separate the promising modes of analysis from those that should be avoided. And finally, the chapter provides illustrations of various approaches, with discussion of both the promise and perils of such work.

Health Policy and the Growth of Globalism in Health Care Commentary

There can be little doubt about the salience of health and health care policy on the public agendas of contemporary nations.[2] Even the most casual inspection of national debates supports this conclusion, and it applies to nations as diverse as Nigeria and Norway, Germany and Greece, Thailand and the Netherlands. The particular topics at issue range widely, from AIDS to ambulatory care and from managing end-of-life care to using preventive medicine and traditional public health measures. But for reasons we shall address in connection with advanced industrial nations, the salience of the broad subject of health policy is not in dispute.

Nor, it should be added, can anyone escape cross-national commentary about health and health care—what Rudolf Klein has vividly described as the "bombardment of information about what is happening in other countries" (Klein, 1995). Indeed, the most obvious task facing anyone interested in the subject of global health comparison is how to make sense of the volume of information crossing borders. One might observe that a substantial imbalance now exists between the magnitude of cross-border information flows about health care and the capacity to make sense of that information, let alone draw useful policy and managerial lessons from it. The very speed of communications *about* developments globally makes defensible cross-national lesson drawing more difficult.

Making sense of global developments themselves (learning about them), then, is a challenging task. And the task of drawing lessons from them is even more difficult because comparative policy studies are subject to two lesson-drawing fallacies. One we can call the World Cup fallacy—the notion that cross-national learning is like picking the best soccer team. The idea is to find the best model (management technique, organizational form, or payment policy) from around the world and transplant it elsewhere. But this approach is quite unrealistic. No institution, policy, or program is transplantable in this simplistic way. Yet there continues to be a market for one-size-fits-all reforms that attracts consulting contracts, articles, speeches, and many conferences on the state of medical care.

The second fallacy reflects the opposite danger, that is, the misleading idea that because nations (cities, neighborhoods, families) always differ in some respects, there is no way they can learn policy lessons from each other. This we can describe as the fallacy of comparative difference; it can be put syllogistically: (1) there is no way to learn from another nation where there are differences; (2) there are always differences across nations; therefore (3) there can be no policy learning across borders. Though seldom put so starkly, this provincial claim is a familiar weapon in the health policy wars of many nations, particularly well illustrated in American debates over universal health insurance. Between these two extremes lie other uses to which comparative analysis can be put. But even the most sensible efforts to learn from the experience of others raise a number of issues, which I discuss in the sections to follow.

Health Policy, National Schemes, and Global Forces

Health reform, one is often told, is now a global trend. According to one European health newsletter, for example, "Countries everywhere are reforming their health care systems" (Hunter, 1995, p. 1). Such global enthusiasts go on to claim that "there cannot be a country in the world [that] is not at least raising questions about the cost of delivery of health care." We are then led to the conclusion that "what is remarkable about this global movement is that both the diagnosis of the problems and the prescription for them are virtually the same in all health care systems" (p. 1).

It is hard to imagine a more misleading description of health policymaking globally. Indeed, within this brief paragraph are two misconceptions that "global marketeers" in health care regularly promote. First, the marketeers assume that the diagnoses and remedies associated with so-called health reform have the same meanings in different settings. This view is, a priori, implausible, and we shall see that it is empirically unsustainable. Second, there is the presumption that because the problems are similar and the remedies analogous, cross-national learning is largely a matter of establishing a database and information network on health system reform. This trivializes both the need to understand the differing contexts of health policymaking and the real threats to mislearning that make appeals to easy cross-national transfer of experience seem so naive.

Nonetheless, as we have noted already there is little doubt about the globalization of commentary in the world of medical care. Why has that come about in recent decades? And what does such speculation suggest about more promising forms of international intellectual exchange about health care?

The rise of comparative inquiry is undeniable in North America and Western Europe since the stagflation of the 1970s. Canada's form of universal health insurance—a model of achievement for many observers—has been the subject of considerable intellectual scrutiny and the destination of many policy travelers in search of illumination. Yet a majority of its provinces in the decade after 1985 felt sufficiently concerned about the condition of Canadian Medicare (and general fiscal pressures) to set up royal commissions to chart adjustments. The United States was perhaps most obvious about its medical care worries in the early 1990s; the Clinton administration's proposal for universal health insurance excited extraordinary political controversy, substantial international interest, and considerable myth making about international experience with health insurance.

There has been continuing international interest in Dutch policy disputes, largely centered on claims about euthanasia. But changes in the competition policies of the European Union have forced Holland (and other EU members) to consider more carefully how and why their health care practices differ from those of their European neighbors. One could continue with examples of policy controversies in Germany (burdened by the fiscal pressures of unification), in Great Britain (preoccupied with intentions to change the "internal market" of the Thatcher years), and so on.

The puzzle is not whether there is widespread interest in comparative health policy but why that is happening now. Why has international evidence (arguments, claims, caricatures) become more prominent in this round of "reform" than, for example, during the fiscal strains of the early 1970s? What can be usefully said not only about the substance of the experience of different nations but also about the political processes of introducing and acting on policy change? These issues are bluntly stated in order to distinguish these comments from the casual presumption, noted earlier, that there is a global discussion of the *same* problems and the *same* remedies.

This last point should be stressed. The presumption that the diagnoses and remedies for health policy are similar is widespread. The Hunter argument summarizes this familiar view clearly: there are "common pressures to contain costs, attempts to keep pace with demographic and technological changes, and the need to improve the performance and quality of care provided to service users" (Hunter, 1995). This diagnosis, of course, is not only commonplace but also undifferentiated. Every health care system in the postwar world has addressed them but has formulated the problem differently, with differing weights and emphasis. As for remedies, the globalist view is that contemporary "reforms share a number of common elements: a separation of purchaser and provider functions, the introduction of market principles based on the notion of managed competition, and an emphasis on clinical effectiveness and on health outcomes" (Hunter, 1995).

Here again is the triumph of faddish commentary over analytical clarity. There is no doubt that such phrases as *market principles, payer-provider splits,* and *managed competition* came into widespread use in the last quarter of the twentieth century (Ranade, 1998). But with important exceptions, the use has been largely by parties critical of the welfare state, ideologically celebratory of market allocation, and appealing to business and managerial convictions more than scholarly evidence. The reference to interest in "health outcomes" is perhaps the most obvious example of renaming what any competent medical policymaker has been interested in. Equally, the appeal to the idea of "managed competition" is an example of a slogan being substituted for thought. Competition is regulated (well or poorly), not managed, whereas human resources can be managed. So it was that the real policy idea—regulating competition and managing human resources more sensibly—got reduced to a slogan that misleads.

Why the Increased Attention to Global Developments?

There is a simple answer to this question. Medical care policy came to the forefront of public agendas during the late 1980s and early 1990s for one or more of the following reasons. First, the financing of personal medical care became a major financial component of the budgets of mature welfare states.[3] When fiscal strain arose, as during the prolonged recession of those years, policy scrutiny, not simply incremental budgeting, was the predictable result. Second, mature welfare states had, under almost all circumstances, less capacity for bold fiscal expansion in new areas. This meant that the management of existing programs (in new ways perhaps but in changing economic circumstances) necessarily came to occupy a larger share of the public agenda. Third, there was what might be termed the wearing out (perhaps wearing down) of the postwar consensus about the welfare state, namely the effects of more than two decades of fretfulness about the affordability, desirability, and governability of the welfare state since the early 1970s.[4]

Begun in earnest during the severe shortage of oil and gasoline in 1973 and 1974, sustained by stagflation, and bolstered by electoral victories (or advancement) of parties opposed to the welfare state expansion, critics assumed a bolder posture, and mass publics came increasingly to hear challenges to programs that had for decades seemed sacrosanct.[5] From Mulroney to Thatcher, from New

Zealand to the Netherlands, the message of "necessary change" was heard. Accordingly, when economic strain reappears, the inner rim of programmatic protection—not interest group commitment but social faith—is weaker, and the incentives to explore transformative but not fiscally burdensome options become relatively stronger. Such developments help to explain the clear international pattern of welfare state review (including health policy) over recent decades—a review that intensified as recession moved across national borders in 1990.[6]

Even accepting this contention, the question still remains: Why was there such increased attention in these reviews to other national experiences? The widespread proclivity to turn to the American health care experience seems particularly puzzling to those who, preoccupied with health care problems in the United States, are disposed to seek relevant lessons from others. It is not clear what American experience (lagging as it is on coverage and cost control) can teach others about economy and effectiveness in the delivery of medical care. Nonetheless, a globalization of inquiry has undeniably occurred and includes considerable interest in American innovations, particularly those thought to be managerial and exportable.

Times of policy change sharply increase the demand for new ideas, or at least new means to old ends. Just as many American analysts turned to Canada's example, so Canadian, German, Dutch, and other intellectual entrepreneurs in recent years turned their attention internationally. It is apparent why that is so from the concerns expressed at international meetings. Conferees express interest in getting better policy answers to the problems they face at home. They want to find a balance between "solidarity and subsidiarity," to maintain a high-quality health system in times of economic stress. Optimistic queries can be heard, such as "What are the optimum relations between patients, insurers, providers, and the government?" This common type of questioning may simply be mind stretching, that is, an effort to explore what is possible conceptually or what others have achieved. But if it is understood as the pursuit of the best model, absent further exploration of the political, social, and economic context required for implementation, it is wishful thinking.

Many such international conferences see the opportunity for an informational version of this intellectual stretching: quests for exchange of "policy information" of various sorts without commitment to policy importation, exchanges of views with kindred spirits, and explicit calls for stimulation to generate thoughts about specific initiatives. All these represent the learning that anthropologists have long extolled, namely, understanding the range of possibilities and seeing one's own circumstances more clearly by contrast.

But what about drawing policy lessons from such exercises? What are the rules of defensible conduct here, and are they being followed? The truth is that whatever appearances might suggest, most policy debates in most countries are (and will remain) parochial affairs. They address national problems; they emphasize historical and contemporary national developments in the particular domain (pensions, medical finance, transportation); they embody conflicting visions of what policies the particular country should adopt. Only rarely are the experiences of other nations—and the lessons they embody—seriously considered. When cross-national comparisons are employed in such parochial struggles, their use is typically that of policy warfare, not policy understanding and careful lesson drawing. And there are fewer local, knowledgeable critics of ideas about "solutions" abroad.

In the world of American medical debate, the misuse of British and Canadian experience surely illustrates this point. The National Health Service from the late 1940s to the late 1970s represented what "government medicine" and "rationing" could mean. In recent years, myth making about Canada has dominated the distortion league tables in North America. The parochialism of national debates remains dominant.

The reasons are almost too obvious to cite. But clearly, policymakers are busy with day-to-day pressures. Practical concerns incline them, if they take the time for comparative inquiry, to pay more attention to what appears to work, not to academic reasons for what is and is not transferable and why. Policy debaters— whether politicians, policy analysts, or spokespersons for interest groups—are in struggles, not seminars. Like lawyers, they seek victory, not illumination. For that purpose, compelling stories, whether well substantiated or not, are more useful than careful conclusions. Interest groups, as their label suggests, have material and symbolic stakes in policy outcomes, not reputations for intellectual precision to protect.[7]

None of these considerations are new or surprising. But the increased flow of cross-national claims in health policy generates new reasons to reconsider the meaning of cross-national policy learning.

Cross-Border Learning: Learning About and Learning From

There is a sharp distinction, too seldom made, between learning about and learning from cross-national experience. Accurate description is of course the necessary condition for learning about anything. Characterizing national systems, however, is not as simple as it is sometimes portrayed. Not only are the dimensions to be described not obvious but medical care arrangements are in a constant state of flux. And the meaning of apparently similar terms (hospital, doctor, nurse) differs cross-nationally. Getting reasonably comparable portraits is a challenge—one that has been done with great effort and skill by the OECD under the leadership until very recently of Jean-Pierre Poullier. As Chapter Two shows, the product of those efforts is a database that allows cross-national characterization of a quite reliable sort.

Descriptive efforts, comparative or not, do not entail any particular policy conclusion. As I have already noted, some of the most fascinating uses of cross-national portraits have to do with clarification, not policy transplantation. That is to say, one can understand a national system more clearly through comparison. Anyone interested in comprehending American medicine can do so illuminatingly by contrasting its cost experience in the postwar period with Canada's. Broadly comparable from 1945 to 1970, the United States and Canada diverged sharply in per capita outlays from 1970 to the present. And because hospital and physician utilization rates are now lower in the United States, the explanation cannot lie in those two measures. But again, the comparison, whether across quite different or quite similar systems, for this purpose is one of clarifying what is at work, not what remedies work.

By contrast, there are two strong bases for drawing policy lessons from the experience of other nations. One deals with lessons from studies of quite similar systems. Where conditions are broadly comparable—economically, politically, culturally—one can be reasonably confident that a particular policy innovation in one site is at least possible in the other (or others). That is to say, the policy might well be implementable, and, roughly speaking, the results in country A are likely to be the consequences in similar country B, or C, or D. In short, structural similarity and policy transplantability are closely linked. (The Nordic nations, to an outsider, appear to provide many instances of this process.)

But with this form of learning come constraints. Promising, appealing, compelling policy "answers" may, for instance, lie elsewhere, in a very different sort of society. What follows from that finding? No conclusion at all follows, only an understanding of that fact. Of course, that is another way of saying that learning about other national experiences is not the same as learning from them.

There remains, however, one other form of lesson drawing that is rare but powerful. Some describe the inquiry as "generalization from the widest variety of cases"—the very opposite of a "similar system" design. If a policy generalization holds over many divergent cases, some powerful factor is at work, something policymakers and administrators ignore at their (and their constituents') peril. The logic is straightforward: if Q follows from policy X in countries A to T, why should nation Z believe its experience will be different? Just as the most similar design narrows the range of findings, so too does the most different design narrow the scope. But in the latter instance, the narrowing is not of countries but of the likelihood that there will be a large number of such transplantable generalizations. One striking example of such a generalization is this: the costs of implementing new policies are always much larger than those estimated by their advocates—a claim substantiated in a very diverse range of national experiences in medical as well as other policy areas. Another illustration of such broad generalizations applies to the likelihood of wholesale transformations of the ways doctors are paid—a familiar yearning of health policy analysts. This, it turns out, is almost never a practical option. If accepted, this lesson from international experience has great practical importance for debates about and proposed reforms of payment policy.

A variety of myths, however, easily prevent the learning of lessons from other countries' experience in financing and delivering medical care. For example, as the last industrial democracy without universal health insurance, the United States has the advantage of being able to learn from nearly a century of experience elsewhere with national health insurance. Yet the American debate has been characterized not by cross-national learning but largely by myths about foreign experience regularly repeated by critics of national health insurance. This section of the chapter provides a number of illustrations of the barriers to cross-border learning—illustrations drawn from the experience of Canada and the United States since 1970.

Canada's Experience

Canada's path to and experience with universal health insurance is an obvious subject of inquiry for the American analyst seeking to use a most-similar system design. The United States, after all, shares with Canada a common language and English political roots, a comparably diverse population with a similar standard of living, increasingly integrated economies, and a tradition of fractious but constitutional federalism that makes North American political disputes similar though not identical. Moreover, until Canada consolidated its national health insurance in 1971, North American patterns and styles of medical care had been nearly identical.[8]

If public financing of medical care has worked fairly well in Canada, it seems reasonable that it should work in the United States as well. That, at least, was the plausible premise of most of the favorable American commentary about Canada's national health insurance program. That was also the premise of Australian planners who examined Canada's national program while designing what they called Medibank. However, claiming that it is possible to learn from the experience of others is not to say that simply importing another country's institutional form of universal health insurance is a good idea. Even if the public were supportive, the most enlightening comparisons seldom convince the skeptical that a "foreign" program, whatever its virtues, can simply be transplanted—with identical results—to native soil.

No system of medical care financing is free of problems or easily administered. A gap between medical wishes and medical facts is unavoidable. The relevant inquiry is whether the problems associated with one system are more serious than those linked to another. And, of course, this is the challenge that many chapters of this volume address when considering the serious problems of transformation in eastern Europe, when dealing with the huge population of Brazil, or when restructuring Israel's medical arrangements amidst enormous tension and intermittent violence.

There is much confusion everywhere. Consider the significance of managing medical care under public auspices and through public budgets. Some Canadians, for example, came to believe in the 1990s that all would be well if only there were private arrangements to augment the squeezed public system. But the productivity and growth of any Canadian economy does not depend on how much medical finance flows through the public sector. Medical services represent current consumption and therefore drain resources from investment, research, and the promotion of productivity no matter whose budget they go through.

For the control of costs, however, it does matter which budget medical care goes through. As the financial experiences of most OECD nations during the 1980s and 1990s unambiguously show, governments are *capable* of controlling medical costs (see Chapter Two). Business firms probably cannot; at least, the American experience suggests that they seldom have. The international relevance of American experience in the period between 1970 and 1990 is precisely that it offers an object lesson in the failure of privately based controls on medical care (Macke, 1991). It is worth remembering that in 1970 the United States spent about 7 percent of the GNP (gross national product) on health care. A quarter century later, the United States spends about 15 percent—nearly twice the level of Germany and one-third more than Canada, while U.S. patients face the highest out-of-pocket charges in the world. Keeping this in mind will be important as reports of U.S. success stories with managed care and competition continue to be distributed widely in the global marketplace of ideas.

Crisis mongering in a number of industrial democracies has led in recent years to suggestions that health insurance be privatized. In the United States during the early 1990s, ironically, this emerged just as Americans looked elsewhere for models of how to control a system that seemed out of control. For those who accepted the "underfunding and privatization" view of national health insurance, the model was the United States, not Europe or Canada. Yet the American model hardly suggested how to free up resources to improve international competitiveness.

Likewise, it is worth remembering that the OECD nations share a number of economic troubles, none of which would be improved by moving toward an American style of health outlays and financing. These nations are rightly concerned about lagging productivity and, from a worldwide standpoint, modest levels of economic growth. Future economic competitiveness will depend on investment in human as well as physical capital. Current consumption must be restrained if non-inflationary investment is to have a future. The current U.S. savings rate is low by any standard, whereas the Canadian rate is not impressive, except by comparison to the United States. Japan and Germany have higher savings rates, to be sure, but economic productivity throughout the OECD world is of concern. Coping with the pressure of increasing medical costs is crucial for the future economic health of all the countries represented in this book. Doing so on the basis of mythical pictures of foreign experience is the danger, not the answer. Avoiding that danger means that care must be taken to interpret the many selective and sometimes seductive glances across national borders.

Myths About National Health Insurance

Distorted analyses of foreign systems have led to the dissemination and sometimes wide acceptance of a number of myths. The myths that focus either on the performance of national systems or on whether any foreign experience, no matter how good, can find a home in another setting, need to be examined. As evidence of effects, comparisons between the United States and Canada will be used.

Myth 1. National health insurance leads to bureaucratic red tape and high administrative costs. This assertion is not true in Canada, Australia, or Sweden; nor is it true in most of the sickness insurance arrangements of Holland, Germany, and France. Doctors and hospitals in Canada, for example, receive all their payments from one source—a provincial ministry. They do not have to keep track of the eligibility requirements or definitions of insured services in hundreds of insurance plans. Canadian patients never have to file claims, much less deal with incomprehensible forms. By contrast, Americans have to file multiple, complicated claims, as do most physicians. The European sickness fund systems are more expensive administratively than those of Australia or Canada but are not as administratively costly as arrangements in the United States. Here is the triumph of cliché over fact, a concrete example of which follows.

In the British Columbia office of one primary physician, an observer reports that total staff time spent on billing for 150 patient visits per week is two hours. The physician is paid twice a month, with turnaround time between two and four weeks. For this physician, the total of unpaid bills after ninety days comes to about $42. A Canadian practice of the same size as the American observer's (400 patient visits per week) would require about six hours in personnel time per week plus $500 per month in computer charges for a total billing cost of under

$800 per month—roughly 50 cents per visit. In the American doctor's own practice, 400 patient visits per week consume 2.5 staff persons plus another full-time equivalent in receptionist, office manager, and physician time, dealing with 450 insurance companies and costing a total of $10,000 per month—or something over $6 per visit.[9]

Myth 2. *National health insurance interferes with the doctor-patient relationship.* One AMA advertisement attacking national health insurance asked in the early 1990s, "Elective surgery—shouldn't it be up to you?" The ad implies that government health insurance typically reduces the ordinary citizen's freedom of choice. It was a thinly veiled message to those Americans with broad insurance coverage: experience abroad shows that you will have less choice with national health insurance.

The irony, of course, is that this same message will hold little appeal to the millions of Americans without the money or coverage to obtain elective surgery. Nor is it likely to appeal to Americans whose choice of doctor is increasingly limited by their health maintenance organizations (HMOs) or by lower reimbursement for visits to out-of-plan doctors (under preferred provider organizations or PPOs). Under the rubric of "managed care," many such plans limit elective surgery, require second opinions, or require approval by an insurance company administrator. Here again, fact and fancy hardly intersect.

Myth 3. *National health insurance leads to long queues for treatment.* Every country, including the United States, has long waiting lists for elective procedures and sometimes even essential ones. The important question is, What is the impact on patients' well-being? Americans being treated in hospital emergency rooms, particularly in big cities, often wait hours for critical care. Private hospitals routinely turn away uninsured patients, dumping them on the public sector. Estimated at 250,000 annually in the United States, these economic transfers often result in serious delays in treatment, cause long-term harm, and occasionally cost patients their lives, although federal law now requires hospitals to ensure that patients are in stable condition before being transferred elsewhere.

When most Canadians are sick or injured, they receive care in a timely manner. Indeed, the overall rate of hospital use per capita is considerably higher in Canada than in the United States, as is the ratio of general physicians and family practitioners to the population as a whole. Nonetheless, long waiting lists have developed for some services, particularly for open heart surgery and magnetic resonance imaging. These delays reflect managerial problems and labor bottlenecks as much as chronic shortages of facilities. If they involve patients in urgent, life-threatening conditions, there is political outrage. Open heart surgery is currently the most controversial example. Government officials in British Columbia watched their waiting list for cardiac surgery grow to more than five hundred during 1990; in response they purchased surgery from Seattle hospitals with excess beds and heart surgeons.

Myth 4. *National health insurance lowers the quality of medical care.* If quality is defined as easier access (for those who are insured) to complex technologies, regardless of their effectiveness, or if quality is defined by the technologies and facilities available to the most privileged members of a population, then the United States certainly has medical care of higher quality than Canada. But if quality is defined by some measure that reflects both the effectiveness of treatment and the respect and consideration shown to patients—all patients, not just the affluent and insured—then America ranks lower than other OECD countries (including Canada) that have national health insurance. And if consumer satisfaction is the basis for judgment, then both polls and political behavior give a big edge to Canada.

Myth 5. *National health insurance leads to rationing.* Critics warn that Canada rations medical care. If by *rationing* one simply means limiting services, every country in the world rations health care. The question is how rationing is done and how much it is done. The United States limits services by ability to pay and, accordingly, shows significant differences in access to medical care by race, class, and employment circumstances. By contrast, Canada and most other developed countries attempt to provide more uniform access to the entire population. Medical care depends more on a professional assessment of medical need than on insurance status.

Rationing, in this context, is another name for allocation. Whether it is objectionable depends also on the extent of free choice and the distribution of control. Americans in HMOs and other systems of managed care face systems of corporate rationing; the rules for rationing are matters of business strategy. To be sure, some employees in the United States are offered a choice among such plans, but they are hardly in a position to know much about how the HMOs control spending. They have no way of knowing, for example, whether an HMO might deny them referral to a specialist in the event of a rare disease or difficult procedure. Because Canadians have free choice of physician, they do not have to worry about that kind of rationing. And whereas the rationing choices of an American HMO are private, Canada's choices about spending on hospitals and other health services are publicly debated and democratically decided. If Canadians come to feel that they should spend more on high-technology services, their system allows them to do so efficiently and equitably.

Myth 6. *National health insurance causes an exodus of physicians.* Some Canadian physicians were coming to the United States long before Canada introduced national health insurance. Emigration did not significantly increase thereafter. Indeed, the ratio of physicians to population has steadily increased and actually grown closer to the American level. In 1987, the United States had 234 doctors per 100,000 people, whereas Canada had 216.

Stories about deep discontent among Canadian physicians are much exaggerated. Physicians were the highest-paid professionals in Canada prior to the introduction of universal medical insurance; they still are. Provincial medical associations and ministries of health negotiate budgets annually. Because much of the bargaining for resources and control gets carried out in the public arena, these negotiations are contentious, with provincial ministers of finance typically forecasting imminent bankruptcy and medical associations threatening dire service cutbacks if they don't get more money. The media, always hungry for conflict, seize on the extremes of these positions. Although such controversies sell newspapers, they do not mean the Canadian system is about to collapse.

Myth 7. *The United States and Canada are too different to borrow from each other.* According to those skeptical about health insurance, Canadians have altogether different political attitudes than Americans—a claim said by some to be supported by Seymour Martin Lipset's *Continental Divide* (1990). According to Lipset, Canadians respect government more than do Americans—a contention symbolized by the difference between the Canadian founding document and the U.S. Declaration of Independence. Canadians are committed to "peace, order and good government" whereas the American creed is an individualistic "pursuit of happiness." But Lipset's book does not, in fact, substantiate assertions about the character, depth, and significance of Canadian and American distinctiveness. Rather, Lipset observes that Canada and the United States "resemble each other more than either resembles any other nation" and at the same time still differ in some important aspects.

The misuse by some skeptics of Lipset's North American comparisons highlights the importance of not reading out of context, as well as of understanding a basic rule of comparative scholarship. Lipset's study was an effort at detailed comparison of closely linked neighbors, not of cross-cultural variations on a broad international scale. This sort of "narrow" comparison is destined to bring out dissimilarities, whereas "broad comparison brings out similarities" (1990, p. 225). Given the narrow comparison Lipset has undertaken, any similarities he finds must be quite strong. Lipset makes no claim for the broader significance of the differences he identifies. Nor, for the purpose of learning about health care in Canada, should we.

Myth 8. *Government in the United States is too corrupt, too subject to interest group pressure, and too incompetent for centrally administered, Canadian-style health insurance to work.* This claim reflects ignorance of Canadian history and current events. Public confidence in Canadian government had been severely shaken over the past decade by defense procurement and influence pedaling scandals that match American miseries over savings-and-loan bail-outs or fraud in the U.S. Department of Housing and Urban Development. None of this has touched Canadian health care, just as U.S. scandals have left the Social Security Administration unscathed. Corruption is not an exclusively American product, nor is competent public administration an exclusively foreign invention.

In both countries, the politics of group and institutional fragmentation frequently produce either incoherence or paralysis in policy formation. The primary difference is that in Canada this fragmentation tends most often to be expressed in regional and intergovernmental conflict, whereas in the United States it is expressed in the separation of powers and in the tension between the executive branch and a highly decentralized congressional system. Citizens of both countries now express considerable dissatisfaction with the accountability, responsiveness, and effectiveness of government.

Corrective Measures and Comparative Value

In the determined pursuit of reform in the way medical care is financed, delivered, and evaluated, attention must be focused on the hard questions:

- How to raise the funds to pay for medical care
- How to distribute this financial burden fairly
- How to place defensible borders on whatever is spent
- How to ensure results that are reasonably reliable and acceptably administered

By themselves, code words like *market, managed care,* and even *national health insurance* provide no answers to these questions.

In the discussions of reforms in the United States during the early 1990s, it would have been useful to have had less mythology about American uniqueness and more willingness to learn what others can teach. The aim ought to have been drawing on foreign (and historical) experiences and setting about the serious work of devising suitable financing arrangements for the present. Nothing in the United States makes a universal health insurance scheme impossible to implement. However, propaganda that was funneled through a largely ignorant media scared politicians far more than their constituencies would wish. And so it was that the great debate over national health insurance—revived by the Clinton administration in 1993—died a quiet and disappointing death in the summer of 1994.

The fate of American health reform in the Clinton administration is not the subject of this section. It is, instead, simply an illustrative case of cross-border learning, though needed and available, being both wildly unreliable and unhelpful. The hope for this volume is that such nonlearning will be less evident in the future.

Notes

1. An illustration is those who contrast tax-supported regimes with social insurance regimes—a comparison sometimes presented as the Beveridge model (first introduced by the United Kingdom and the USSR, followed by the Scandinavian countries, New Zealand, Australia, Canada, as well as parts of U.S. social policy) versus the Bismarkian model (introduced in Germany and adopted by the Netherlands, Austria, France, Belgium, and Japan). These two models are characterized by a series of distinguishing features:

   Eligibility: citizenship (all citizens) or employment (workers and their families) as the main eligibility criterion

   Universalism: universalistic welfare state programs versus expanded welfare state coverage by the aggregation of discrete programs

   Administration: administration by government or by intermediary work-related institutions

   Channeling of funding: contributions levied through general taxation or earmarked taxes versus income-related contributions and employers' contributions

   Contracting: public officials managing money and contract negotiations versus publicly controlled decentralized intermediary organizations

2. Readers might be puzzled by my reluctance to use the term *health reform*. That arises from discomfort with the marketing connotations of *reform*. I prefer to think of reform as simply change, which can be beneficial or a burden and thus avoids the misleading presumption that reform must be improvement.

3. Technically, this statement is not true, as is evident in the sickness fund financing of care in Germany, the Netherlands, and elsewhere. But because mandatory contributions are close cousins of "taxes," budget officials must obviously treat these outlays as constraints on direct tax increases. Moreover, the precise level of acceptable cost increases is a regulatory issue of great controversy.

4. The bulk of this ideological struggle took place, of course, within national borders, free from the spread of "foreign" ideas. To the extent similar arguments arose cross-nationally, most represented "parallel development." But there are striking contemporary examples of the explicit international transfer and highlighting of welfare state commentary. Some take place through think-tank networks; some occur through media campaigns on

behalf of particular figures; some take place through academic exchanges and official meetings. Charles Murray—the controversial author of *Losing Ground* (1984) and coauthor of *The Bell Curve* (1994)—illustrates all three of these phenomena. The medium of transfer seems to have changed in the postwar period. Whereas the Beveridge Report would have been known only to social policy elites very broadly, however much they used it, the modern form seems to be the long newspaper or magazine article and the interview in the broadcast media.

5. For an elaboration of this point, see Marmor (1994), pp. 179–194.

6. Again one must distinguish between common pressures and common definitions of problems or remedies. The fact that welfare states everywhere faced strains does not entail a common definition of either problem or solution in health care matters. Canada and the United States faced quite similar fiscal strains over this period, but the policymaking debate differed enormously and results were vastly different.

7. The political fight over the Clinton health plan vividly illustrates these generalizations. The number of interest groups with a stake in the Clinton plan's fate—given the nearly $1 trillion medical economy—was enormous; there were more than 8,000 *registered* lobbyists alone in Washington, and thousands more trying to influence the outcome under some other label. The estimates of expenditures on the battle are in the hundreds of millions of dollars; one trade association (the Pharmaceutical Manufacturers' Association) spent $7 million on public relations in 1993.

8. This similarity of care had been the case for so long that until well after World War II, Canadian regulators used the U.S. Joint Commission on Hospital Accreditation to judge the credibility of their hospitals and medical schools.

9. The example is taken from a lengthy discussion in "Global Health Policy Reform" (C. Altensetter and J. W. Bjorkman, 1997).

References

"Global Health Policy Reform: Misleading Mythology or Learning Opportunity." In C. Altenstetter and J. W. Björkman (eds.), *Health Policy Reform: National Variations and Globalization*. Hampshire, England: International Political Science Association/Macmillan, 1997.

Hunter, D. "A New Focus for Dialogue." *European Health Reform*, 1995, *1*, 1.

Klein, R. "Background Paper." Paper presented at the Four-Country Conference on Health Policy, Feb. 23–27, 1995, The Hague, Netherlands.

Lipset, S. M. *The Continental Divide: The Values and Institutions of the United States and Canada.* New York: Routledge, 1990.

Macke, K. *Commentary on Canadian Health Insurance: Lessons for the United States.* Report to the Committee on Government Operations, U.S. House of Representatives, June 18, 1991. Washington, D.C.: U.S. Government Accounting Office, 1991.

Marmor, T. R. *Understanding Health Care Reform.* New Haven, Conn.: Yale University Press, 1994.

Ranade, W. (ed.). "The Procompetitive Movement in American Medical Politics." In *Markets and Health Care: A Comparative Analysis.* Reading, Mass.: Addison-Wesley, 1998.

Tuohy, C. *Accidental Logics: The Dynamics of Change in the Healthcare Arena in the United States, Britain and Canada.* New York: Oxford University Press, 1999.

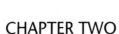

CHAPTER TWO

TRENDS IN EXPENDITURES, ACCESS, AND OUTCOMES AMONG INDUSTRIALIZED COUNTRIES

Gerard F. Anderson, Peter Sotir Hussey

Countries can compare their performance relative to other countries by using international data. Cross-sectional comparisons give an indication of where countries are doing well and where additional attention is needed during the most recent year. Comparisons of longitudinal data allow the evaluation of how a country's policies are influencing health care costs, access to health care services, and health care outcomes relative to other countries over many years.

As each nation crafts its policies for the organization, financing, and delivery of health care, comparisons with other countries can provide benchmarks (for example, see Davis, 1999; U.S. General Accounting Office, 1994; Rock, 1999). Although comparability problems in international comparisons of health care systems limit the ability of researchers and policymakers to reach definitive conclusions, the analysis of international health data raises a number of interesting questions for further research. This chapter creates a context for the rest of the book by comparing levels and trends in health spending, insurance coverage, and outcomes in twenty-nine industrialized countries.

This chapter is a revision of an article, "Health Spending, Access, and Outcomes: Trends in Industrialized Countries," by Gerard F. Anderson and Jean-Pierre Poullier, that first appeared in *Health Affairs*, 1999, *18*(3), 178–192. Copyright 1999, 'The People-to-People Health Foundation, Inc., Project HOPE.' http://www.projhope.org/HA

Every year the Organization for Economic Cooperation and Development (OECD), which includes the most developed and industrialized democracies, publishes the most complete data set available for comparisons of health care in developed countries.[1] This chapter relies primarily on these OECD health data, which cover the organization's twenty-nine member countries.

In the first section of the chapter, levels and trends of total health care spending are examined, revealing that health expenditures have been increasing since 1960 in all OECD countries, although at slightly different rates. Some factors (population aging, per capita income) that are correlated with increasing health expenditures are discussed briefly, followed by a closer examination of the most prominent outlier of health care spending—the United States.

The second section is devoted to insurance coverage and describes how all but three of the twenty-nine OECD member countries have universal, government-guaranteed health insurance coverage. The following three sections examine the share of health resources allocated to hospital services, physician services, and pharmaceuticals. The final section concludes with a comparison of available health outcome measures.

Overview of Health Expenditures

Table 2.1 presents data on per capita spending for health care services in 1997.[2] Expenditures were adjusted using purchasing power parities—a commonly used method to adjust for cost-of-living differences across countries.[3] Total health spending includes expenditures on hospitals, physicians, nursing homes, pharmaceuticals, therapeutic appliances, biomedical research and development, public health, administration, construction, and other services.

Health Expenditures Per Capita

Health expenditures per capita varied considerably across the twenty-nine countries in 1997, ranging from a high of $4,095 in the United States to a low of $259 in Turkey.[4] The United States was a clear outlier; the country with the second-highest level of expenditures per capita was Switzerland at $2,611. The median level of expenditures per capita for all twenty-nine OECD countries was $1,760.

Health expenditures per capita have been growing since 1960 in all twenty-nine countries. Table 2.1 shows the growth in per capita health expenditures, adjusted by purchasing power parities from 1960 to 1997 for Canada, Japan, the United States, and the OECD median.[5] Although the level of health expenditures per capita varies considerably across countries in any particular year, all

TABLE 2.1. HEALTH CARE SPENDING IN TWENTY-NINE COUNTRIES.

	Expenditures Per Capita on Health (US$ equivalent)			Percent of GDP Spent on Health		
	1960	1990	1997	1960	1990	1997
Australia	94	1,320	1,909	4.9	8.2	8.4
Austria	64	1,205	1,905	4.3	7.2	8.3
Belgium	53	1,247	1,768	3.4	7.5	7.6
Canada	109	1,695	2,175	5.4	9.2	9.2
Czech Republic	—	575	943	3.0	5.4	7.2
Denmark	67	1,424	2,042	3.6	8.3	8.0
Finland	54	1,292	1,525	3.9	8.0	7.4
France	72	1,539	2,047	4.2	8.9	9.6
Germany	90	1,602	2,364	4.8	8.7	10.7
Greece	21	702	1,196	3.1	7.6	8.6
Hungary	—	510	642	—	6.1	6.5
Iceland	50	1,374	1,981	3.3	7.9	7.9
Ireland	35	759	1,293	3.8	6.7	6.3
Italy	49	1,321	1,613	3.6	8.1	7.6
Japan	26	1,082	1,760	3.0	6.1	7.2
Korea	—	401	870	—	5.2	6.0
Luxembourg	—	1,495	2,303	—	6.6	7.0
Mexico	—	210	363	—	3.6	4.7
Netherlands	67	1,326	1,933	3.8	8.3	8.5
New Zealand	90	937	1,357	4.3	7.0	7.6
Norway	46	1,365	2,017	2.9	7.8	7.5
Poland	—	216	386	—	4.4	5.2
Portugal	—	614	1,148	—	6.4	7.9
Spain	14	815	1,183	1.5	6.9	7.4
Sweden	89	1,492	1,762	4.7	8.8	8.6
Switzerland	87	1,760	2,611	3.1	8.3	10.0
Turkey	—	171	259	—	3.6	4.0
United Kingdom	74	955	1,391	3.9	6.0	6.8
United States	149	2,798	4,095	5.2	12.6	13.9
OECD median	67	1,247	1,760	3.8	7.5	7.6

Source: OECD (1998) and subsequent updates.

countries showed increasing health expenditures per capita between 1960 and 1997, although at different rates. Between 1960 and 1997, the OECD median level of health expenditures per capita increased at an average rate of 9.2 percent per year. In the United States, expenditures per capita increased at the same rate. For comparison purposes, the average annual increase between 1960 and 1997 was largest in Spain (12.7 percent) and smallest in New Zealand (7.6 percent).

Policymakers are generally more interested in recent trends. Between 1990 and 1997, the annual rate of increase in health care spending per capita was half the rate it had been between 1960 and 1990 in most countries. Between 1990 and 1997, median health expenditures per capita in the OECD increased an average of 5.0 percent per year, compared to 10.2 percent between 1960 and 1990.

Percentage of GDP Spent on Health

A common method of comparing the level of health care spending across countries is to examine the proportion of the gross domestic product (GDP) spent on health care services. The percentage of GDP spent on health care in 1997 varied from a high of 13.9 percent in the United States to a low of 4.0 in Turkey. The median OECD country spent 7.6 percent. Only three countries spent 10 percent or more of their GDP on health care: Germany, Switzerland, and the United States. Two OECD countries spent less than 5 percent of their GDP on health care: Mexico and Turkey.

One reason for focusing on the percentage of GDP spent on health care is what economists call opportunity costs. The larger the proportion of GDP that is spent on health care services, the smaller the proportion that is available for other goods and services. For this reason, many countries have tried to maintain the percentage of GDP spent on health care at a constant level.[6] Between 1960 and 1997, health spending grew faster than GDP in all twenty-nine countries.[7] Ireland, New Zealand, and the United Kingdom were the most successful in containing the growth of health spending as a percent of GDP, and the United States was the least successful during this time. Recently however, some countries have been able to limit the rate of increase in health care spending to the rate of increase in GDP or below. In Denmark, Finland, Ireland, Italy, Norway, and Sweden, the percentage of GDP spent on health care actually declined from 1990 to 1997. Other countries were less successful in limiting the rate of increase. Between 1990 and 1997, the percentage of GDP spent on health care increased fastest in the Czech Republic, Germany, Portugal, Switzerland, and the United States.

Factors Related to Health Expenditures. One possible contributing factor to rising health expenditures is population aging. The percentage of the population over age sixty-five in OECD countries has been increasing steadily since 1960 (data not shown), and some have suggested this will have a major impact on health care systems. For countries with available data, health expenditures for individuals age sixty-five and over are three to five times as great as those for individuals under age sixty-five (data not shown). A cross-sectional analysis, however, shows that the relative size of the population over age sixty-five in a country was not strongly correlated with total national health expenditures in 1996 (coefficient of correlation = 0.44). Furthermore, economists have found that population aging is not likely to be a significant determinant of the growth of total health expenditures over time (Barros, 1998; Leu, 1986). These findings suggest that most of the international differences in the level of total health expenditures may not be due to the relative size of the elderly population.

Two factors that are strongly associated with average health expenditures per capita are (1) per capita income and (2) GDP per capita. Health expenditures per capita were correlated with per capita income in the OECD countries in 1997 (correlation coefficient = 0.70) and even more highly correlated with GDP per capita (correlation coefficient = 0.88). Previous studies examining the same data for different years concluded that the income elasticity of health expenditures across countries is greater than one; in economic terms, health care is a luxury good (Leu, 1986; Newhouse, 1977). In other words, as a country's income increases, it spends an increasingly larger share of its income on health care.

Health Expenditure Trends in the United States. It should be recognized that, relative to other industrialized countries, the United States has always had high levels of health expenditures. As early as 1960, the United States was spending almost 50 percent more per capita than any other OECD country. From 1960 to 1997, the rate of growth of health spending per capita in the United States was similar to the rate of growth in the median OECD country. During the 1990s, however, health spending per capita grew more rapidly in the United States than the median OECD country, in spite of the proliferation of managed care and federal and state governments' attempts to slow the rate of increase in Medicare and Medicaid costs.

Possibly more significant from a public policy perspective, however, is the rapid growth in the percentage of the GDP spent on health care in the United States. Between 1960 and 1997, the percentage of GDP spent on health care increased 8.7 percentage points in the United States, compared to 3.8 percentage points in the median OECD country. Much of the growth in the percentage of GDP spent on health in the United States is attributable to slow growth in GDP and not rapid growth in health spending, however. Between 1960 and 1997, the GDP of the median OECD country grew by an average of 8.4 percent per year, compared to 7.7

percent per year in the United States.[8] Per capita health expenditures, however, grew at roughly the same rate in the United States as the OECD median.

Insurance Coverage

Most OECD governments ensure that individuals have health insurance coverage through a variety of mechanisms, most commonly through national health insurance or social insurance.

In 1997, at least 99 percent of citizens in twenty-four of the twenty-nine countries had health insurance coverage that was guaranteed by the federal government (data not shown). In 1960, seven countries already had passed legislation assuring 100 percent of their citizens' health insurance coverage. Between 1961 and 1997, an additional seventeen countries passed similar legislation. Of the five remaining countries, Germany and the Netherlands do not require their most affluent citizens to purchase health insurance; however, nearly all do purchase private health insurance. Therefore, these countries have achieved universal health insurance coverage. Mexico, Turkey, and the United States are the only three OECD countries that did not have universal health insurance coverage in 1997.[9]

Hospital Data

The median OECD country spent 43.2 percent of its health care resources on hospitals in 1996 (see Table 2.2). Denmark spent the highest percentage (62.7 percent), whereas Austria spent the lowest (20.9 percent).[10] The OECD median expenditures on hospital services per capita were $692 in 1996. The United States had the highest per capita spending on hospitals ($1,646), whereas Turkey spent the least ($67). The OECD median was $692. Hospital spending per capita is the result of three factors: admission rates, average length of stay, and expenditures per day.

Admission Rates

There is wide variation in the proportion of the population admitted to the hospital for inpatient care during the year across the twenty-nine countries. Approximately one in four citizens of Austria, Finland, and Iceland were admitted to the hospital during 1996. The OECD median was approximately one in six. Fewer than one in ten Japanese and one in seventeen Mexicans were admitted to the hospital as inpatients in 1996. The percentage of the population admitted

TABLE 2.2. HOSPITAL SPENDING AND SELECTED CHARACTERISTICS IN TWENTY-NINE COUNTRIES.

	Per Capita Spending on Hospitals (US$ equivalent)	Percent of Total Health Spending on Hospitals	Percent of Population with Inpatient Admission	Average Length of Stay	Hospital Days Per Capita	Magnetic Resonance Imagers per Million Population	CT Scanners per Million Population	Employee per Bed
Australia	767	43.2	16.5	15.5	2.6	2.9f	18.4e	2.3
Austria	365	20.9	25.1	10.5	2.6	7.4	23.9	1.9
Belgium	692	40.5	20.0	11.3	2.2	3.3f	16.7e	1.5b
Canada	918	44.5	11.0	10.5	1.9	1.3f	7.9f	2.7e
Czech Republic	252	27.9	22.3	12.3	2.6	1.1	7.1	1.6
Denmark	1,131	62.7	19.5	7.3	1.7	2.5a	5.8a	3.2e
Finland	564	40.8	25.7	11.6	3.2	2.4a	9.0a	2.1e
France	902	45.6	22.5	11.2	2.6	2.3	9.4	1.1
Germany	796	35.0	20.9	14.3	2.8	5.7	16.4	1.5
Greece	261e	41.1e	15.0f	8.2	1.2	1.2	6.1	1.4e
Hungary	306	57.5	23.4f	10.8	2.5	1.4	5.1	0.5e
Iceland	1,039	54.9	27.0	18.0	4.5	7.4	14.9	—
Ireland	692g	54.2g	15.2	7.0	1.1	0.3a	14.3	1.8
Italy	743	46.9	16.2f	9.8	1.6	3.5f	17.5f	2.2
Japan	463f	28.5	9.3	43.7	4.1f	18.8	69.7	0.9
Korea	185	34.4	6.3f	13.0	0.8	4.7	16.3	0.8
Luxembourg	703	32.9	19.0	15.3	2.8	2.6a	15.7a	—
Mexico	118d,p	36.2d,p	5.8	4.1	0.2	0.2a	2.1a	—
Netherlands	954	53.4	11.1	32.5	3.6	3.9f	9.0d	2.2
New Zealand	573	45.1	13.8	6.5	1.5	2.7	7.7	—
Norway	679f	37.5f	15.3	9.9	4.5	0.7a	11.6a	3.5
Poland	170	45.9g	11.6f	10.6	2.6	0.2	0.4	1.0
Portugal	396	37.0	11.4	9.8	1.1	2.8	12.0g	2.6
Spain	501	45.0	10.0	11.0	1.1	3.2	9.0	2.6e
Sweden	665f,p	41.9f,p	18.1	7.5	1.3	6.8f	13.7d	—
Switzerland	1,231	—	15.0	15.0	2.7	7.4d	17.7d	2.0c
Turkey	67	28.8	6.3f	6.3	0.4	0.3a	1.6a	1.6e
United Kingdom	521f	42.0	16.0	9.8	1.7	3.4f	6.3d	3.5
United States	1,646	42.2	12.2	7.8	1.1	16.0f	26.9d	3.9
OECD median	692	43.2	16.0	10.6	2.2	2.8	11.6	2.0

Source: OECD (1998) and subsequent updates.

a1990; b1991; c1992; d1993; e1994; f1995; g1997; Ppublic expenditures only.

to the hospital has changed in some countries and remained relatively stable in others since 1960 (data not presented). Canada and the United States were the only two countries with data available where the percentage of the population admitted to the hospital actually declined from 1960 to 1996.[11] The inpatient admission rate nearly doubled in the United Kingdom, Austria, Finland, Hungary, Italy, and Turkey.

Average Length of Stay

In the median OECD country, the average inpatient stay was 10.6 days in 1996 (see Table 2.2).[12] The range was from 43.7 days in Japan[13] and 32.5 days in the Netherlands to less than 7.0 days in Mexico, Turkey, and New Zealand. The average length of inpatient stay in the median OECD country declined between 1960 and 1996 from 27.0 days to 10.6 days.

Inpatient Days per Capita

Inpatient hospital days per capita are a function of both admission rates and length of stay. In 1996, the United States had 1.1 inpatient hospital days per capita (see Table 2.2). Only Korea, Mexico, and Turkey had fewer inpatient hospital days per capita.[14] The OECD median was 2.2. Iceland and Norway had the highest number of inpatient hospital days per capita (4.5).

Hospital Expenditures per Day

The United States had the highest hospital expenditures per day by a wide margin (see Table 2.2).[15] In 1996, average hospital expenditures per day in the United States were $1,128. The countries with the second and third highest expenditures per day were Denmark at $632 and Canada at $489.[16] The OECD median was $227.

Intensity of Hospital Service

Two commonly accepted rationales for high hospital costs are technology and intensity of service (Newhouse, 1993). Table 2.2 shows the number of magnetic resonance imagers and scanners per million people in 1996. Japan had the most MRIs per capita, followed by the United States. Japan also had the most scanners per million population, followed by the United States and Austria. A widely used proxy for intensity of service is the number of full-time equivalent hospital employees per bed.[17] The number of hospital employees per bed in 1995 was highest in the United States at 3.9 (see Table 2.2). The OECD median was 2.0. The only other countries with more than three employees per bed were Denmark, Norway, and the United Kingdom.

Physician Data

In 1996, spending on physician services accounted for between 10 and 20 percent of health care resources in most countries. The median OECD country spent 15.4 percent of health care expenditures on physician services. In 1996, expenditures per capita on physician services in the United States were $761. The country with the second-highest level of expenditures per capita on physician services was Japan at $542. The median OECD country spent $295 per capita on physician services, and Greece spent only $114 per capita.

Number of Physicians

Training the appropriate number of physicians is a major public policy issue in many countries. In the median OECD country, there were 2.8 physicians for every 1,000 persons in 1996—an average of 1 physician for every 357 people. Countries with relatively high physician-to-population ratios included Italy (5.5), Spain (4.2), and Hungary (4.2). Countries with relatively low physician-to-population ratios were Korea (1.1), Turkey (1.1), Mexico (1.5), and the United Kingdom (1.7).

Physician Visits

In most OECD countries, there are 5 to 7 visits per person to the physician each year. Countries with a high number of physician visits per capita included Japan (15.8) and Hungary (14.8). Countries with relatively few physician visits per capita were Mexico (2.1) and Sweden (3.0).

Physician Incomes

Nearly half of the OECD countries have data available on physician incomes (see Table 2.3).[18] Of countries with data available in 1996, physician incomes were much higher in the United States ($199,000) than any other country.[19] In the United States, physician incomes increased faster than inflation during the period from 1960 to 1996.[20] In most other OECD countries with available longitudinal data, physician incomes have either kept pace with inflation or only slightly exceed the rate of inflation. In Australia and France, physician incomes actually declined in real terms from 1960 to 1996.

	Per Capita Spending on Physician Services (US$ equivalent)	Percent of Total Health Spending on Physicians	Physicians per Thousand Population	Physician Visits Per Capita[b]	Pharmaceutical Expenditures Per Capita (US$ equivalent)	Percent of Total Health Spending on Pharmaceuticals
Australia	307[a]	19.2	2.5	6.6	202	16.8
Austria	265	15.2	2.8	6.3	247	20.8
Belgium	315[f]	—	3.4[b]	8.0[d]	306	9.0
Canada	298	14.5	2.1	6.5[e]	258	11.7
Czech Republic	—	—	2.9	—	234	9.9
Denmark	139	7.7	2.9	5.4	165	14.1
Finland	—	—	2.8	4.1	209	12.7
France	237	11.8	2.9	6.5[e]	337	26.3
Germany	375	16.4	3.4	6.4	289	15.2
Greece	114[a]	18.0[a]	3.9[b]	—	236	17.9
Hungary	—	—	4.2[b]	14.8	172	17.9
Iceland	291	15.4	3.0[a]	4.8[a]	312	—
Ireland	120[a,f]	—	2.1	—	126	11.4
Italy	320	20.2	5.5	—	284	10.9
Japan	542[b]	34.4	1.8	15.8	349	13.0
Korea	121[b]	25.1[b]	1.1[b]	9.5	—	7.6
Luxembourg	274	12.8	2.2[b]	—	250	—
Mexico	—	—	1.5	2.1	—	31.6
Netherlands	154	8.7	2.6[c]	5.7	193	9.2
New Zealand	132[d]	11.1	2.1	—	194	15.2
Norway	—	—	2.8	5.4	174	12.5
Poland	—	—	2.4	3.2	—	16.5
Portugal	—	—	3.0	—	282	—
Spain	—	—	4.2	—	223	16.5
Sweden	187[a]	12.2[a]	3.1	3.0	218	26.6
Switzerland	446	17.9	3.2	—	190	25.9
Turkey	—	—	1.1[b]	—	—	8.8
United Kingdom	184[a]	15.5	1.7	5.9	218	28.5
United States	761	19.5	2.6	6.0	344	20.0
OECD median	295	15.4	2.8	5.9	234	15.9

Source: OECD (1998) and subsequent updates.

[a]1994; [b]1995; [c]1990; [d]1993; [e]1996; [f]public expenditures only.

Pharmaceutical Data

There is general uniformity in the level of spending per capita on pharmaceuticals in the OECD in spite of wide differences in total health spending (see Table 2.3). The median OECD country spent $234 per capita on pharmaceuticals in 1996. The range was from $126 in Ireland to $349 in Japan.

There is much greater variation in the percentage of health care resources spent on pharmaceuticals than in pharmaceutical expenditures per capita. Switzerland and the United States spent the smallest percentage of health care resources on pharmaceuticals in 1996, and Turkey and Hungary spent the largest. Generally, there is an inverse relationship between per capita income and percentage of the health care dollar spent on pharmaceuticals.

Health Status and Outcomes

Comparisons of outcomes using international data have numerous problems. It is widely recognized that most standard outcome measures such as longevity or infant mortality are only crude proxies for health status and are not very sensitive to changes in the health care financing and delivery system (Kindig, 1997). Research is continuing on the development of better outcome indicators. Some researchers are trying to develop or refine a health status measure that summarizes the health status of a country using a single indicator. These include quality-adjusted life years (Weinstein and Stason, 1977), disability-adjusted life years (Murray, 1994), health-adjusted life years (Wilkins and Adams, 1983), years of healthy life (Erickson, Wilson, and Shannon, 1995), health expectancy (Robine and Ritchie, 1991), active life expectancy (Katz, Branch, and Branson, 1983), potential years of life lost (Romeder and McWhinnie, 1977), and others.[21] In addition, a number of health status measures have been adapted for use in other languages and cultures. At the same time, other researchers and countries have decided that a single aggregate indicator cannot possibly summarize the health status of a population and have been developing systems of multiple indicators (Roos, Black, Frohlich, and De Coster, 1996).[22]

Unlike longevity and infant mortality, most of these measures are still in development or are not collected routinely in many countries. Because of the current scarcity of data that can be used to compare health status internationally, analysts must rely on available indicators as a proxy for health care outcomes. For better comparisons of health outcomes at the population level, it will be necessary to expand data collection efforts that reflect the health status of the population and are sensitive to interventions in the health care financing and delivery system. Better data will allow countries to evaluate the impact of countrywide interventions on health status. Until these data are available, comparisons will have to rely on the standard measures (see Table 2.4).

Life Expectancy

In 1996, life expectancy for women at birth ranged from a high of 83.6 in Japan to a low of 70.5 in Turkey. For women aged sixty-five, life expectancy ranged from a high of 21.5 years in Japan to a low of 15.9 in Hungary.[23]

Life expectancy for males at birth was 6.3 years shorter than for females in the median OECD country in 1996. The country with the longest life expectancy at birth for males was Japan at 77.0 years; the shortest was Turkey at 65.9 years. For men at age sixty-five, life expectancy ranged from a high of 16.9 years in Japan to a low of 12.1 years in Hungary.

Life expectancy has been increasing steadily since 1960. Between 1960 and 1996, life expectancy for females at birth in the median OECD country increased 7.6 years, while for males it increased 6.5 years (data not presented). Turkey had the largest increase for both males and females at 19.4 and 20.8 years, respectively. Hungary had the smallest increase for males at 0.7 years, and the Czech Republic had the smallest increase for females at 3.8 years.

At age sixty-five, the median OECD life expectancy increased 4.0 years for females and 3.0 years for males from 1960 to 1996. Japan had the largest increase for both men and women at 7.4 and 5.3 years, respectively. Poland had the smallest increase for females at 1.9 years and Hungary the smallest for males, where life expectancy at sixty-five actually decreased by 0.2 years from 1960 to 1996.

Infant Mortality

Another available outcome indicator is the infant mortality rate. In 1996, the OECD median infant mortality rate was 5.8 deaths per 1,000 live births (see Table 2.4). Hungary, Korea, Mexico, Poland, Turkey, and the United States had the highest infant mortality rates in 1996. From 1960 to 1996, the infant mortality rate declined in all countries (data not presented). In the OECD median country, the decline was 21.6 per 1,000 live births.

Potential Years of Life Lost

A more sophisticated measure of longevity is potential years of life lost (PYLL).[24] This indicator sums the number of years people died prior to age seventy due to causes for which mortality is considered preventable. Examples of "preventable"

TABLE 2.4. POPULATION HEALTH STATUS IN TWENTY-NINE COUNTRIES.

	Percent of Population Aged 65 and Over	Female Life Expectancy at Birth in Years	Male Life Expectancy at Birth in Years	Female Life Expectancy at 65 in Years	Male Life Expectancy at 65 in Years	Infant Mortality per Thousand Live Births	Potential Years of Life Lost per 100,000 Life Years Females[a]	Potential Years of Life Lost per 100,000 Life Years Males[a]
Australia	12.0	81.1	75.2	19.6	15.8	5.8	3,103	5,193
Austria	14.7	80.2	73.9	18.8	15.3	5.1	3,248	6,321
Belgium	15.9	81.0	74.3	19.7	15.3	6.0	3,526	6,259
Canada	12.0	81.5	75.4	20.2	16.3	6.0	3,284	5,451
Czech Republic	12.5	77.2	70.5	16.5	12.9	6.0	4,233	8,935
Denmark	15.5	78.0	72.8	17.7	14.2	5.2	4,058	6,217
Finland	14.4	80.5	73.0	18.7	14.6	4.0	2,856	6,217
France	15.4	82.0	74.1	20.6	16.1	4.9	3,092	6,861
Germany	15.6	79.9	73.6	18.6	14.9	5.0	3,337	6,505
Greece	16.0	80.4	75.1	18.6	16.1	7.3	3,165	6,317
Hungary	14.1	74.7	66.6	15.9	12.1	10.6	6,334	145,19
Iceland	11.5	80.6	76.2	19.1	16.2	3.7	2,520	3,928
Ireland	11.4	78.5	73.2	17.4[a]	13.7[a]	5.5	3,444	5,795
Italy	16.3	81.3	74.9	19.6	15.7	5.8	3,144	5,951
Japan	14.6	83.6	77.0	21.5	16.9	3.8	2,399	4,443
Korea	6.1	77.4[a]	69.5[a]	16.9[a]	13.2[a]	9.0	3,251	7,403
Luxembourg	13.7	80.0	73.0	19.2[a]	14.7[a]	4.9	3,015	6,303
Mexico	4.1	76.5	70.1	18.8	15.5	17.0	5,872	9,945
Netherlands	13.3	80.4	74.7	18.6	14.4	5.2	3,262	5,139
New Zealand	11.3	79.8	74.3	19.0	15.5	7.4	4,775	7,342
Norway	15.6	81.1	75.4	19.5	15.5	4.0	3,070	4,968
Poland	11.5	76.8	67.8	16.8	13.0	12.3	5,361	12,103
Portugal	14.8	78.5	71.2	17.7	14.3	6.9	4,117	9,234
Spain	15.5	81.6	74.4	19.8	15.8	5.0	3,056	6,940
Sweden	17.5	81.5	76.5	19.7	16.1	4.0	2,631	4,305
Switzerland	14.9	81.9	75.7	20.3	16.3	4.7	2,948	5,527
Turkey	5.2	70.5	65.9	—	—	42.2	—	—
United Kingdom	15.6	79.3	74.4	18.4	14.7	6.1	3,616	5,690
United States	12.7	79.4	72.7	18.9	15.7	7.8	4,591	8,401
OECD median	14.4	80.3	74.0	18.9	15.5	5.8	3,256	6,281

Source: OECD (1998) and subsequent updates.

mortality are motor vehicle accidents, adverse effects of pharmaceuticals, and cirrhosis of the liver. In 1995, the range of PYLL for women was from 6,334 years per 100,000 life years in Hungary to 2,399 years in Japan (see Table 2.4). The rate in the United States was 4,591 years. For men the range was from 14,519 years in Hungary to 3,928 years in Iceland.

Conclusion

Health expenditures per capita and health expenditures as a percentage of the GDP have gradually increased in all countries since 1960, although some countries have been much more successful than others in controlling the rate of increase in health care spending. The rate of growth in health care spending has slowed down in the 1990s in most industrialized countries. In 1997, at least 99 percent of citizens had health insurance coverage guaranteed by the federal government in twenty-four out of twenty-nine OECD countries, with Mexico, Turkey, and the United States having the most uninsured citizens. Countries use hospital, physician, and pharmaceutical services in very different ways, spending different proportions of their health care spending on these services and providing access in different ways. Outcomes gradually improved from 1960 to 1997 in all countries, although the rates of improvement vary considerably across the twenty-nine OECD countries.

Trends in health care spending and outcomes in the median OECD country established in the 1990s are likely to continue in the period from 2001 to 2005, although actions by some countries could affect their relative ranking. In most countries, the proportion of health care resources spent on hospitals will continue to decline, with the ambulatory and post-acute sectors growing.

Notes

1. Data presented here are based on OECD data for 1998, in some instances updated from the initial release available on CD-ROM. For further information, contact the OECD Information Center, 2001 L Street NW, Suite 605, Washington, DC, 20036-4922. Phone: (202) 785-6323; fax: (202) 785-0350; e-mail: washington.contact@oecd.org
2. International comparisons of the level of health spending must take into account that countries include slightly different services in the health sector and that numbers are continually being revised as new information becomes available. Some of the numbers for 1996 are estimates.
3. Purchasing power parities adjust for differences in cost of living across countries by comparing prices for a fixed basket of goods and services. The basket of goods and services used here is broad-based, not health-based.

4. For ranking purposes, data from recent years are sometimes substituted if data for the desired year are missing for a particular country, rather than omitting the country completely from the analysis. For example, purchasing power parities have not been calculated for the Czech Republic, Hungary, and Poland for 1997, so the figures for health expenditures per capita for 1996 were used.

5. The median was chosen because outliers influence it less than the mean. The median is calculated based on the countries for which data are reported in that year. In some years that will not include all twenty-nine countries.

6. For example, the Maastricht Treaty requires countries to limit their public finance deficit to less than 3 percent of GDP in order for the country to be eligible for the Euro. This placed considerable pressure on countries to control health expenditures in order to keep the public finance deficit low.

7. Change in the percentage of the GDP spent on health care reflects the change in GDP as well as the change in health care expenditures. GDP grew in all OECD countries from 1960 to 1997, although at different rates. The countries with the most rapid growth in GDP in the period from 1960 to 1997 were Greece, Ireland, and Turkey. Countries with relatively slow growth were Sweden, Switzerland, and the United Kingdom. The OECD median GDP grew seventeenfold from 1960 to 1997. The rate of growth of GDP in the United States was fourteenfold, or twentieth out of twenty-four countries during the time period.

8. Growth in GDP could not be calculated for the Czech Republic, Hungary, Korea, Mexico, and Poland.

9. "Universal health insurance coverage" is used here to indicate that at least 99 percent of the population has health insurance coverage.

10. This may be an accounting issue for Austria. An upward revision is likely and is expected to bring Austria into the 40 percent range.

11. In Canada, the inpatient admissions rate declined from 15.0 to 11.0 percent of the population from 1960 to 1996. In the United States, the decline was from 13.9 to 12.2 percent. Inpatient admissions data were available for fourteen countries for 1960 and 1995 or 1996.

12. A portion of the variation in length of stay could be attributable to differences in how the term *hospital* is defined.

13. Part of the explanation for the much longer average length of stay in Japan is the lack of a fully developed nursing home industry. Among the countries reporting data on nursing home beds, Japan has one of the lowest numbers of nursing home beds per capita. As a result, patients requiring long-term care may be treated in acute care hospitals. In Japan, 45 percent of inpatients over age sixty-five remain in the hospital for more than six months. See Ikegami (1996), p. 9.

14. Ireland, Portugal, and Spain also had 1.1 inpatient hospital days per 1,000.

15. In most countries, hospital-based physicians are salaried employees of the hospital, and their costs cannot be separated from the other expenditures. Only the United States separates physicians' fees from other hospital expenditures when a patient is treated in the hospital. If physicians' fees were included in hospital expenditures, hospital expenditures per capita and hospital expenditures per day would be even higher.

16. Denmark's hospital expenditures per day may be high because nursing homes were not included in some calculations. The OECD definition of "inpatient" includes nursing homes.

17. Sometimes the figures reflect total employees and not FTE employees per bed.

18. Physician incomes after practice expenses and malpractice insurance but before income tax. The data are typically collected from surveys of physicians and may not include the full universe of physicians reported in column 3 of Table 2.4.

19. Physician incomes are also lower in Japan and Hungary, but the data may not be accurate and thus are not reported.
20. Physician incomes were adjusted for inflation using the all-items Consumer Price Index.
21. Quality-adjusted life years measure quality and length of life by taking the sum of the products of length of life in years and a value weight reflecting health-related quality of life. "Disability-adjusted life years" measures expected healthy life lost using life tables, adjusted for the value of time lived at different ages, then adjusted for time lived with a disability using a disability severity index. "Health-adjusted life expectancy" is the product of life expectancy and a value weight reflecting health-related quality of life. Health expectancy, or healthy life expectancy, combines mortality and disability data to measure life expectancy free of disability. "Active life expectancy" measures the expected duration of life with functional well-being by combining life-table techniques with the index of activities of daily living (ADL). "Potential years of life" measures premature mortality by summing years of life lost before age seventy due to causes for which mortality is considered preventable.
22. The United Kingdom is piloting an information system that will allow comparison of health status along a number of dimensions. Other attempts are under way in Australia, Canada, the Netherlands, and New Zealand, and other countries.
23. Life expectancy at age sixty-five is probably lower in Turkey, where it is not calculated.
24. The OECD defines "potential years of life lost" as a summary measure of premature mortality providing an explicit way of weighting deaths occurring at younger ages that are considered preventable. The calculation for PYLL involves adding up deaths occurring at each age and multiplying this by the number of remaining years to live until a selected age limit. A limit of seventy years was chosen for the calculations in OECD (1998).

References

Barros, P. "The Black Box of Health Care Expenditure Growth Determinants." *Health Economics,* 1998, *7*(6), 533–544.

Davis, K. "International Health Policy: Common Problems, Alternative Strategies." *Health Affairs,* 1999, *18*(3), 135–143.

Erickson, P., Wilson, R., and Shannon, I. "Years of Healthy Life." In *NCHS Healthy People Statistical Notes,* no. 7. Washington, D.C.: U.S. Public Health Service, 1995.

Ikegami, N. "Overview: Health Care in Japan." In N. Ikegami and J. C. Campbell, *Containing Health Care Costs in Japan.* Ann Arbor: University of Michigan Press, 1996.

Katz, S., Branch, L., and Branson, M. "Active Life Expectancy." *New England Journal of Medicine,* 1983, *309*(20), 1218–1224.

Kindig, D. A. *Purchasing Population Health.* Ann Arbor: University of Michigan Press, 1997.

Leu, R. E. "The Public-Private Mix and International Health Care Costs." In A. J. Culyer and B. Jonsson (eds.), *Public and Private Health Services.* Oxford: Blackwell, 1986.

Murray, C.J.L. "Quantifying the Burden of Disease: The Technical Basis for Disability-Adjusted Life Year." *Bulletin of the World Health Organization,* 1994, *72*(3), 429–445.

Newhouse, J. P. "Medical-Care Expenditure: A Cross-National Survey." *Journal of Human Resources,* 1977, *12,* 15.

Newhouse, J. P. "An Iconoclastic View of Health Cost Containment." *Health Affairs,* 1993, *12*(Suppl.), 152–171.

Organization for Economic Cooperation and Development. *OECD Health Data, 1998.* Washington, D.C.: Organization for Economic Cooperation and Development, 1998.

Robine, J. M., and Ritchie, K. "Healthy Life Expectancy: Evaluation of a Global Indicator of Change in Population Health." *British Medical Journal,* 1991, *302,* 457–460.

Rock, A. "Revitalizing Health Care from the Federal Perspective." Presentation at the Canadian National Healthcare Leadership Conference and Exhibition, June 7, 1999. [http://www.hcc.gc.ca/english/archives/speeches/7june99mine.htm]

Romeder, J.-M., and McWhinnie, J. R. "Potential Years of Life Lost Between Ages 1 and 70: An Indicator of Premature Mortality for Health Planning." *International Journal of Epidemiology,* 1977, *6,* 143–151.

Roos, N., Black, C., Frohlich, N., and De Coster, C. "Population Health and Health Care Use: An Information System for Health Policy Makers." *Milbank Quarterly,* 1996, *74*(1), 3–29.

U.S. General Accounting Office. *Long-Term Care: Other Countries Tighten Budgets While Seeking Better Access.* Washington, D.C.: U.S. General Accounting Office, 1994.

Weinstein, M., and Stason, W. "Foundations of Cost-Effectiveness Analysis for Health and Medical Practices." *New England Journal of Medicine,* 1977, *296*(13), 716–721.

Wilkins R., and Adams, O. B. "Health Expectancy in Canada, Late 1970s: Demographic, Regional, and Social Dimensions." *American Journal of Public Health,* 1983, *73,* 1073–1080.

THE GROWING ROLE
OF PRIVATE INSURANCE

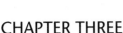

CHAPTER THREE

CRITICAL ISSUES IN EVALUATING GLOBAL MARKETS

Howard A. Kahn, Margaret Ware

Managed care grew rapidly in the United States in response to a unique combination of conditions and influences. What drove health cost-containment efforts in the 1970s through the 1990s were circumstances quite different from those being faced in other countries today. People around the world may and should look to the U.S. stockpile of tools, techniques, and products that evolved over the last twenty-five years, but these cannot be viewed as the final answer. They are a starting point; the underlying learning must be used to build new applications in other countries. In addition, new capabilities such as the Internet create innovations that must become incorporated in the next generation of health care financing solutions.

Despite all the publicized successes, insurers and managed care organizations (MCOs) have made mistakes when introducing new products and services in the past, and these mistakes must be considered in future efforts. Failing to analyze an environment enough to properly select and shape a tool before introducing it in a health care system or analyzing an environment only through North American frames of reference is often at the root of the problem. Based on Aetna

This article is adapted with permission from "Crossing Borders: Considerations in Delivering Health Insurance Products and Services," *Managed Care Quarterly*, 1999, 7(2), 57–64. ©1999 Aspen Publishers, Inc.

International's experience with health-related operations in many countries (Argentina, Brazil, Chile, Colombia, Hong Kong, Indonesia, Malaysia, Mexico, New Zealand, Peru, Philippines, Thailand, and Venezuela), we believe that it is important to study the local environment of a country and to understand and respond to the demands and needs of that country's government, consumers, providers, and purchasers.

For any new health business venture, the goal is to supply the kind of care and financing that will meet the specific demands of the target population. In order to balance supply and demand, entrepreneurs must be wary of any instability in an existing system. Although such instabilities create opportunity for entrepreneurs, they also constitute a challenge for health care management in general. Inevitably, an aging population combined with advancing medical technology creates imbalances in what might otherwise have been a stable system. The large number of diverse players involved in a system further increases the potential for instability.

Before any discussion of health insurance and delivery system alternatives can take place, then, one must look at major factors influencing the existing system, with a goal of more consciously directing health spending. Such factors include (1) the government's role and plans for reform, (2) health care funding sources and uses, (3) consumer expectations and preferences, (4) the local medical provider infrastructure, (5) the health information structure, and (6) the local culture. Following is a brief review of key considerations.

Government's Role and Plans for Reform

Governments play several roles to varying degrees within the health care system: they may employ clinicians, own and run facilities that provide care directly, set spending levels, negotiate health budgets, regulate care delivery, and act as a financial intermediary. Goals and agendas determine whether and where a government will address pressures on a system and set the tone for public and private initiatives.

A government can be central to shaping a private company's opportunities, or it can be just a bit player. India is perhaps the best example of a country in which the government plays a central role. At this writing, no private firms, local or foreign, are licensed to sell insurance in that country, but the government has stated its intention to open the market soon. Understanding the current and anticipated role of the government is imperative to success in India.

Understanding the government is no less important in a country such as Brazil, where the private health insurance sector is lively and growing. The Sul America-Aetna joint venture, the largest health insurer in Brazil, continues to grow as local businesses shift health care to companies with financial strength and a recognized brand. In anticipation of government regulation to increase capital reserves, an effort to strengthen the financial status of the health insurance sector triggered this "flight to quality." At the same time, small local competitors were handicapped.

Although the citizens who use public health systems usually hold strong views of those systems, opinions can change. In response to privatization in Spain, for example, considerable effort has been made to improve service in the public system, so that many believe competition from the public system now inhibits private market growth. In Thailand, the public system is well regarded, and employers are under strong competitive economic pressure; these factors make using corporate assets to fund rich programs of private health benefits for their employees relatively unattractive at this time. The biggest perceived need in that country may be for the private coverage of accidents and catastrophic dread diseases, which could be available as riders to individual insurance policies.

Health Funding Sources and Uses

In fact, emerging markets often respond initially to individual consumer needs for protection against accidents and catastrophic medical episodes. Depending on government policy, mandatory plans or sponsored programs with more comprehensive coverage may evolve. In many markets, larger employers have informally sponsored self-insured, self-administered programs and have provided an internal set of services for employees. Companies with such self-contained programs have found it impossible to stay abreast of developments such as an improving country infrastructure and more sophisticated forms of treatment. In some countries, then, administrative services only (ASO) contracts or third party administration (TPA) may be a desirable alternative because the burden of keeping up with changes is shifted to the TPA.

Consumer Expectations and Preferences

Many emerging markets and industrialized, socialized markets are predominantly driven by the individual rather than by the employer. Given that, understanding the real and perceived needs of consumers is critical at the earliest stages. In India, for example, consumers appear to be most interested in hospitalization coverage because ambulatory (domiciliary) care is viewed as affordable and available, whereas private hospitals require advance payment for services (literally a pay-as-you-go service, often on a day-by-day basis). Further, the quality of facilities in

India varies considerably. A full managed care program may simply miss the perceived need of many consumers.

Culturally accepted patterns of care in many other countries involve strong preferences regarding pharmacy—whether allopathic, ayurvedic, or oriental. In China, for example, medical costs are much more heavily weighted toward pharmacy than toward hospital care, as in the United States. The lack of facilities is probably part of the reason for this, but the availability of and historical reliance on respected traditional herbal medicines and noninvasive treatments is also a factor. Pharmaceutical preferences are also strong in France, where consumers have been noted to express a belief that they have not been properly treated if they leave a doctor's office without a prescription. A French survey reported in *EIU Healthcare Europe* (Wyke, 1997) found that almost four in ten consumers had acquired at least one pharmaceutical product in the prior month. Correspondingly, France has the second-highest drug consumption rate per person in Europe. Furthermore, the social security system reimburses more than 75 percent of France's pharmaceutical industry domestic turnover. The government must struggle with the trade-off between controlling national spending on drugs and supporting its French pharmaceutical industry, which employs more than 85,000 people. Entrepreneurs must be mindful that the interplay between government and consumer agendas shapes viable private opportunities.

The Local Medical Provider Infrastructure

Configuration of the provider community affects medical supply and demand and largely determines how health care is delivered locally; this in turn affects private health care and private insurance opportunities in a market. Many doctors can be found in cities, but there is a severe shortage of specialists and rural physicians. Private hospitals are allowed, but the majority of people rely on public facilities, so physicians often split their practice between public and private facilities, each for part of the day, and also hold private office hours. Access is affected by the limitations of public transportation and by word-of-mouth referrals to physicians with the "right touch." All of these circumstances must be considered when negotiating contract fees with providers, deciding if and where to add new medical facilities, and determining which providers to include in contracted networks.

If a country's basic medical infrastructure is still developing, the strongest added value from a new insurer might be credentialing based on quality. In the case of an unregulated hospital environment, consumers might highly value facility credentialing or selective contracting based on the prescreening of providers (for example, a threshold of quality might include twenty-four-hour physician access for emergencies and a minimum volume for certain procedures). In the United

States, Aetna U.S. Healthcare selectively contracts for many advanced procedures based on quality of outcomes, which is, in turn, closely related to volume (Gordon and others, 1995). In some environments, this could mean credentialing only certain institutions, based on volume.

The mix of public and private facilities and the mix of facility types have an impact on access patterns of consumers. In India, for example, the government provides all outpatient and inpatient care without charging patients for services used. As in many developing countries where the infrastructure does not meet the demand, waits for both primary and secondary care are long. Small private hospitals often provide primary and secondary treatments as well, but patients pay for that out of pocket. Although medical capacity in India does not meet the population's need, the private capacity in major cities is greater than what is needed by those who can afford to pay. Individuals who do access the private system are concerned that they will suffer unnecessary invasive treatments, not because of medical need but solely because they are able to pay for them.

The Health Information Structure

In the United States, the AMA's CPT codes and the World Health Organization's ICD coding systems are used universally. Many countries are without such a common uniform data structure, however, and hospitals often develop unique means of describing what has been done. Diagnosis information may not be required or collected by payers yet. Before techniques of health management are implemented, such information must be either collected regularly or somehow discerned from available data describing types of illnesses and treatments.

The Local Culture

Any discussion of health insurance and delivery system alternatives must recognize the many complicating social and cultural factors in health status: wealth, level of urbanity, education, social structure, cultural values, diversity, and behaviors. At some level, one needs to understand the cultural perspective dominant in the target-market segment and the expectations held by both providers and patients.

In Indonesia when a person is hospitalized, family members often attend the individual in assigned shifts around the clock, bringing food from home and providing care. Consumers therefore place a high value on the location of facilities, as well as on its reputation for quality because transportation obstacles might make a distant facility inaccessible to the family members caring for the patient.

Attitudes toward elders may affect health care utilization patterns, for example. Although elders are respected members of extended families in most emerging market countries, these elders are often reluctant to drain family resources that could be used by younger generations. They might choose to die at home with dignity, surrounded by family, rather than to buy expensive private medical treatments for fatal conditions. Introducing full health insurance coverage in such countries could result in higher costs than expected.

As another example, physicians in Hong Kong often dispense drugs directly; they generally dispense only a two- to four-day supply of antibiotics and expect a revisit. Patients expect the physician's continued personal attention as a measure of quality of care. In addition, doctors believe that if they were to dispense a ten-day prescription, patients would discontinue the drugs when symptoms abated and sell any remaining medication. To change that pattern of care overnight would confuse physicians and disappoint patients who are accustomed to frequent contact with providers during an episode of illness. Using managed care tools to compare provider performance against local standards of care could help build a more effective network, however.

Cautions and Considerations

We have provided some conceptual framework and examples of how health systems tend to find their own idiosyncratic structure. Innovative utilization management solutions may add the most value where supply and demand are currently mismatched. In addition, business people should be alert to the potential problems discussed in the sections to follow.

Fraud

All countries with a significant informal economy (Italy, Greece, Brazil, China, and India, for example) tend to face the issue of fraud—an issue that presents a challenge for insurance operations in these markets. However, the strongest forms of managed care that tightly integrate care and financing may be the solution to this problem because fraud can enter these systems in fewer places. For example, giving providers fixed payments for care of a given population decreases the tendency for collusion between providers and consumers seeking coverage for family members and friends who are not covered.

Funding Application

One purpose of a copayment is to focus consumer awareness on the cost of treatments. In France, over 80 percent of the population has private insurance covering copayments and hence bear no personal responsibility for them. As a result, copayments are not an effective consumer motivator, which is consistent with the considerably higher pharmaceutical consumption by those who have complementary insurance.

Lack of Benefit Funding Rules

In many Asian countries, plan sponsors have self-insured, self-administered programs that allow them discretion at "point of benefit." Insured programs require fixed coverage, which would force purchasing sponsors to give up their case-by-case discretion—something they are reluctant to do (as in Indonesia, for example).

Low Benefit Limits

Where sponsors do not want or need to fund comprehensive coverage, they may cover a low level of expenses equated to primary care. Or they may cover a middle layer of exposure, leaving small, affordable amounts and very high amounts uncovered. In either case, a low coverage limit thwarts care coordination and disease management, handicaps efforts to control secondary and tertiary expenses (where most of the money is spent), and in general inhibits efficient allocation of medical resources (as in Malaysia and India, for example).

Stovepiped Budgets

Lack of integrated funding for primary as opposed to tertiary care prevents spending on primary care to generate greater savings in tertiary care. It also inhibits coordination across episodes of care (as in Canada, Germany, and Hong Kong, for example).

Unrelated, Bundled Products

Health care is not always a stand-alone product. In some countries, it is a loss leader component that is bundled with other coverage in a benefits package, making it difficult to compete profitably in health on a stand-alone basis (as in Portugal, Spain, and Greece, for example).

Shortage of Private Suppliers

In some markets, private providers are simply too few to serve a significant privately insured population. In these countries, either the private insurance market will be slow to develop or an insurer must learn how to interface with public providers (in Australia, Poland, Spain, and Sweden, for example).

Delays in Implementation of Public Policy

Changes in public policy nearly always take longer to effect than the government's publicly announced schedule for the change. In Argentina, India, Mexico, and New Zealand, among many others, announced changes have not been implemented, and legislators and regulators struggle with new obstacles and resistance from negatively affected sectors. In some cases, the government has even changed hands, either in due process (as in France, Germany, and Venezuela) or from instability (as in India), as interest groups use political pressures to redirect policies.

Lack of Entrepreneurial Initiative

It is important to realize that behind the managed care movement in the United States were the myriad techniques discovered and developed because of the entrepreneurial culture here. In such a culture, problems are seen as opportunities, and problem solving is applied with change-generating momentum to the issues of imbalances within a system. What the U.S. managed care movement can export is exactly that entrepreneurial culture and flair, supplemented by some experiences that have worked and lessons learned from some that have failed under one set of circumstances.

Conclusion

The challenge in structuring the next evolution of health care products is to borrow selectively from the successes in the United States and other local national systems and to learn from the mistakes, both from indemnity and managed care experiences. To find opportunities as an entrepreneur, one must look at the lessons learned in a variety of systems around the world. A successful business proposition can only be developed, however, with careful consideration of the local target environment. Ultimately, a market-based approach—not a product-based approach—is necessary. A successful solution is market specific, borrowing from the best available U.S. competencies and adapting them to the local environment.

References

Gordon, T., and others. "The Effects of Regionalization on Cost and Outcome for One General High-Risk Surgical Procedure." *Annals of Surgery,* 1995, *221*(1), 43–49.

Wyke, A. *EIU Healthcare Europe.* London: Economist Intelligence Unity, 1997.

CHAPTER FOUR

WHEN MANAGED CARE DOESN'T TRAVEL WELL

A Case Study of South Africa

Brian S. Gould

In 1995 United HealthCare had a rare opportunity. The company was at the top of its game in the United States, and the global business environment now invited the expansion of its core products internationally. Favorable economic and political trends were motivating prospective foreign partners to seek the company out, hoping to be chosen. For its first international venture, United selected South Africa and spared neither expense nor effort in showing what enlightened managed care could accomplish. However, one trend had not been anticipated: the global mass market for publicity. In this case the constant drumbeat of anti–managed care stories and opinions moved faster and with more impact than even the largest American health care company could cope with.

Background

As the end of 1993 neared, United HealthCare Corporation (later renamed the United HealthGroup) felt it was ready to take on the challenge of international expansion. The company, having survived a near-death experience in the late 1980s, was again enjoying conspicuous success in the U.S. market. During the period between 1990 and 1993, United had increased its health plan enrollment by almost 100 percent to 2.4 million people. It owned nine health plans, managed nine others, and held purchase agreements that would shortly add several more. During the same three-year period, United increased the enrollment in its managed care specialty businesses. These include a collection of ancillary service companies primarily marketed to larger employer groups: a pharmacy benefit management company (PBM), geriatric services, mental health services, utilization review, employee assistance, workers' compensation, and a transplant specialty network. Enrollment grew from 7.7 million to 33.5 million people—a gain of 335 percent. And the growth was profitable. In 1993 revenues were over the $3 billion in U.S. dollars, with operating income of US$335 million. With no debt, the company was cash-positive and was building extensive reserves. At that time, United was in the midst of negotiating to sell its most successful specialty company, Diversified Pharmaceutical Services (a pharmacy benefit management firm, or PBM), to the United Kingdom's SmithKline Beecham PLC for US$2.3 billion. (As products, PBMs developed and managed drug formularies, generic drug substitution programs, drug utilization review programs, and in some cases mail order programs for chronic medications.)

It is understandable, therefore, that United was feeling particularly confident, resource rich, and literally ready to tackle the world. United's president and one of those chiefly responsible for its remarkable turnaround, William McGuire, felt the company was ready to act on his vision that its expertise in successfully managing diverse health care systems was an exportable asset. But the strategic question was still an open one: Could United achieve business success with managed care in non-U.S. markets?

United felt particularly well suited for this pioneering role. After all, it had never been a doctrinaire or model-driven company in its approach to managing care. On the contrary, its broad acquisition experience had been instructive as to the marketing advantages of accepting local preferences about such issues as how open or closed to make the provider network, the formats for provider payments, and the style of the medical management program. In its role as frequent acquirer of various regional health plans, United had enjoyed great success by avoiding programmatic regimentation, relying instead on a trio of core competencies: (1) strong centralized financial management, (2) an efficient and automated claims-driven data system, and (3) a doctor-friendly but expert medical management capability. United was able to offer managed care coverage in a broad variety of products attuned to local market preferences, including preferences for HMOs, PPOs, or point-of-service "wraparounds," for primary care gatekeeper or open models, and for capitated or fee-for-service physicians. There was no "United model" per se, only a polymorphous spectrum of plans designed to be competitive in each local market on price, features, and performance.

United's International Vision

In the immediate aftermath of the cold war, the entire world seemed to embrace the concepts of American-style capitalism, democratization, and privatization (or at least its stepchild, deregulation). In the industrial countries prosperity and freedom brought along a growing middle class (that is, families with discretionary income), a graying population (the consequence of lower birth rates), and an ever-increasing demand for more health care. These demographic and political trends, particularly in areas where one encountered an abundant supply of providers, created frequent health care financing "crises"—an environment clearly favorable to our concepts of managed care.

Although the literature on international health has tended to focus on such issues as comparisons of the major systems of health care financing or cultural attitudes toward disease, United considered most of these to be largely tangential to the real issues of improving health care cost-effectiveness. It took the view that as long as a health care system was based on Western-style scientific and technical medicine, it would tend toward significant waste and inefficiency in its delivery. The reasons for this were rooted in technical specialization, causing organizational fragmentation and redundancy. But the antidote was similarly generic. The efficiency and cost-effectiveness of the health care system could always be improved if a few key environmental variables were present. Examples include putting suitable information technology in place, improving data standardization, letting providers and payers be independent but cooperative, motivating patients to become involved in their own clinical outcomes, and (most critically), obtaining the necessary governmental approvals.

United had long understood that, contrary to popular perception, the core goals of managed care have little to do with any particular mechanisms of risk sharing or utilization control. "Managed care" does not really require any particular model of capitation, gatekeeping, or medical management per se to be effective. Instead, managed care is built on a foundation of four objectives that can be pursued in various ways, depending on the profile of local priorities and the preferences of the participants in the local health care system:

- Reducing prices through volume contracting
- Reducing variation in treatment patterns
- Reducing the need for services through prevention and early identification of acute conditions
- Reducing transaction costs through information technology

One of the secrets of United's considerable domestic success had been its efforts to adapt its products and managed care programs to such local preferences. In going international, we concluded that those "local differences" would be greater in scale and significantly more difficult to identify, understand, and adapt to but would represent an essentially similar process to the one with which United was already familiar.

What we could see as we surveyed the world was (1) health care financial pressures and rising demand everywhere, (2) a large number of countries in the process of privatizing state health care systems in the name of reform, and (3) the availability of a new generation of powerful, affordable, and easily available information technology. By mid-decade, distributed client-server, PC-based systems could easily deliver the computing power of the pricey and difficult-to-support mainframes of only a few years earlier.

For its part the world seemed intrigued, even infatuated, with managed care. As anticipated, the problem of increasing medical inflation seemed to be universal, but so was the availability of the requisite technology for managed care programs: the PC, the telephone, and the fax machine. It was ironic that we were being sought out as rescuers by delegates from other countries, and our health care systems were being held up as models in the U.S. political debate over universal coverage. It seemed that the United States, burdened with a notoriously expensive private health care system, had pioneered something unique: a data bridge between the utilization of clinical services, the cost of services, and the circumstances under which they were being used.

We considered this interest to be consistent with our view of managed care—that it was merely the application of the scientific tradition to ordinary medical practice, always stressing the importance of objective findings in assessing the appropriateness of medical treatment (particularly the indications so important for so-called evidence-based medicine and the outcomes measurements for determining their effectiveness).

Although the technique was broadly applicable, and if correctly applied would lead to valid conclusions, the methodology was essentially statistical and therefore vulnerable to criticism from more passionate and less numeric quarters. If the U.S. managed care industry had accomplished a lot with its statistical modeling, connecting the hard financial and administrative costs of health care with the more complicated clinical data of "indications" and "outcomes," it seemed rather tone deaf to the public relations weaknesses introduced with the technique.

The reality is that, regardless of country or culture, health care is always very personal, intimate, and emotional. People do not simply seek treatment to obtain pills or procedures. They also seek reassurance from *their* doctor, a most trusted source, a comforting touch, or simply a place in which it is safe to be weak and afraid. In its focus on population-level data and unconscious discounting of subjective issues such as discomfort, inconvenience, and personal preference in its outcomes data, managed care made the mistakes of underweighting qualities of care that are highly valued on an individual level. Thus managed care seemed to be excessively interested in efficiency and profits over doing good. Despite having a demonstrable impact in finally bringing the problem of medical inflation under control, by mid-decade it did not require any particular creativity to write human interest stories portraying managed care as fearsomely antihumanistic. People were ready to believe that was true.

Unfortunately, the crescendo of anti–managed care criticism was heating up in the United States just as the technology was being discovered internationally. In many respects, managed care was the ideal answer to the central political problem of universal health care systems: On what basis should care be denied to an individual? Certainly U.S. managed care companies had nothing to teach foreign health systems about cost control. In both their nationalized and private forms, international health care had long relied on blunt mechanisms for cost control such as strict coverage limits, fee schedules, global budgeting, and even direct rationing of services of a type unknown in the United States (for example, "No one over the age of X is eligible for a kidney transplant"). It was the U.S. managed care movement that created the technology that made reimbursement decisions based on clinical criteria (for example, medical appropriateness) practical on a large scale for the first time. It then became politically attractive to use managed care to control utilization and conserve resources in other places. It was the implied promise of preserving access to "everyone who would benefit" from health care services while still controlling costs. The savings would come out of waste and inefficiency rather than from patients who would benefit from treatment. And, unlike so much health policy theorizing, the experience of the large U.S. employers who had adopted managed care coverage programs a decade earlier seemed to confirm that this approach actually worked in the real world.

The key requirement was that the program making such determinations be able to meet the high level of information intensity required for adjudication in real time with acceptable validity. Judging the "medical appropriateness" of specific services given to real patients implies the availability of large amounts of data about actual clinical findings, patient history (such as responses to alternative treatments in the past), relative costs, risks, and even convenience, not to mention a good deal of skill. United had the expertise, experience, and technology to do that.

United had been regularly receiving delegations visiting from around the world, trying to learn more about its techniques for incorporating clinical evaluations into actual insurance operations. As market conditions generally improved around the world, the global opportunity became irresistible.

Market Selection

On New Year's Day in 1994, United responded by formally creating its new Global Services Division. But now it needed to decide exactly where to go and precisely what it could sell.

The range of choices was overwhelming. Beginning in London (not atypical for American companies first starting international activities) and in quick succession, we evaluated and rejected the acquisition of a U.K. private medical insurance company, a hospital-prepaid health care joint venture in Shanghai, numerous entreaties to license our systems, and an Italian joint venture with a large and venerable multiline insurer there. By the end of the year, we had recognized that the easiest foreign entry would be into the market most like our own. With regard to health plans, that meant going to South Africa.

Why South Africa?

South Africa mirrors many of the health care characteristics of the United States: coverage is principally financed through employer-sponsored private comprehensive insurance; doctors and hospitals legally operate as private, independent businesses; and the overall system maintains a first-class standard of clinical care. A U.S. practitioner could parachute into any South African hospital or medical office and start practicing immediately without difficulty. The annual premium cost for a family of four in Johannesburg is similar to a comparable family living in a U.S. city.

Although there are exceptions, that family is usually white, not black. South Africa remains a double country with a dual culture. As the South Africans themselves say, their country is a place where the first world and the third world coexist. In this dualism, South Africa presents dramatically opposite health care challenges.

The great mass of its population needs greater access to basic health care services. Yet it is estimated that in 1992, 64 percent of that nation's total health care expenditures were directed at the 17 percent of the population with private health insurance. Worse, medical inflation in that sector is maintaining double-digit annual rates (Benatar, 1997). Even though premiums for private insurance are comparable to those in the United States, the uninsured must rely on an underfinanced, overwhelmed public health system and often go without professional attention, even for serious illnesses.

But given its customer base, the South African insurance industry has been more concerned with exploding costs than increasing access to care. In this effort they held a very positive, even idealistic view of managed care's capabilities and were eager to import it. In fact, one large health insurer, The Southern Life Association, Ltd., had contacted United for that purpose as early as 1992. South Africa's insurance industry had already begun to experiment with preferred provider contracting and limited utilization review, promising employer-purchasers some relief from continuous cost escalation. The delegation from Southern described an attractive market opportunity for a U.S. company capable of providing expert assistance and systems. Sounding a great deal like U.S. conditions a decade earlier, one that managed care had helped bring under control, the opportunity was attractive.

Timing Was Critical

Doing business in South Africa during the apartheid era, though, was simply out of the question. United staff was able to offer some pointers and suggestions on an informal basis, but serious consideration of anything more was deferred until the election of 1994 brought constitutional reform and an end to the embargo. With the rest of the world, United cheered the peaceful arrival of the "New South Africa" and wasted no time in putting a business plan together.

When discussions with Southern Life resumed in 1994, they were different in two fundamental ways. First, United was now interested in pursuing a true joint venture with Southern to create a new South African managed health care company, not limiting itself to merely being a systems vendor or a consultant. We had come to think that beyond computer systems and fee schedules, the success of managed care programs depended on the hundreds, perhaps thousands of individual decisions made each day by the entire staff. Each one would require expertise, thoroughness, and sensitivity. And training an entire staff in how to do it would require sustained, on-site, hands-on involvement. United either wanted to go into the managed care business in South Africa, or not go at all.

The second change was that Southern was now joined in the project by Anglo American Corporation, South Africa's huge mining and financial services conglomerate. Anglo American is perhaps the largest and most dominant company in modern South Africa, and certainly it is one of the country's major employers. Their interest in the health insurance business had roots in two interests: (1) controlling the escalating costs of their own employee health plan and (2) a desire to funnel whatever economies they could achieve into at least partial funding for a major expansion of their program. They wanted to offer coverage for the first time to thousands of low-wage, mostly nonwhite mine workers and dependents. They also thought that if this voluntary, progressive move was successful, it would create a business opportunity in offering the same plan to other employers.

For United HealthCare it was a chance to enter its first foreign market partnered with its largest employer and third largest insurer.

Going Global

For United HealthCare, a company with neither international experience nor tradition, this was all unchartered territory. The joint venture structure was easy to describe: the South African partners would provide local market expertise, actuarial expertise, and the all-important relationships with providers, customers, and regulators. United would provide systems, U.S.-proven managed care programs, and technical expertise. In the early years, the Americans and the South Africans would share responsibility for product design, marketing, and management, with the Americans in charge. Later the company would be entirely managed by South Africans. Above all, the United executives cautioned themselves not to make the classic mistake of trying to recreate U.S.-style HMOs and force them into an unwilling foreign market.

Transferring Expertise

The plan for transferring expertise ten thousand miles relied on five main conveyance mechanisms:

1. *The development of a totally new information system.* The system would be based on existing United technology, would fully exploit small system network architecture for lower implementation and maintenance costs, and provide greater programming flexibility for transnational applications. We were able to successfully transfer all the sophisticated business functionality of United's legacy COBOL mainframe systems to a modern table-driven, hub-database, client-server system that would use small servers and PC workstations. Country-specific "reprogramming" could then be as easy as replacing one data table with another.

2. *A comprehensive Managed Care School curriculum for foreign staff.* The curriculum was to be taught by seasoned United operations personnel in Minneapolis and on location at several of our HMOs.

3. *An Ambassador Program that would temporarily take experienced personnel off-line on a scheduled basis.* The program would permit subject matter experts from all over

United's operations and program areas to visit South Africa for two weeks to a month in order to train their joint venture (JV) counterparts before returning to resume their regular responsibilities. A continuing long-distance support and mentoring relationship could then be maintained via phone and e-mail.

4. *American staff to conduct an annual audit of the South African programs, operations, and technology.* This would ensure the JV's continuing conformance with target levels of performance.

5. *To field an exceptional team of expatriate managers to start the JV.* This was most critical. Led by Kathy Walstead-Plumb, veteran senior head of United's Group Services Administration division and now the first female CEO of an Anglo-American subsidiary in its history, a team of seven experienced executives and their families would relocate to Johannesburg for up to two years. These would be the experts on whom the new company would rely for its program design, operations implementation, contract development, installation of computer and telephonic information systems, and recruitment and training of staff. In short, these would be the people who would personify United and carry it to South Africa. They would make it all work.

Reality Sets In

The early stages of the project were pure excitement. The new system was using all the hot technology of the moment. Staff on both sides of the Atlantic were infected with the spirit of nation building and considered themselves committed to a grand cause. The new health plan would offer better benefits, affordability, and customer service than anything previously available in South Africa. The goals were high, but the workers were motivated and hard working. They expected it to be hard and felt ready for the struggle.

A Long Development Cycle

Simply negotiating the contractual framework for a three-party transnational joint venture took the better part of a year; repeated trans-Atlantic red-eye flights were followed by marathon legal sessions. The "simple" systems rewrite eventually went over budget and behind schedule, but not by much. The hardware specifications for running the new client-server system had to be upgraded twice before performance was acceptable. (Not an insignificant specification change in a country where computer hardware imports were subject to a 100 percent tariff.)

Then the expatriation of seven executives and six families proved to be the most complicated set of personnel actions in the history of the company. And finally, just before the JV's launch, Southern Life's existing health plan company, AMA, began to come apart and had to be prematurely merged into the new company, significantly adding to the management burden of the start-up.

System Implemented Successfully

Nevertheless, on October 1, 1996, only three months behind schedule but well under budget, Southern HealthCare JV commenced operations with considerable fanfare. Despite its rushed development and the usual shake-down problems aggravated by sheer physical distance and a seven-hour time difference, the new information system had been successfully debugged and installed. A total staff of six hundred people had been trained and were ready to go; four hundred of those presented a training challenge because they had been involuntary transfers from the unsuccessful company, AMA. Finally on January 1, 1997, Southern HealthCare successfully completed the simultaneous "big bang" conversion of Anglo's 135,000-member employee health plan. After years of theorizing and hard work, it was a heady moment of triumph.

Negative Physician Response

Unfortunately, there was not to be another one. In the five-year period from 1992 to 1997, attitudes about managed care had changed quite a lot in South Africa. Doctors were no longer curious about the American trend. They were not interested in Southern HealthCare JV's plans for managed care in South Africa. The doctors already felt they knew what was coming, and they had made up their minds not to like it at all. At provider meetings, someone always had several anti–managed care editorials and horror stories clipped from the pages of the *New York Times* and *USA Today*. Following dramatic readings, everyone present would vow not to let the same atrocities "happen here." Southern HealthCare began to be publicly accused of "medical imperialism" and, most sensationally, "medical apartheid." (Similar sentiments can be seen in Perez-Stable, 1999.) The expatriated United executives were commonly referred to as the Minnesota Mafia. (Later they would be credited for doing more for physician unity in two years than the South African medical society had been able to accomplish in a century.)

Provider Boycotts

The contract for pharmaceutical benefits management in the Southern Health-Care program was held by Interpharm, SmithKline's South African subsidiary that was acquired from United. Unfortunately, it would be abandoned after several months of successful boycott by most of the pharmacies in the country. Pharmacies were refusing to fill Southern HealthCare–insured prescriptions without cash or a credit card at the point of service, rendering the benefit of much less value.

Immediately after that crisis was settled (essentially by Southern HealthCare agreeing to pay list price for pharmaceuticals), the surgical specialty society led a similar boycott of its own, covering all but emergency cases. And then, once the surgeons were placated by agreeing to their contract demands and higher reimbursement levels, the primary care physicians began subjecting Southern HealthCare members to an appointment slowdown.

Bad Press

Stories about how American managed care was not working in South Africa became a staple of the daily newspapers. New member sales were nonexistent. The staff soldiered on, but their initial spirit of innovation and nation building was irretrievably lost. The much-needed product that had been planned for low-wage employees was now impossible—no black doctors were willing to join the Southern HealthCare network. By January 1998 a new South African CEO was named, and the Americans returned home.

The Joint Venture Is Abandoned

Later that year Anglo American made an independent business decision to divest all of its non-mining businesses. Southern Life would be sold, its interest in Southern HealthCare taken over directly by Anglo, only to be resold (with United's shares as well) to a competitor. In late 1997 and based in part on this disappointing experience, United HealthCare made its own policy decision to limit new international ventures to consulting contracts. (Support for existing overseas operations, such as the United joint ventures in Hong Kong and Lisbon, was continued, and they are reportedly continuing to do well today.)

Lessons Learned

United and Client Were Overcommitted

It is clearer in retrospect than it was at the time that we made the mistake of trying to do too much. Despite an excellent plan for creating a state-of-the-art health plan in a minimum amount of time, the project was rejected by the people it was intended to serve. In spite of the joint venture structure, the company was always perceived by the South Africans as American and foreign, not local. With surprising rapidity, managed care transformed from a political remedy to a demonized target deserving broad political criticism. The expected cooperative relationship with providers (raising their fees for practicing good medicine but getting them out of the pharmacy business) failed from the start. One would wish to be able to list at least a few small counterbalancing triumphs, no matter how small. But if they occurred they remain obscure.

Ultimately, health care depends on relationships of trust and confidence to a degree that is perhaps unique in business. Ultimately, one is not buying a product but the treatment of a loved one. So a health care program that is distrusted and lacks the support of the community's practitioners has no chance. We had misread the market for an American-style managed care program, and from the time planning started until the JV went live, it had turned actively against us.

Physicians and Pharmacies Felt Threatened

In analyzing this disappointing outcome, three overlooked differences from the U.S. environment stand out for comment. The war over pharmaceuticals, for example, was most unusual and completely unanticipated. In the United States there had been very little real resistance to managed care evidenced by pharmacists or pharmacy chains. In fact, in 1998 one large retail chain, Rite Aid, acquired its own PBM, PCS. Within the U.S. pharmacy industry, the PBMs, although sometimes administratively irksome, have been credited with having had the salutary effect of moving prescription drugs under insurance benefits for the first time. This, of course, insulated consumers from the economic impact of significant drug cost increases and had the net effect of expanding the market for higher-priced pharmaceuticals.

In South Africa, in contrast, the distribution of pharmaceuticals is quite different than in the United States, with an enormous wholesale-to-retail markup. In addition, many physicians earn a sizable percentage of their incomes by dispensing medication in the office. Approximately 30 percent of South Africa's total health care expenditures are prescription drug costs, versus only 10 percent in the United States. By simultaneously attacking both the pharmacy markups and physician dispensing, Southern HealthCare miscalculated, appearing to threaten both groups of professionals (plus their wholesalers) at the same time.

In addition, the government demurred on its earlier intention to use this opportunity to tighten physician dispensing and improve patient safety by forcing compliance with regulations on labeling and inventory controls, much the way it is done in the United States. The government appeared to back off after this policy change was successfully portrayed as being particularly onerous to black patients and their doctors, for whom conveniently located retail alternatives are often unavailable. Without government support, Southern HealthCare had no hope of successfully challenging the practice.

In a small country like South Africa, it is not particularly difficult for an angry, oppositional group of a few hundred people to organize over a weekend into a successful boycott. One boycott will then inspire other emulators on other, similar issues. That is exactly what happened. The American executives had never had to deal with anything like this before, even in small communities.

Employer Support Is Required

A second mistake was failing to recognize the eventual importance that not having an active employer lobby in South Africa would have. Unlike the United States, the South African employers as a group never argued for the growing unaffordability of health coverage and the necessity of managed care. They informally complained about the cost of health insurance of course, but they never cut back their paternalistic health plans or made their plight a political issue. So later, any pain associated with the managed care concept was seen as having been "caused" by Southern HealthCare, not by continual medical cost escalation or employer purchasing decisions. Again, a solitary vendor perceived as promoting an unpopular product has little chance of gaining either political or public support.

Black Physicians Are Essential

Finally, the failure of Southern HealthCare to gain the support of the black physicians was a mistake of major proportions. South Africa is a country in self-conscious transition from being unfairly racially segregated to equitably integrated. In the current milieu, the issue of who is to be included or excluded from any social program or institution is always a sensitive issue and always carries an emotional charge. Somehow, despite the reality of its American-style, equal-opportunity hiring and promotion practices and its hopes for bringing insurance benefits to thousands of heretofore uncovered employees, Southern HealthCare became perceived as being on the wrong side of that divide. The black doctors would not join.

Moreover, without meaning to, in our lack of familiarity with the implications of "two countries in one land mass," we violated one of the foundational prerequisites for managed care's success that we knew so well: the reliance on provider overcapacity. Although we were focused on the U.S.-like white health care system, we failed to give the black doctor shortage the importance it deserved. There was no overcapacity of physicians in the black South Africa. Those who are there work all day every day, tending to the constant tide of black patients needing care. There is little motivation for these doctors to network, bargain on fees, or negotiate about treatment plans. They need respite, not more practice volume.

Eventually we learned that without the support of the community of black physicians, the new government would not get involved in supporting managed care reforms.

In the end Southern HealthCare had many enemies, few friends, and no market. Its American technology and management practices were magnificent, but their benefits could not be demonstrated.

The Market Prefers Something Different

Given the political debate over managed care that is now raging in the United States, a sidebar from the South African experience should not go unnoticed. While Southern HealthCare's experiment with managed care was struggling and ultimately failing, a new local entrant into the South African market, Momentum Health, Ltd. (now renamed Discovery Health, Ltd.) quietly grew from its own start-up in 1995 to more than 500,000 insureds today. This is amazing growth, even by U.S. standards, and Momentum accomplished it by offering an innovative, *consumer-friendly,* medical savings account product. Competitively priced, offering excellent coverage (including unique personal fitness and well-being benefits), and enjoying favorable provider relations, it is now the undisputed market leader in that country. And as a business it is impressively profitable. Perhaps there is a domestic lesson here.

References

Benatar, S. "Health Care Reform in the New South Africa." *New England Journal of Medicine,* 1997, *336*(12), 891–895.

Perez-Stable, E. J. "Managed Care Arrives in Latin America." Letter to the editor. *New England Journal of Medicine,* 1999, *340*(14).

CHAPTER FIVE

THE ROLE OF REGULATION
IN GLOBAL MANAGED CARE

Lynn Shapiro Snyder, Leslie V. Norwalk

Every country in the world is grappling with the basic problem of providing medically necessary services to its citizens at a reasonable price. Beyond this basic goal is the desire to improve the health of the population and to prevent the delivery of unnecessary health care services.

Private sector innovation is helping both public and private payers achieve these goals through new types of financing and delivery systems. The managed care industry throughout the world has evolved precisely to achieve the payer's and consumer's objectives of access to quality health care at an affordable price.

However, local governments have an obligation to protect the health and welfare of their citizens and often regulate the activities of the private sector. Government regulators throughout the world are at different stages of developing ways to ensure that the public interest is protected through the regulation of the health care industry generally and managed care health benefit products in particular.

The regulatory schemes that are developed reflect the wide variety of managed care products available. For example, at one end of the spectrum is a managed indemnity product, which would include PPOs. At the other end of the spectrum is a closed-panel HMO. For purposes of this chapter, any health benefits product that combines financing and delivery, including PPOs and HMOs, is referred to collectively as an MCO (managed care organization).

The objective of any managed care regulatory scheme is universal. Such schemes address common areas of public interest relating to the MCO's function as both insurer and health care provider. These areas include but are not limited to the following: premium rating, fiduciary responsibilities, investments, protection against insolvency, limitation of enrollee liability, coordination of benefits, contents of the evidence of coverage and other enrollee marketing materials, quality assurance, utilization review, enrollment period, and confidentiality of medical information.

Generally speaking, the looser the managed care product, the less stringent the regulatory requirements. The converse also is true. In other words, the more insurance risk a company accepts and the greater the restrictions on accessing providers of health care, the more oversight regulators will demand.

Often, MCOs are reluctant to expand their operations across borders, whether those borders are state or federal boundaries. This reluctance stems from a number of real and perceived barriers to entry into "foreign" markets.

One of the key barriers to expansion across borders is the need to master a new and perhaps more stringent government regulatory scheme for the operation of the MCO in the new jurisdiction. However, our extensive experience as U.S. health lawyers representing a wide variety of health care clients throughout the world has shown that certain universal concepts are consistently the subject of the health regulatory environment. These universal concepts include consumer protection, fiscal solvency, and adequate disclosure, as well as the constant tension between free market prices and regulated prices for payment of medically necessary health care services.

When confronting a new territory, an MCO first should examine the government regulatory scheme that is a condition precedent to operating in that new jurisdiction. The scheme should be viewed as a starting point and not an end point. Even when confronted with a hostile or complicated regulatory scheme, there may be opportunities to encourage regulators to consider new types of regulatory schemes based on the experience the MCO may have had in its domestic jurisdiction.

This chapter can be used by private payers to educate existing or future regulators of MCOs outside the United States about the ways in which U.S. regulators have addressed certain universal issues that have confronted the managed care industry in the past. This advocacy piece could be useful, especially when approaching regulators that have not yet established a comprehensive managed care regulatory scheme or where such a regulatory scheme is in its infancy.

Although this chapter focuses on the U.S. managed care industry's experience, it could serve as a model for the creation or modification of a health regulatory scheme across borders for new types of health care providers or payers. Other possible topics could include the regulation of new types of providers such as freestanding ambulatory surgery centers or new types of technology such as mail order pharmacies and Internet prescribing activities. Suffice it to say that this chapter is just one example of the way the U.S. health regulatory scheme for a health care product or service (that is, for MCOs) can be used by the private sector to modify a foreign health regulatory environment in order to create a regulatory scheme across borders that satisfies the concerns of both the private and public sectors.

Regulatory Barriers

The topics discussed in the sections to follow have been identified as key health regulatory barriers to the expansion of managed care in countries other than the United States. The experiences of the managed care health regulatory environment in the United States can serve as a public policy resource for businesses seeking to promote managed care enterprises throughout the world.

Advertising by Health Practitioners

The ethical codes of numerous professional groups, including medical associations, establish constraints on the types, modes, and content of advertising. Such limitations are based on the ostensible rationale that advertising by professionals is undignified and lowers the esteem in which the profession is held by the public.

In the United States, restraints on advertising in the medical profession were promulgated by state regulatory bodies and by private medical associations. Successful challenges to these advertising restrictions have been based on two different legal theories: (1) commercial speech is protected by the First Amendment to the Constitution[1] and (2) advertising restrictions are a violation of state and federal antitrust laws.[2]

Prohibitions on Fee Splitting

Many states in the United States have enacted fee-splitting statutes that operate to preclude kickback or other illegal remuneration arrangements. Fee splitting generally occurs when a physician or other health care professional refers a patient to another health care provider and then collects from the recipient health professional a portion of a fee paid by the patient for the referred services. However, several states that otherwise prohibit fee splitting still allow the sharing of fees by physicians in a group practice setting or when the fee is really for an administrative service rendered and represents the fair market value for such services. Other states take a broader view of the fee-splitting proscription, prohibiting health care providers from paying fees to anyone, whether or not a source of patient referrals, based on the fees associated with patient services.[3]

Capitation or Other Prepaid Fee Arrangement

The inappropriate use of medical services can be costly and raises concerns about the quality of care. U.S. managed care organizations employ various techniques that are intended to make inappropriate care less likely, including payment methods such as capitation and other incentive arrangements for physicians.

The phrase *physician financial incentive arrangements* may be loosely defined as compensation arrangements between a managed care plan and its physicians that are intended to encourage physicians to control the services provided to plan enrollees. Such incentives can take many forms. For example, capitation payments that shift financial risk to physicians are sometimes used. Such risk-shifting capitation arrangements can be for primary care only or may include referral services.

In the United States, a physician's acceptance of the prepayment of fees for services is generally permitted as a form of pricing risk rather than insurance risk. Once multiple health care providers are involved in a single capitation, the issue of insurance risk becomes more relevant. In any event, the United States does regulate such incentive arrangements to some extent.

Although physician financial incentive arrangements may be designed to improve the quality of care by reducing unnecessary or inappropriate services, they also can have the potential to reduce quality by causing physicians to withhold beneficial treatment. Like fee-for-service, these arrangements can create a potential conflict between providers, financial interests, and patients' medical needs. Although fee-for-service can lead to the overprovision of services, managed care physician incentive arrangements can lead physicians to limit services inappropriately. Concerns about tying treatment decisions to financial rewards have been expressed by members of the medical community, consumer advocacy groups, and others. Therefore, some states have enacted laws to prohibit or limit the use of physician financial incentive arrangements in managed care plans. Other state laws have been enacted to help ensure that managed care enrollees are made aware of their physicians' financial incentive arrangements and that physicians are not prevented by plans from disclosing this information. Federal law regulates physician financial incentive arrangements for Medicare beneficiaries (generally those persons who are disabled or sixty-five years old or older.)[4]

Managed care plans also may use methods other than physician financial incentives to control costs and the use of services. These methods include selecting providers to participate in the network whose practice patterns seem to share the plan's cost-control goals, and requiring physicians to obtain the plan's preapproval when ordering expensive services such as hospital and specialty care.

Consumer advocates, the medical community, and others have expressed concerns about these controls as well. Concern has been expressed that a patient's choice of providers may be restricted because of a limited selection available in the number and types of providers participating in a managed care plan's network. There also is concern that controls used by plans to limit the number of patient visits to hospitals and specialists may inappropriately restrict patient access to needed medical care. In addition, concerns have been raised that the threat of contract termination or nonrenewal can be used to influence and restrict physicians' health care decisions.

Some states have enacted a variety of laws to address such concerns. These laws are intended to help ensure that managed care patients receive access to appropriate medical care. For example, some of these laws provide managed care plan enrollees with a greater choice of and access to providers both within and outside plan networks, limit the influence that plans have over physicians' medical decisions, allow physicians to discuss freely all treatment options with their patients, and protect physicians from having their contracts inappropriately terminated or not renewed so they are not unduly influenced in their decisions about the need for medical care.

Anti-Kickback Laws

The federal government prohibits individuals from paying or receiving any remuneration "in return for referring an individual to a [health care provider] for which payment may be made in whole or in part under a Federal healthcare program."[5] Several statutory exceptions are set forth in the anti-kickback statute,[6] and the U.S. Department of Health and Human Services (HHS) also has promulgated "safe harbor" regulations that protect individuals who perform the activities enumerated in such regulations.[7]

Many states also prohibit licensed health care professionals (that is, physicians, pharmacists, or nurses) from offering, delivering, receiving, or accepting any monetary payment or other consideration for the referral of patients.[8] However, payment for services other than for referrals of patients may be permitted, provided the payment is commensurate with the value of the services furnished.[9] Additionally, some states provide statutory exceptions for referrals made in the context of a prepaid health plan.[10]

Corporate Practice of Medicine Prohibitions

In the United States, the practice of medicine is typically regulated by state medical boards. Many states prohibit a corporation from engaging in the practice of medicine. This prohibition is in the form of state statute or state case law. This means that corporations that are not solely made up of professionals are prohibited from hiring physicians to provide medical services. However, most states exempt hospitals and HMOs from this prohibition.[11]

Pharmacy Ownership

A few states prohibit physicians (or any other person authorized to write a prescription) from owning a pharmacy.[12] Likewise, a professional corporation is proscribed from holding a pharmacy license.[13]

Drug Formularies

A few states have statutes that, depending on the facts, may forbid pharmacists, pharmacies, and hospitals from participating in certain rebate arrangements. For example, a rebate may not be generated to a managed care plan from drug manufacturers based on purchases made at the pharmacies participating in the managed care plan's pharmacy network.[14] This prohibition is premised on the idea that pharmaceuticals should be included on a managed care plan's formulary based solely on the drug's efficacy and cost-effectiveness.

Physicians in some states are prohibited from receiving any incentive from a managed care plan to prescribe from the formulary. Moreover, state pharmacy statutes may prohibit licensed pharmacists from receiving compensation for a referral.[15] This could prohibit a managed care plan from sharing rebates with network pharmacies. In addition, a few states have laws prohibiting hospitals from entering into compensation arrangements with pharmacies.[16]

Most state insurance laws prohibit an insurer from either (1) executing a contract or agreement relating to an insurance policy that has not been expressly disclosed in the insurance policy itself or (2) offering an undisclosed rebate, refund, or other consideration as an inducement to insurance. Although disclosure of the rebate may reduce exposure under some of these state statutes, the statutory language in several states expressly requires the disclosure of a rebate arrangement in the insurance policy itself, irrespective of whether it is a marketed feature.[17]

Many state anti-kickback statutes forbid the drug rebates with or without disclosure, although arguments do exist that the rebate is being paid in return for the education of physicians, pharmacists, and patients as to the efficacy of certain products that have been selected for inclusion in the formulary rather than for physician referrals. Those physicians would (so the argument goes) exercise independent medical judgment and at no time would receive incentives from a managed care plan provider to prescribe from the formulary.

Confidentiality

Most states and some federal statutes protect the confidentiality of patient medical records information. This confidentiality extends to the physical record as well as to the information contained in such a record. The basis for confidentiality of patient records information stems from a variety of sources. For example, state statutes and case law governing health care providers, such as the medical practice acts of many states, specify that physicians who fail to abide by the laws governing the confidentiality of patient medical records are guilty of unprofessional conduct and may be subject to disciplinary action by the state licensing board.[18] Some states have expanded the duty of confidentiality to other health care providers.[19] The patient-physician privilege in many states also typically prohibits physicians and other practitioners from disclosing to third parties information they acquired through their professional relationship with a patient.[20]

States may also have statutes directed at specific types of medical records information, such as mental health records,[21] alcohol and drug abuse treatment records,[22] and AIDS-related records information.[23] States have found that patients may have a state constitutional right to confidentiality,[24] an implied covenant of confidentiality that derives from the nature of the patient's relationship with a physician or other health care provider,[25] or the fiduciary nature of such relationships.[26]

Preferred Provider Arrangements

In the United States preferred provider arrangements evolved out of a consumer demand for greater choices and an employer's demand for cost containment; in most cases the employee consumes the health care services yet the employer pays the bill. Initially, there was little state regulation of preferred provider arrangements because they were viewed merely as discount arrangements and bill-paying organizations. However, as these MCOs began to be more powerful in the marketplace and to use more managed care utilization control techniques, the need for regulation became more apparent. At this time, there is a model PPO Act. The National Association of Insurance Commissioners (NAIC), which is responsible for this model act, has also been developing a model MCO act that is designed to increase the amount of regulation as risk assumption increases.[27]

Provider Networks and Antitrust

The mere formation of provider networks by entrepreneurs does not raise antitrust concerns at the outset. The situation is different if the network's owners are themselves providers from the same marketplace. Due to arguments by interest groups such as the American Medical Association (AMA) that physicians and other providers were being discouraged from forming provider-controlled networks because of the antitrust risks involved, the U.S. Department of Justice and the Federal Trade Commission jointly released new health care antitrust guidelines.[28] Arguing that provider networks can benefit consumers by introducing more effective quality assurance and utilization review techniques, the AMA urged the antitrust agencies to take steps to clarify that the creation of provider-controlled managed care networks can be beneficial to consumers and, as a result, should be encouraged.

In order to achieve this result, the government agencies have specified in these guidelines that the integration necessary to bring provider-controlled networks within the rule of reason is not limited to integration through shared financial risk and can include substantial clinical integration. The guidelines focus on whether the network, if it does not involve the sharing of substantial financial risk, contains programs in areas such as utilization management and quality assurance that genuinely will yield increased efficiencies. Nonetheless, the guidelines make clear that programs purporting to be utilization management or quality assurance, but in reality add little of value to the network from a payer's perspective, will not enable the network to escape per se condemnation as an illegal price-fixing arrangement among competitors.

Patient and Provider Protection

Many states have passed measures designed to safeguard patient rights. Some of these measures require a managed care plan to disclose to its enrollees the managed care plan's cost-control features, such as the financial incentives offered to physicians for withholding services or avoiding referrals.[29] Similarly, managed care plans that have a risk-sharing agreement with the Medicare program or the Medicaid program cannot operate a physician incentive plan (PIP) unless that PIP meets certain specified criteria.[30]

Managed care plans often develop PIPs as part of their provider reimbursement scheme. In the Medicare managed care context, however, these managed care plans must comply with certain federal restrictions imposed on PIPs. The PIP rules apply only to PIPs that base compensation (in whole or in part) on the use or cost of services furnished to Medicare beneficiaries or Medicaid recipients. Additionally, PIPs apply to subcontracting arrangements.[31] PIPs that affect only commercial enrollees of managed care plans are not regulated by the federal statute.

President Clinton recently proposed that the U.S. Congress pass a Patient's Bill of Rights, which would provide consumer access to detailed information about the quality of health plans, hospitals, and physicians. The Patient's Bill of Rights would also provide consumers the right to access emergency health care services when and where the need arises. Moreover, the proposal would give consumers the right to fully participate in decisions related to their health care. The Patient's Bill of Rights would grant consumers the right to communicate with health care professionals in confidence and to have their medical records kept confidential. Finally, President Clinton's proposal would ensure that consumers have a right to a fair and efficient process to appeal to an independent body any decision that denied patient care.[32]

Role of Associations in the Managed Care Regulatory Environment

The American Association of Health Plans (AAHP), an association of over 1,000 managed care organizations, requires managed care plans joining or renewing membership in the organization to adopt AAHP's patient-centered policies. AAHP's Philosophy of Care includes the following tenets: patients should have the right care, at the right time, in the right setting; all health care professionals should be held accountable for the quality of the services they provide and for the satisfaction of their patients; patients should have a choice within their health plans of physicians who meet high standards of professional training and experience; health care decisions should be the shared responsibility of patients, their families, and health care professionals; consumers have a right to information about health plans and how they work; working with people to keep them healthy is as important as making them well; and access to affordable, comprehensive care gives consumers the value they expect and contributes to the peace of mind that is essential to good health.

The National Association of Insurance Commissioners (NAIC) is an association of insurance regulators from all fifty states. The primary responsibility of state regulators is to protect the interests of insurance consumers, including enrollees in MCOs. Insurance departments regulate the national insurance business on a state-by-state basis. Thus, state insurance regulators created the NAIC to address the need to coordinate the regulation of multistate insurers. The NAIC provides a forum for the development of uniform state insurance policies. The NAIC develops model laws, regulations, and guidelines that in turn may be adopted by the states.[33] The states may either adopt the model laws intact or modify them to meet their specific needs and conditions.

Gag Rules

Federal and state laws, as well as medical associations (including the AMA) prohibit managed care plan contract provisions that prevent physicians from making statements that could undermine a patient's confidence in a plan's policies or coverage. Physicians are also prohibited from informing patients about physicians or facilities not included in a plan or referring a patient for a second opinion.[34]

Freedom of Choice

As of April 1996, at least twenty-four states had laws requiring managed care plans to accept any provider willing to agree to and abide by the terms of a plan's contract. Approximately fourteen of these laws have been enacted since 1992. The intent of these any-willing-provider laws is to restrict plans from excluding providers from their networks and to provide enrollees with greater freedom of choice. Most laws apply only to certain types of providers—typically pharmacists—but several more recent laws include physicians and other types of providers.

Other state laws have been enacted or proposed to ensure that managed care plan enrollees have access to providers outside their plans' networks. For example, New York passed a law in 1995 requiring that plans allow certain enrollees to use nonplan providers, although the enrollees would have to pay higher deductibles and copayments.[35] Greater enrollee access to providers, including specialists, has been provided by a variety of other types of laws enacted and proposed in some states. Some states have also enacted laws to help ensure that enrollees are not denied necessary medical care because of decisions by plan representatives who are not licensed physicians.

Conclusion

These are just a few examples of the way in which the experience in the United States can be used to facilitate a more favorable regulatory scheme across borders that satisfies the concerns of both the private and public sectors.

Notes

1. See *Zauderer* v. *Office of Disciplinary Counsel,* 471 U.S. 626, 638: "Commercial speech that is not false or deceptive and does not concern unlawful activities . . . may be restricted only

in the service of a substantial government interest, and only through means that directly advance that interest."

2. See American Medical Association, 94 F.T.C. 701, 1110 (1980), enforced, 638 F.2d 443 (2d Cir. 1980), aff'd by equally divided court, 455 U.S. 676 (1982): the AMA "has simply not demonstrated that a broad ban [on advertising] is necessary to ensure that advertising is nondeceptive and that solicitation is inoffensive to vulnerable classes of consumers."

3. See, for example, 225 Ill. Comp. Stat. 60/22A(a)(14): physicians are proscribed from "[d]ividing with anyone other than physicians with whom the licensee practices in a partnership, Professional Association or Medical or Professional Corporation any fee, commission, rebate or other form of compensation for any professional services not actually and personally rendered."

4. 42 U.S.C. §1395mm(i)(8)(B); 42 C.F.R. §417.479(b).

5. 42 U.S.C. §1320a-7b(b); 42 C.F.R. §1001.951.

6. 42 U.S.C. §1320a-7b(b)(3); 42 C.F.R. §1001.952.

7. 42 C.F.R. §1001.952; 56 Fed. Reg. 35,932 (July 29, 1991); 61 Fed. Reg. 2,122 (Jan. 26, 1996).

8. See also *Annotated Guidelines on Gifts to Physicians from Industry,* American Medical Association, Council on Ethical and Judicial Affairs, Oct. 9, 1991.

9. See Cal. Bus. & Prof. Code §650.

10. Cal. Health & Safety Code §445.

11. See, for example, Cal. Health & Safety Code §1395(b): a health care service plan "shall not be deemed to be engaged in the practice of a profession, and may employ, or contract with, any professional licensed . . . to deliver professional services"; 65 Op. Cal. Att. Gen. 223 (1982) (noting several exceptions to the corporate practice doctrine).

12. See Cal. Bus. & Prof. Code §4111(a): the Board of Pharmacy is prohibited from issuing or renewing "any license to conduct a pharmacy to any of the following: (1) A person or persons authorized to prescribe or write a prescription . . . (2) A person or persons with whom a person or persons specified in paragraph (1) shares a community or other financial interest in the permit sought."

13. See Cal. Bus. & Prof. Code §4111(a)(3): "Any corporation that is controlled by, or in which 10 percent or more of the stock is owned by a person or persons prohibited from pharmacy ownership" is also prohibited from holding a pharmacy license.

14. See, for example, Ariz. Comp. Admin. R. & Regs. R4-23-404: a pharmacist may not accept or deliver "any unearned rebate, refund, commission, preference, patronage dividend, discount, or other unearned consideration" as "compensation or inducement for referring patients, clients, or customers to any person."

15. See, for example, Ariz. Rev. Stat. Ann. §32-1927(B)(3)(a): Arizona law provides that a pharmacist's license may be revoked for "paying rebates or entering into an agreement for payment of rebates to a medical practitioner or any other person in the health field"; Nev. Rev. Stat. Ann. §639.264: the Nevada Pharmacy Act specifically prohibits discounts to any person as compensation or inducement to such person for referring prescription patients; Cal. Bus. & Prof. Code §650.

16. Maryland explicitly forbids a hospital from receiving a rebate or other consideration from a "provider of drugs, prescriptions, or pharmaceutical services." Md. Code Ann., Health Gen. §19-357. Hospitals in Arizona are also expressly barred from directly or indirectly offering or implying an offer of rebate of fee-splitting to another licensed person; Ariz. Rev. Stat. Ann. §36-407(D) (1993). Illinois has a comparable statute, 225 Ill. Comp. Stat. 85/23.

17. See, for example, Ariz. Rev. Stat. Ann. §20-451: no person shall give, directly or indirectly, "any rebate, discount . . . or any valuable consideration or inducement whatever, not specified in the policy of insurance."
18. See, for example, Cal. Bus. & Prof. Code §2263; 225 Ill. Comp. Stat. 60/22-A(30); Pa. Stat. Ann. §§455.241 & 422.41; 49 Pa. Code §16.61(a)(1).
19. See, for example, Cal. Civ. Code §§56 et seq.
20. See, for example, Cal. Evid. Code §994; Fla. Stat. §80.503 (regarding psychiatrists); 735 Ill. Comp. Stat. 5/8-802; N.J. Stat. Ann. §2A:84A-22.2; N.Y. Civ. Prac. L. & R. §4504(a); Ohio Rev. Code Ann. §2317.02(B)(1); Pa. Stat. Ann. tit. 42, §5929.
21. See, for example, Cal. Welf. & Inst. Code §§4514 & 5328; 740 Ill. Comp. Stat. 110/5; N.J. Stat. Ann. §30:4-24.3; N.Y. Mental Hyg. Law §33.13; Ohio Rev. Code Ann. §5122.31; Pa. Stat. Ann. tit. 50, §§4605(5) & 7111; Tex. Health & Safety Code Ann. §611.002.
22. See, for example, 20 Ill. Comp. Stat. 301/30-5(bb); N.J. Stat. Ann. §26:2B-20.
23. See, for example, 410 Ill. Comp. Stat. 305/1 et seq.; N.J. Stat. Ann. §26:5C-5 et seq.; N.Y. Pub. Health Law §2782; Tex. Health & Safety Code Ann. §81.101 et seq.
24. See for example, *Wood* v. *Superior Court*, 212 Cal. Rptr. 811 (Cal. Ct. App. 1985).
25. See, for example, *Doe* v. *Roe,* 400 N.Y.S.2d 668 (N.Y. Sup. Ct. 1977).
26. See, for example, *Alexander* v. *Knight,* 177 A.2d 142, 146 (Pa. Super. Ct. 1962); *Piller* v. *Kovosky,* 476 A.2d 1279 (N.J. Super. Ct. Law Div. 1984).
27. See NAIC Model Preferred Provider Organization Act.
28. Statements of Antitrust Enforcement Policy in Health Care, Aug. 28, 1996.
29. See, for example, Cal. Health & Safety Code §1367.10; Va. Code Ann. §38.2-3407.10(C)(4)(A).
30. 42 U.S.C. §1395mm(i)(8)(B); 42 U.S.C. §1396b(2)(A)(x).
31. 42 C.F.R. §417.479(b).
32. White House, "President Clinton Endorses Consumer Bill of Rights and Calls for Immediate Action to Implement," press release, Nov. 20, 1997.
33. See NAIC Model Health Maintenance Organization Act.
34. See, for example, the Health Care Financing Administration, Operational Policy Letter no. 44 (Nov. 25, 1996); statement by the American Medical Association Council on Ethical and Judicial Affairs, Jan. 1996; White House, "Remarks by the President on Medicaid Gag Rule," press release, Feb. 20, 1997.
35. N.Y. Pub. Health §4403(6)(a).

EMERGING DEVELOPMENTS

CHAPTER SIX

ACCREDITATION AND GLOBALIZATION

K. Tina Donahue

The globalization of business and improved communications alone will have a profound impact on cross-border issues, including health—a highly personal issue for each of us. Citizens will begin to demand more information about and accountability for health care, which will drive evidence-based practice and accurate measurement of quality and performance. Health care delivery foci will shift from acute to primary care settings; government's role will change from health service provider to steward, driving the formalization of minimum standards for health care by country. The number of country-specific accreditation schemes will increase at the same time international health care organization accreditation is tested and implemented.

This chapter provides an overview of the state of the art in international health care organization accreditation. Knowledge of global health care markets includes concern about the quality of health care being delivered and how it is measured everywhere on our shrinking globe.

The chapter first provides an overview of the changing international landscape as it relates to health system quality and accreditation issues. A brief history of the evolution of accreditation and its links to political, social, and economic situations is provided in descriptions of a few country-specific accreditation schemes.

International accreditation is described as recent and continuing evolution. The need for and challenges inherent in implementing a universally applicable set of standards for hospitals and the debate around this challenge is also discussed.

And finally, predictions on policy changes based on the chapter's conclusions give the reader a glimpse into the new millennium. Whether as a clinician, manager, insurer, or government official, we, as citizens of the world, should find this directional piece of vital interest.

World Overview

Sweeping economic, political, and social changes worldwide over the last ten years have prompted many countries to examine their respective health care systems as a public good. There is widespread agreement that escalating health care costs are consuming increasing proportions of the GDP. Key health care experts and economists as well note a general trend toward privatization of health delivery systems and a movement from regulatory approaches to quality- and measurement-oriented approaches for improving health care. Significant change is driven by leaders and decision makers whose knowledge and support of quality initiatives are essential for successful reform. Thus, relentless education about mechanisms to improve care is essential at every level of the health care system.

Countries are accepting the imperative to control costs but not at the expense of improving access and quality for citizens in need of health care. These objectives conflict and stimulate more competition for resources but also provide incentives for creative approaches to achieving more accessible, higher-quality, and more cost-effective health care (Donahue and O'Leary, 1997).

Forces for Change

Forces for change aim to introduce new payment schemes, shift or reduce capacity for care, and set minimum quality standards. The role of government in health care systems is shifting as well, retaining responsibility for providing citizens with overall health services but shifting accountability for the quality and cost of services to public and private providers.

Physicians are seeking to define more clearly the scientific bases for clinical care to enable the practice of truly evidence-based medicine. Outcomes, population-based, and operational measures are sought out and used more frequently. The public in developed nations is demanding accountability and information from the health system. In addition, hospital CEOs in developed and developing countries are seeking a means to differentiate their organizations in their national and international markets. Many look to accreditation as the tool to demonstrate their hospitals are high-quality, efficient care providers.

This new era emphasizes more effective health care financing and delivery systems as means to health sector reform, underscores the importance of quality, and drives the development of health care evaluation systems (Donahue and Janeski, 1998). In this context, health care organization accreditation is seen as a powerful tool to effect health system change.

Developments by Country

At the turn of the last decade, five established and country-specific health care organization accreditors existed in the United States, Canada, Australia, New Zealand, and the United Kingdom. At the turn of the last century, we observe the number of established and new accreditation schemes at no less than thirty-two in twenty-six countries and counting (Rooney and van Ostenberg, 1999).

World regions represented in that group include the Americas, Western, Central, and Eastern Europe, the New Independent States, Asia, Pacific Rim, Middle East, and Africa (see Figure 6.1). Although these facts demonstrate that reform initiatives frequently lead to exploring accreditation as a tool to improve or maintain quality in a cost-managed environment, it is also known that a universally accepted accreditation scheme was *not* used in each country or region. A few examples of accreditation activity around the world follow.

Zambia. Zambia, a developing country of 9 million people located in southern central Africa, developed and launched an accreditation system in 1999. The system was part of a major health reform initiative begun in the mid-1990s. This program, sponsored by the U.S. Agency for International Development (AID) Quality Assurance Project and administered by the Ministry of Health, was one of the first of its kind to be attempted in a developing country. Its standards were written to focus on the nation's most pressing health problems, specifically, management of childhood illnesses, preventive childhood health care, maternal and infant care, HIV-AIDS prevention, and treatment of epidemic diseases such as tuberculosis and malaria.

Czech Republic. The Czech Republic's accreditation program originated as a government function in the early 1990s but was moved into the private sector to allow for an accreditation program free from the pressures of the political process. The program focus is hospital-specific, but standards have also been written for specialty delivery services such as kidney dialysis centers. The standards of several established accreditors were used as a guide to develop the Czech standards for accreditation.

FIGURE 6.1. COUNTRIES WITH ESTABLISHED AND NEW HOSPITAL ACCREDITORS.

North America
Canada
United States

South America
Brazil

Western Europe
France
Netherlands
Spain
United Kingdom

Central and Eastern Europe
Czech Republic
Hungary
Lithuania
Poland
Romania

Newly Independent States
Kyrgyzstan
Ukraine

Asia and Pacific Rim
Australia
China
Japan
Korea
Malaysia
New Zealand
Philippines
Taiwan

Middle East
Saudi Arabia

Africa
Egypt
South Africa
Zambia

Source: Rooney and van Ostenberg, 1999.

The Foundation of Avedis Donabedian (FAD), a private nongovernmental organization (NGO) in Barcelona, Spain, established a joint accreditation program in 1998 with the U.S.-based Joint Commission International Accreditation (JCIA). FAD used the U.S. standards of the Joint Commission on Accreditation of Healthcare Organizations (JCAHO), translated to Spanish for application in Spanish hospitals.

Kyrgyzstan. Kyrgyzstan's Ministry of Health developed its accreditation program in the mid-1990s for hospitals with funding from a U.S. AID health markets reform project. An early version of U.S. structurally oriented standards was revised for adaptation in Kyrgyzstan's hospitals. Lack of ongoing fiscal support for the accreditation program has halted progress.

Australia and New Zealand. The Australia and New Zealand programs are well-established NGOs and have evolved over the last twenty years into contemporary-standards-based programs. Their more recently evolved standards are less focused on structural issues and more focused on patient-centered functions. The Australians have had some success in incorporating the use of clinical indicators into the program. A growing number of accreditation experts around the world support the use of indicators as a more effective means of measuring the results of standards application and other improvement tools.

Brazil. With funding from the private sector, Brazil has developed and plans to launch in 2000 an NGO accreditation program. The standards were originally adapted from the U.S. JCAHO standards but eventually incorporated the new JCIA standards. The latter decision was made anticipating that the JCIA standards would eventually become a universally accepted set of standards for hospitals. The Brazilian government is also planning to mandate accreditation but has not yet specified how hospital accreditation will be carried off or what entities may provide the service.

United States and Canada. The U.S. and Canadian accreditation programs are the longest-tenured schemes, having been established in the 1950s. Both are NGOs whose contemporary accreditation services and decisions are accepted by federal, state, and provincial governments in lieu of government certification. Both are working toward incorporating the use of indicators into their respective accreditation processes. In fact, the Joint Commission conducted research on the development of reliable and valid indicators for use in an accreditation system and plans to have an accreditation system fully incorporating the use of indicators within ten years.

International Accreditation

Although the details of the world's country-specific accreditation schemes are far too extensive to describe here, attention must be given to a series of issues evolving across the globe that are common to those planning to use accreditation as a tool for reform. The International Society for Quality in Health Care (ISQua) launched a program called Agenda for Leadership in Programs for Healthcare Accreditation (ALPHA) to further the development of a global approach to aligning health care standards and accreditation processes. The initiative is structured as a federation of health care organization accreditors and currently constitutes the world's health care accreditation experts (International Society for Quality in Health Care, 1999).

These experts have noted that the key variables in accreditation programs from country to country are driven by social structures, societal values, and other cultural, political, economic, and technological realities. Culture, in particular, has much to do with what is valued in health care because health is one of our most personal interests. For example, people in developing countries may value access to potable water, whereas people in developed countries value the availability of organ transplants. Thus the expectations for standards and what is evaluated will vary among cultures, nations, and regions. Based on an assessment of its own characteristics, a new national accreditor could draw components from other systems and adapt these to reflect its own priorities (what is valued). The objectives and expected outcomes of the accreditation system must be clear. Any combination of the following (the list is not all-inclusive) may be acceptable:

- Improve quality
- Reduce cost
- Increase efficiency
- Strengthen public confidence
- Improve management
- Educate
- Rationalize payment schemes
- Provide comparative data

One of the first challenges faced by new accreditors, and indeed all health care professionals, has been defining, in English, key basic evaluation terms such as *accreditation, certification,* and *licensure,* not to mention the challenges inherent in translation to other languages (Donahue and O'Leary, 1997).

It is this diversity that prompted the world's accreditation experts to establish ALPHA and charge it to develop an international framework of principles that could be used to guide development and refinement of country-specific health care organization standards (see Figure 6.2). It was assumed these principles would need to apply, regardless of the state of evolution of the standards over time. In addition, a set of standards for health care accreditation bodies to be used by ALPHA for peer assessment of these accreditors was developed, as well (see Figure 6.3).

JCIA was the first entity to take the then-draft ALPHA principles and develop an international set of standards for hospitals (see Figure 6.4). An international task force consisting of accreditation and quality experts from seven world regions and ISQua completed the development of the standards and the entire international accreditation program in mid-1999. The standards were published in November 1999; shortly thereafter, the first JCIA hospital surveys were conducted in South America and the Middle East. Prior to the establishment of

FIGURE 6.2. ISQUA DRAFT PRINCIPLES FOR STANDARDS.

1. Key concepts which underpin all standards regardless of how their content is presented, should be required.
2. The type of standards is clearly defined.
3. The scope of standards is clearly defined.
4. The content of the standards is comprehensive and clearly structured.
5. Standards are formulated through a well-defined process.
6. Standards are amenable to measurement of performance.

Source: International Society for Quality in Health Care, 1999, pp. 4–5.

FIGURE 6.3. CATEGORIES OF ISQUA DRAFT STANDARDS FOR HEALTH CARE ACCREDITATION BODIES.

1. Corporate governance and strategic directions
2. Organization and management performance
3. Human resource management
4. Surveyor selection, development and deployment
5. Financial and resource management
6. Information management
7. Survey management
8. Accreditation process
9. Standards development
10. Education and information

Source: International Society for Quality in Health Care, 1999, pp. 6–14.

the JCIA program, no international scheme constructed specifically for hospitals had existed.

The task force aimed to develop an accreditation relevant to and effective in virtually all nations—a formidable challenge, given the diversity encountered in health care systems and in worldwide accreditation work. Yet that work also pointed to a common set of standards JCIA could consider core-essential standards in a universally applicable accreditation scheme; they are so designated in the new international standards manual released in November 1999. The international standards were developed to meet a need for health care quality guidelines at international, national, and organizational levels worldwide. JCIA accreditation could be used as a third-party evaluation adjunct to existing national accreditation schemes or as primary in countries devoid of an accreditation scheme.

FIGURE 6.4. JOINT COMMISSION INTERNATIONAL ACCREDITATION STANDARDS FOR HOSPITALS CATEGORIES.

Section I:	Patient-centered standards
	Access to care and continuity of care
	Patient and family rights
	Assessment of patients
	Care of patients
	Patient and family education
Section II:	Health care organization
	Management standards
	Quality management and improvement
	Prevention and control of infections
	Governance, leadership, and direction
	Facility management and safety
	Staff qualifications and education
	Management of information

Source: Joint Commission, 2000.

A set of supporting principles underpinning the accreditation scheme, which helped ensure it would be an independent, objective process, included that the scheme should

- Be highly credible and unbiased
- Represent the broadest possible consensus
- Be used positively to encourage improvement
- Be relied on by key health system stakeholders

Thus, in addition to guidance from an international task force, the standards and other accreditation components were reviewed by key stakeholders in more than fifteen countries, discussed by focus groups in seven world regions, and evaluated in four test accreditation surveys in Latin America, Western Europe, and the Middle East.

In order to develop a set of universally applicable hospital standards, the process focused primarily on (1) systems, processes, and outcomes basic to meeting patients' needs for safe and effective care anywhere, (2) use of equivalencies in how each standard could be met respecting cultural values, and (3) developing a system that would allow for production and appropriate use of valid comparative information about accredited organizations (Donahue and Schyve, 1999). The JCIA standards were shown in test surveys to have applicability in different cultures with different country-specific laws and regulations. This is due to the focus of each standard on the principle as opposed to the evident structure or process (Donahue and van Ostenberg, forthcoming). Implementation of the JCIA program will further test the theory of "universal applicability."

Accreditation experts worldwide are debating the merits of various evaluation systems for use in their respective settings. In order to make clearer the overlap and gaps in comparing JCIA standards with other sets of standards used in hospitals around the world, the first edition of the JCIA Standards for Hospitals contains an appendix comparing the JCIA standards, JCAHO U.S. standards, European Foundation for Quality Management (EFQM) criteria, U.S. Baldrige criteria, and ISO 9000 standards.

The European Commission funded a project named External Peer Review Techniques Project (ExPeRT) from 1996 through 1999, to research the scope, mechanisms, and use of external quality schemes in the improvement of health care. The project identified four models: (1) *visitatie* (developed and used in the Netherlands), (2) accreditation, (3) EFQM, and (4) ISO and national variants of each. The strengths and weaknesses of each approach were analyzed in terms of their respective reliability and validity. The report concluded that many features identified could be incorporated into a convergent model for Europe. It proposed additional descriptive research aimed at demonstrating the relative effectiveness and efficiency of the models. Controlled trials of program operation and impact could provide more specific answers to long-standing questions about the effects on patient processes and outcomes (Shaw, 2000).

Accreditation system effectiveness research is currently being conducted in Zambia and the KwaZulu Natal Province of South Africa under the U.S. AID Quality Assurance Project II. The Zambia research protocol measures the impact of the hospital accreditation program, launched at the end of 1999, on indicators of quality care. These indicators relate to the country's focus on specific health issues, for example, pediatric pneumonia and diarrhea mortality. The South Africa research protocol also measures the impact of its five-year-old NGO accreditation program in hospitals and clinics never before accredited. The quality indicators used relate to the common clinical interventions provided to patients at those hospitals and clinics.

These research projects, to the best of our knowledge, are the first anywhere in the world to examine prospectively, and by means of rigorous study design, the effectiveness of hospital accreditation on indicators of care. We anxiously await the results.

How to Proceed

Florence Nightingale, at the end of the nineteenth century, was the first health professional to measure performance for improvement—a controversial issue then and now. The art and science of performance measurement continues to evolve and be debated. In July 1999, the Joint Commission's First World Symposium on Improving Health Care Through Accreditation was held in Barcelona, Spain, and attended by 250 representatives from more than fifty countries.

Four controversial accreditation issues were debated and voted. Issues and results were as follows:

1. Opinion was mixed on the proposition that no single set of quality standards is appropriate for universal use in health care organizations. In addition, strong support was shown for basing standards on scientific evidence rather than expert opinion.
2. There was a wide range of opinion on the extent to which health care financing mechanisms provide the primary incentives and disincentives to deliver high-quality care. Most voters believed that, over time, accreditation enhances efficiency.
3. On the issue of whether effective health system reform must be legislated and encompass reliance on the private sector, more than half of voters agreed that reform must be legislated. However, voters strongly supported government reliance on independent NGOs for accreditation services and holding virtually all health system stakeholders accountable for care.
4. Voters overwhelmingly supported the proposition that an accreditation system that includes professional credentialing and evidence-based practice will improve health care outcomes. Attendees strongly favored combining certification of health professionals with accreditation of organizations, and expressed near unanimity that accreditation standards should require health care organizations to evaluate best practices and research data, seeking out evidence of effectiveness (Ente, 1999).

The diverse opinions expressed on these important questions reveal further the complexities in health reform and underscore the need for a multifaceted approach to health care reform and improvement. Figure 6.5 offers a simple graphic suggesting the challenges faced in any health care system attempting reform for better health service. What is needed to achieve the objective and sustain improvement is an integrated, systems-based approach that weaves together the key components necessary for a better health system.

FIGURE 6.5. ACCREDITATION AS THE HUB OF A QUALITY HEALTH CARE SYSTEM.

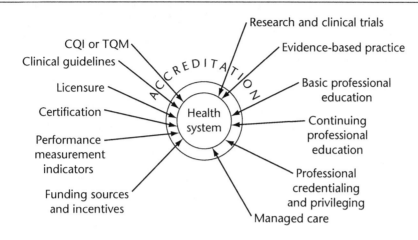

Predictions

If in the coming five years the information explosion profoundly affects every aspect of our lives, we can expect it to affect our health systems as well. Citizens will demand accountability; they will expect and have access to health care organization and even individual practitioner evaluation results, although the accuracy of that information cannot be predicted. As our knowledge of performance measurement and the use of comparative data evolve, the accuracy of the data will improve. However, only a few systems will begin to produce credible data for international comparison.

Health reform initiatives will bring new payment schemes in an attempt to link quality (performance) with reimbursement. Some countries will attempt some degree of health systems privatization, shifting governments' role from provider to steward and the focus of care from acute settings to primary care settings. More governments will seek to formalize at least minimum standards of performance for health care organizations and begin to put in place quality information mechanisms. These changes will increase the use of operational, disease-specific, and population-based health care measures; one or two will be established, and a few well-funded new accreditors will partially incorporate performance measurement into their programs. The number of country-specific accreditation programs will increase where economic and social systems remain stable.

The scientific basis for clinical care will be more clearly defined worldwide as a better understanding of evidence-based practice is facilitated by the Internet and personal information systems. Health systems will eventually pressure educators of health care professionals to reexamine traditional educational paradigms to accommodate practice in information-rich, performance-based, more tightly managed and patient-focused health systems.

Conclusions

That better health care at a reasonable cost is needed everywhere in our world is a given. Developed and developing nations able to improve access and quality while managing health care economics will have the most successful health systems. Notwithstanding how success is defined, the ultimate outcome measure will be a population whose health consistently improves. Worldwide communications and information availability will cause an exponential increase in our knowledge of performance measurement tools, including accreditation. Decision makers at national levels must recognize that a mechanism to synthesize the diverse components of improvement for the system is needed. Research must be done to determine the effectiveness of various improvement components, including accreditation.

Whether an internationally applicable accreditation scheme is feasible remains to be tested. In the meantime, it is in the best interest of all for our policymakers to continue to provide resources to research and implement the best possible health systems—a public good to which all populations are entitled.

References

Donahue, K. T., and Janeski, J. F. "Overview: The Evolution of International Accreditation and Improvement." *Joint Commission Journal on Quality Improvement*, 1998, *24*(5), 223–225.

Donahue, K. T., and O'Leary, D. S. "Evolving Healthcare Organization Accreditation Systems." *International Hospital Federation 50th Anniversary Commemoration*, Nov. 1997, pp. 128–132.

Donahue, K. T., and Schyve, P. "Accreditation and Globalization." *International Journal for Quality in Health Care*, 1999, *11*(6).

Donahue, K. T., and van Ostenberg, P. "Joint Commission International Accreditation Standards: Relationship to Four Models of Evaluation," forthcoming.

Ente, B. "Joint Commission World Symposium on Improving Health Care Through Accreditation." *Joint Commission Journal on Quality Improvement*, 1999, *25*(11), 602–613.

International Society for Quality in Health Care. "ALPHA—Bringing the World of Healthcare Together!" *ALPHA Agenda*, 1999, *1*(1), 1–16.

Joint Commission on Accreditation of Healthcare Organizations. "Joint Commission International Accreditation Standards for Hospitals." *International Journal for Quality in Health Care,* June 2000.

Rooney, A., and van Ostenberg, P. *Licensure, Accreditation, and Certification: Approaches to Health Services Quality.* Quality Assurance Methodology Refinement Series. Bethesda, Md.: Quality Assurance Project, 1999.

Shaw, C. "External Quality Mechanisms for Health Care. Results of the ExPeRT Project on Visitatie, Accreditation, EFQM and ISO Assessment in European Union Countries." *International Journal for Quality in Health Care,* June 2000.

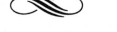

CHAPTER SEVEN

INFORMATION AND COMMUNICATION TECHNOLOGY

Jane Sarasohn-Kahn

Information and communications technologies are the key enablers of the globalization of health care. At a minimum, the convergence of information, communication, and clinical imaging technologies are creating a collective global health care knowledge base. This is a market- and technology-driven phenomenon, and we are well beyond Marshall McLuhan's concept of the global village. Cross-border initiatives—not just nonprofit ventures—are globalizing.

Health Care as a Knowledge-Based Industry

And health knowledge is largely globally transferable. Advances in health care information technology (IT) are narrowing the differences in health care delivery around the world. Whether in technologically advanced countries like Japan, which has been developing applications in medical informatics since the 1960s, or the Asian developing nations, Vietnam and Thailand, certain health care requisites are universal.

The overarching, unifying theme of health care delivery globally is that care needs to be better managed, both in terms of quality and cost. This is the objective of global leadership in the World Health Organization, of national leaders who head Ministries of Health, of regional health departments, and of local providers. The pressure to control health care expenditures tops every political agenda.

Every health ministry or department confronts the same pressing issues—escalating costs, demand for documenting quality of care, and lack of information on effective treatments. There is a growing and shared realization that IT is an essential tool to address these needs. Thus, IT companies active in health care markets have identified the opportunity to go global.

However, exporting health care IT goods and services is not simple. Overseas expansion is as much an exercise in risk management as in marketing strategy. Organizations going to the global market need to be realistic about the key challenges of international business: market access, financial markets, political stability, differences in time horizon, and return-on-investment thresholds.

Erroneous Assumptions About How Sophisticated "They" Are

There are smart cards in Switzerland, paperless hospitals in France, electronic medical records in the United Kingdom, and countless cellular phones in Indonesia and Malaysia. Certain IT applications are more widely distributed outside the United States than at home. For example, Singapore, a much smaller country with a population of only three million, has a number of national health care IT initiatives under way, including becoming the medical hub of Asia through a national intranet, "Singapore ONE." Singapore ONE is an initiative to develop interactive multimedia applications to homes, businesses, and schools throughout the island nation. The project includes a broadband infrastructure level of high-capacity networks and switches, complemented by applications and services that take advantage of the infrastructure's high-speed and high-capacity capabilities. These include health care applications such as telemedicine and continuing medical education. Furthermore, Singapore ONE is working to become a communications hub for the huge Chinese market.

Differences in Time Horizons

Time frames are shaped by politics, cultures, and organizational decision-making structures. Time frames are also influenced by currency fluctuations and political crises. Public sector procurement also has its unique characteristics. By the mid-1990s, the average time a hospital needed to negotiate a supplier contract was more than two years. The market was overcrowded with IT companies bidding unrealistically low in the search for market share.

Market Accessibility

One factor that can prolong the time horizon for an exporter is market accessibility. Some countries have very restrictive entry for foreign technology companies. It takes significant commitment and financial resources to succeed. In much of the world, telecommunications companies remain tightly controlled monopolies where regulations and tariffs inhibit the introduction of contemporary telecommunications applications for the health care setting. In these situations, it is useful to partner or otherwise co-opt the entrenched local player into the market entry strategy.

Labor Markets

One aspect of French and Western European culture that is distressing to many Americans is the ease with which Western European professionals will go on strike. The French, along with Italian and Spanish health care systems, are consistently the most strike-plagued when it comes to their health care sectors. French physicians, residents, nurses, and nonclinical hospital employees strike regularly, often causing significant procedural disruptions.

Lack of Global Strategies

There is no such thing as an effective Pan-European, Pan-Asian, or Pan-American strategy. Thinking in terms of broad regions such as Europe, Asia, Latin America, or even Southeast Asia is difficult. The Philippines has a very different political, governmental, and social context from that of Malaysia; Costa Rica and Argentina are vastly different; the United Kingdom and Italy have very different health care systems; and business and cultural norms are quite dissimilar, even between Mexico City and Guadalajara.

Local Staff

It is not a viable long-term strategy to bring technical experts from home base overseas for more than a year or two; this leads to high costs, personal dislocations, and a lack of local commitment. Instead, you must have internal staff who speak the local language and understand the local culture. Furthermore, by bringing local hires into your organization, you will signal to the marketplace your intention to dig your heels into their soil and commit for the long term. Stories abound about American health care IT companies who played cowboy; they came and went when they couldn't close a contract within twelve months of entering the market.

Cultural Sensitivity

It is extremely important to understand the language and the culture in any marketplace. Cultural sensitivity is a critical success factor for breaking ground overseas. In health care, it's not just sensitivity to the spoken language but to the clinical language as well. For example, we cannot assume that every clinician across borders uses the same coding system. Medical definitions can vary. In some nations, providers are more familiar with the international standard ICD-10 coding system than with the ICD-9 system. Beyond this, clinicians in health care systems outside the United States may not deal with the same level of data granularity (for example, coding sets and procedure-level data).

Need for Privacy

In the United States, legislation is not nearly as sophisticated in the area of data protection, security, confidentiality, and privacy as in Europe. Germany and Scandinavia are perhaps the most advanced in Europe in the area of data privacy. The Health on the Net Foundation (HON), based in Geneva, has advanced a code of ethics called the HONcode and encourages makers of medical and health sites to abide by it and display its logo. The code requires, in part, that sites provide advice only from medically trained and qualified professionals and that they adhere to legal confidentiality requirements of the country or state of origin.

Infrastructure

The major issue with the adoption of communications and information technology is not always the cost. In many parts of the world, what is lacking is infrastructure: reliable electric supplies, telephone lines, and human capital required to maintain the technology. The spread of digital satellite technology is playing a big role in driving down the costs of bandwidth for phone and fax lines, and eventually video.

Wired Hubs

Physical connectivity is growing quickly. Public access to Internet services is now available in the capital cities of forty-two of the fifty-four African nations. FLAG, the "fiber-optic link around the globe," laid 17,000 miles of high-speed cable linking Europe and Asia. Joining FLAG is the $14.7 billion Project Oxygen (so named because project leaders think the capacity to communicate is as important as the capacity to breathe), which plans to unspool ten times as much cable and link 171 countries. Numerous agencies are promoting this development, such as the World Bank's InfoDEV (Information for Development Program), which seeks to fully integrate developing nations into the information economy.

North-South Divide in Health Information

The divide between rich and poor applies to the sphere of health information. By 1999, of Africa's 700 million people, fewer than 1 million use the Internet; about 80 percent of those live in South Africa. Whereas one in six people in the United States or Europe use the Internet, for Africa (excluding South Africa) there is one Internet user for every 5,000 people.

The SatelLife project is seeking to address the health information asymmetry between rich and poor nations. SatelLife's mission is to address what it considers to be the two major problems health care workers in the developing world face: an acute shortage of current health information and isolation of the health professionals from each other. The not-for-profit project provides real-time information on epidemics and disease outbreaks, as well as other crucial health information.

Telemedicine and Telehealth

TeleHealth is shaping the global health care village. The World Health Organization (WHO) has spearheaded a G-7 feasibility study examining global health care applications to improve existing international cooperation in telemedicine, known as the Group of Seven Global Health Applications Project. The delegates on the project—from the United States, United Kingdom, Canada, France, Germany, Italy, and Japan (the G-7 countries, plus Australia)—have agreed on three conditions for fostering telehealth projects:

- The equipment must be affordable; where possible, existing technology should be used.
- A common classification system for diseases and data meanings must exist.
- Patients must be certain their health information is private.

A more ambitious project is the International Extranet Oncology Network, started in 1994. Funded by a G-7 grant, its primary agenda is to improve the detection, diagnosis, and treatment of cancer by encouraging greater cooperation among specialists. The International Extranet Oncology Network links centers of excellence in Milan, Paris, Amsterdam, Berlin, Grenoble, and Oslo. The National Cancer Institute in Amsterdam acts as the central server, picking up specialists' queries, which are then routed to the relevant centers for response. The network will extend to London, and future sites include Tokyo, Moscow, and Stuttgart, Germany. Even though funding for the project has officially ended, the Swiss-based Union International Contre le Cancer (International Union Against Cancer) has agreed to maintain the network.

Telemedicine Outside the United States

Even though telemedicine is not uniformly or universally reimbursed in the United States, reimbursement is standard practice in other nations. It is appropriate and well-entrenched technology in Norway, for example. Although the isolation of many Norwegians inspired the initial use of telemedicine, telemedicine is now integrated into routine health care throughout Norway. Factors that have fostered the growth of telemedicine there include the fact that it is a single health care delivery system, a single legal system (no cross-state licensing issues), and a relatively homogeneous population of patients and physicians.

Global Telemedicine

Increasingly, the U.S. academic medical community is playing a hand in promoting telemedicine abroad. Many American tertiary care centers—including but not limited to the Mayo Clinic, Stanford University Medical Center, and the Cleveland Clinic—have established links overseas to provide medical services and education. While most of these programs are still in experimental stages, they could signal the beginnings of a financially viable telemedicine movement. With the glut of medical specialists in the United States, telemedicine as a means to export U.S. medical expertise is a potential market.

Continuing Medical Education

Continuing Medical Education (CME) has become an international discipline. Several forces are shaping this phenomenon, including cross-disciplinary movements such as evidence-based medicine and common trends in medical education and assessment of professional competence. Movements are under way to develop transnational CME programs. For example, in Europe, the UK-Nordic Medical Educational Trust is bringing together constituents from the AMA, the European Academy of Medical Training, the Norwegian Medical Association, Royal College of Physicians, and the World Federation for Medical Education. These cross-border CME programs have begun to leverage the power of the Internet, multimedia, and broadband networks for the transfer of medical knowledge.

Globalization of Standards

IT standards-setters and implementers the world over are paying attention to each other's efforts. Despite differences in language and form of health care delivery, there is a tremendous amount of collaboration. For health care IT companies with international business, standardization is crucial to globalizing business. Still, there remain differences in health informatics standards across national borders. The health care standards working group, European Committee for Standardization (CEN TC251), liaises with American standards-setting efforts. In addition, the Object Management Group (OMG) has opened up a new Southern Europe liasion office in Milan, and is forming a CORBAmed European chapter to focus on health care's application of CORBA (Common Object Request Broker Architecture) on the Continent. This liaison strategy with the European health informatics community will help to promote standards across borders. Microsoft is also beginning to promote its standard for computing, ActiveX, in Europe, and HL7 has made some inroads in Europe.

Small World

There are clearly global opportunities for companies experienced in delivering IT solutions to health care providers. The advent of the Internet as an infrastructure backbone and the increasing availability of high-speed communications technology worldwide, whether wired or wireless, lessen the technology obstacles to going global. The major challenges to going global in health care IT, in fact, are not technological; they are based on human capital and political constraints.

Countries such as China that are just beginning to automate health care are learning from Western failures in health care IT. Western countries with experience should bring the lessons learned from failures, as well as successes.

As Nicholas Negroponte (1998) has written, "The 'Third World' five years from now may not be where you think it is. There have been many theories of leapfrog development, none of which has yet survived the test of time. That's about to change". This will be true in the global marketing of health care IT. Those organizations willing to do the hard work, take the time required, and make the appropriate investments in terms of money, people, skills, and cultural sensitivity will be those who are successful in helping construct the global health care village.

Asia Pacific Association for Medical Informatics
www.aims.org.sg/apami

National University of Singapore/Medical lnformatics Program
http://medinfo.nus.sg/

Thailand Telehealth
http://h.go.th

European Health Telematics Observatory
http://www.ehto.be

Swiss Society for Medical Informatics
http://www.sgmi-ssim.ch/main_en.htm

International Medical Informatics Organizations
http://www.eur.nl/FGG/MI/organisations.html

International Medical Informatics Association (IMIA)
http://www.imia.org

Pan-American Health Organization, Information Technology
http://www.paho.org/english/hsp/hspita.htm#pro

CommonHealthNet, Global Telemedicine and Healthcare Telecommunication Services
http://griffin.vcu.edu/html/biomede/imednet.html

SatelLife
http://www.healthnet.org/

World Bank Healthcare Group
http://www.worldbank.org/healthreform/

Health Telematics in the Euro-Mediterranean region
http://www.euromednet.ucy.ac.cy/html/body_conclusions.html

G-7 Global Healthcare Applications Project
http://www.ispo.cec.be/g7/projects/g7heal6.html

Global smart card market
http://www.va.gov/card/presentations.htm

United Nations Development Program/Telemedicine
http://www.undp.org

Health on the Net Global Code of Conduct
http://www.hon.ch/HONcode/Conduct.html

Singapore ONE
http://www.s-one.gov.sg/

Reference

Negroponte, N. "The Third Shall Be First." *Wired,* Jan. 1998.

CHAPTER EIGHT

PROJECTING THE IMPACT OF TRADE REGULATIONS

Jan E. Murray, Alexandre Alois Mencik

The market for pharmaceutical products and medical devices has become increasingly an international concern. Historically, decisions about whether and how to regulate the array of drugs and devices have been the responsibility of each nation. Over the last two decades, however, pharmaceutical companies and medical device manufacturers have become multinational in scope, developing, producing, and distributing their products worldwide. For example, as one author notes, even though the United States is the country with the largest pharmaceutical industry in the world, between 1961 and 1987 only 7.5 percent of the new drugs marketed in the United States were marketed first domestically (Domingues-Urban, 1997).

The market represented by the European Union (EU) has become increasingly important for pharmaceutical companies and medical device manufacturers. The EU, with its fifteen member states and more than 370 million people (Kidd, n.d.), is the largest trading economy in the world, accounting for one-third of world trade. The EU pharmaceutical market is the largest in the world, with a market value of US$77 billion and a retail value of more than US$102 billion.[1] The EU legislation is currently applicable in Iceland, Liechtenstein, and Norway, and negotiations for EU membership have already started with six Eastern and Central European countries (Estonia, the Czech Republic, Hungary, Poland, Cypress, and Slovenia). The populations of many of these countries are among the most affluent in the world. Therefore, access to this market by drug

103

and medical device manufacturers headquartered in countries in Asia and the Americas is important, as is access to those markets by EU companies. Consequently, the pharmaceutical and medical device industries have brought considerable pressure to bear on national and international authorities to harmonize and streamline the regulation of their products.

This effort has resulted in significant changes in the approach used by the EU and its member states in the regulation of certain aspects of manufacturing and marketing a drug or device. The process of harmonizing the legislation of the (then) six member states for medicinal products started as early as 1965.[2] This process is well advanced because harmonized requirements now govern the manufacturing, marketing, classifying, labeling, distributing, and advertising of medicinal products for both human and veterinary use.[3] This position was recently consolidated by the creation in 1993 of the European Agency for the Evaluation of Medicinal Products (EMEA), which commenced its operations in 1995. In those areas not governed by harmonized requirements, member states are still free to establish their own requirements.

The scheme for the regulation of medical devices has also been shaped by the effort of the EU to harmonize standards regarding specific regulatory requirements. Today, *directives* (regulations) cover the entire medical devices market, including electromedical equipment,[4] active and implantable medical devices,[5] general medical devices,[6] and in vitro diagnostic medical devices.[7]

When medical devices meet the requirements of these directives, they are "CE marked" (discussed later); member states are then, in principle, prohibited from creating obstacles to their entry on the market within their territories. The member states maintain an important role in determining whether the manufacturing process and resultant devices conform to requirements and, in some instances, in setting standards for these devices.

EU Regulatory Institutions

The EU institutions and agencies involved in the regulation of the manufacture and marketing of medicinal products have evolved over the last twenty-four years, in contrast with the situation applicable to the regulation of medical devices.

The European Commission is the main institution involved in the regulation of medicinal products and medical devices at the community level. It regulates the pharmaceutical and medical device sectors by proposing community legislation, usually in the form of directives, which are adopted by the European Parliament and the Council of Ministers and which must be implemented by the member states within a specific period of time.

In 1975, the so-called pharmaceutical committee was created. It is chaired by a representative of the European Commission and composed of senior experts in public health matters from the member states' administrations. The commission must consult the pharmaceutical committee when preparing proposals for directives in the field of medicinal products.[8] During the same year, the committee for proprietary medicinal products (CPMP) was established. Comprising representatives of the member states and of the commission, the CPMP is charged with delivering a reasoned opinion related to disputes among member states regarding recognition of marketing authorizations granted by other member states (discussed in greater detail later).[9] For those manufacturers of active ingredients and excipients, the requirements for the drug constituents contained in the monographs of the European Pharmacopoeia (EP) of the Council of Europe, to which the EU is a party, are of great significance.

In the medical device sector, two committees essentially assist the commission: (1) the committee on standards and technical regulations[10] and (2) the committee on medical devices.[11] The former committee gives its opinion on all the commission's proposals that are aimed at eliminating barriers to trade due to technical specifications. The latter committee may examine any matter relating to the implementation of the directives relating to medical devices.

The institutional structure just described for the pharmaceutical sector changed with the creation in 1993 of the EMEA.[12] With a total staff of 154 employees by the end of 1998, the EMEA acts as an interface with the national authorities rather than as a centralized organization such as the U.S. Food and Drug Administration. It is, however, a crucial focal point for providing scientific advice in relation to the new system for the authorization and supervision of medicinal products for human and veterinary use.

Each member state also has its own national authority for the regulation of some aspect of both the pharmaceutical and the medical device industries. These national agencies enforce community directives and legislation, set national standards, and implement their own nation's mandates within their borders. For example, for medicinal products the responsible national agency in the United Kingdom is the Medicines Control Agency. The United Kingdom has delegated authority for regulation of certain aspects of medical device assessment to the Medical Devices Agency under the Secretary of State for Health.

Access to the Market for Pharmaceutical Companies

EU legislation regulates the manufacture and import of finished medicinal products. The manufacture of such products in the EU requires manufacturing authorization, even if the products are only exported to countries outside the EU. This obligation extends to the partial manufacture of medicinal products, such as the manufacture of intermediate products and bulk products, and the various processes of packaging and distributing except where such processes are carried out by pharmacists and other authorized persons. A manufacturing authorization is also required for imports coming from non-EU countries into a member state. However, once an authorized medicinal product is legally imported into one member state, it may circulate freely within the EU without the need to obtain an additional authorization.

Although active ingredients and excipients are excluded from the manufacturing authorization process, the manufacturers of such constituents are required by EU legislation to provide detailed information to the manufacturer of the finished medicinal product relating, in particular, to the analytical methods used for controlling the quality of the constituents.[13] The more than 1,400 monographs of the EP greatly assist manufacturers of constituents because they may fulfill most of their reporting obligations simply by referring to the EP monograph in question. However, if a drug constituent is not covered by an EP monograph or a member state believes that the constituent has been manufactured by a method liable to leave impurities not controlled in the EP monograph, the member state may request specifications that are more appropriate.[14]

Regulation of Marketing

EU legislation also regulates the marketing of medicinal products. In the EU, manufacturers of finished medicinal products (including all nonprescription drugs or over-the-counter products) must receive a full authorization in order to place their products on the market of a member state, subject to certain exceptions. These exceptions include certain finished drugs and those manufactured for export only.

When a particular member state has already granted a marketing authorization for a given product, the manufacturer can request the recognition of this authorization by any or all of the member states that have not yet authorized the product. These member states may, however, object to the mutual recognition if their authorities believe that the existing marketing authorization(s) may present a risk for public health.[15] For medicinal products developed by specific biotechnological processes, the manufacturer need only file a single five-year application to the EMEA for an authorization to the entire community market. An extension to the scope of this centralization procedure is proposed in order to allow sponsors of orphan medicinal products to obtain a single community authorization.

In order to obtain a marketing authorization, the person who will place the finished medicinal product on the market must complete a dossier for submission to the competent authority. The dossier must include all particulars and documents necessary to demonstrate the safety, efficacy, and quality of the product. Establishment through EU legislation and the standards of the CPMP has notably harmonized these particulars.

Once the marketing authorization has been granted, the product will be subject to a system of supervision and control. This system is designed to remove from the market any medicinal product whose use proves to be harmful or whose therapeutic efficacy is lacking.[16] Marketing authorizations are granted for a period of five years and may be renewed for five-year periods.

Medicinal products are classified in accordance with basic principles set out in EU legislation that conform to principles adopted under the auspices of the Council of Europe. Member states are free to determine which products may be sold only by pharmacies, and the majority still imposes a prohibition on the sale of both medicinal products subject to medical prescription and nonprescription products in outlets other than in pharmacies.[17]

Labeling, Packaging, and Distribution

The labeling for the outer packaging of a medicinal product (or the immediate packaging) and the leaflet required for the users are also governed by detailed EU legislation. Member states are free to adopt national requirements for labeling. For example, they may require the use of their own official language(s), identification of the price and reimbursement conditions, and determination of the legal status for supplying the medicine to the patient.

Any person engaged in the activity of the wholesale distribution of medicinal products must obtain a license under EU legislation, except if that person holds a manufacturing authorization and only distributes by wholesale the products covered by that authorization. (The use of the term *person* in this text refers also to business entities.) This legislation includes requirements such as the obligation to deliver the product only to authorized wholesalers or other authorized persons. Licensees must also meet certain standards relating to harmonizing good distribution practices. Member states are free to add other requirements to these minimums such as public service obligations (for example, an obligation to stock specific medicinal products or to distribute them). Although in theory each member state is obligated to recognize the license granted by another, wholesalers are often required to obtain a license in each state where they conduct business.

EU legislation regulates the advertising of medicinal products and strictly prohibits the advertising to the general public of products that may only be obtained by prescription or for which no marketing authorization has been granted.

Member states may impose additional restrictions for the advertising of products in their own jurisdictions.

Finally, EU legislation provides a limited regulation of the pricing of medicinal products, resulting in substantial variation among member states in the prices of medicinal products. More significantly, there is considerable divergence among member states about the scope of national health insurance coverage and reimbursement systems for these products.

Access to the Market for Medical Device Manufacturers

Any manufacturer[18] who currently places a medical device or its accessory (except an in vitro diagnostic medical device) on the market of any member state[19] must comply with a series of harmonized requirements, although certain devices have been grandfathered for the next few years.

The manufacturer must first ensure that the medical device meets certain general safety requirements and requirements regarding design and construction that implement specific safety objectives. Medical devices are subject to a system of classification found in the Medical Devices Directive, which includes four product classes: I, IIa, IIb, and III. These classes represent the range of risk inherent in the intended use of the device, with Class I devices posing the least risk. The manufacturer must ensure that the devices have passed through the appropriate conformity assessment procedure, which serves to demonstrate and control conformity with the relevant safety requirements. According to the Medical Devices Directive, a device that falls within Class III must comply with the most comprehensive conformity assessment procedure, which includes premarket authorization by a so-called notified body (the certification organization appointed by a member state to ensure conformity). If the device falls within Class IIa or IIb, the intervention of the notified body is compulsory at the production stage and even, in certain cases, at the design and manufacturing stages. The manufacturer of a Class I device may simply declare that its device conforms to the relevant essential requirements. In all cases, the manufacturer has a certain degree of flexibility because he can generally choose the specific conformity assessment procedure applicable to the device and determine in which member state the device will be certified and by which certification authority.

Once the appropriate conformity assessment procedure has been undertaken, the devices must bear the CE mark *prior* to marketing, which demonstrates their conformity with the requirements of the relevant directives.

Once the device is on the market, it is subject to the medical device vigilance system. This system mandates reporting to the authorities of certain types of incidents and "near incidents" involving the device. As is the case with pharmaceuticals, the EU legislation also regulates the labeling of medical devices. By contrast, to pharmaceuticals, there is no specific EU legislation regulating the distributing and advertising of medical devices.

Efforts to Harmonize Regulation

As indicated earlier in this chapter, several aspects of the regulation of medicinal products have been harmonized at the EU level. However, the process is not complete, and in those instances where the EU has not prescribed requirements, the authorities of the various member states are free to legislate and enforce their own requirements.

For instance, the EU requires manufacturing authorization for the manufacture and import of finished medicinal products but not for the manufacture and import of active ingredients, pharmaceutical excipients, and products for clinical trials. The principles and guidelines of good manufacturing practices (GMPs) are harmonized among the member states, whereas the content of the manufacturing authorization itself is not harmonized. The current exemptions for active ingredients, excipients, and products for clinical trials may end due to proposed EU legislation requiring a manufacturing authorization for "starting materials" (including all active substances and certain listed excipients) and "investigational medicinal products."[20]

The Medical Devices Directive sets out that member states must presume compliance with the safety requirements referred to in the directive for devices that are in conformity with harmonized standards adopted at the EU level.[21] However, only a limited number of harmonized standards have been adopted at the EU level. As a result, manufacturers are often left with the cumbersome obligation of demonstrating compliance with the safety requirements by other means.

Harmonizing Regulations of EU and Non-EU Countries

In the pharmaceutical and devices sectors, harmonization efforts among the EU and non-EU countries, including the United States and Japan, have occurred at two levels. First, the pharmaceutical industry, through certain of its trade associations acting in concert with the relevant authorities of the EU, the United States, and Japan, established the International Conference on Harmonization (ICH; Horton, 1998). One of the primary goals of the ICH is to harmonize requirements for testing drugs and biologicals. It has carried out this work quite successfully, with expert work groups and bi-annual public meetings since 1991. The

ICH is now moving to forge agreement on what information should be presented for obtaining authorization to market products in these countries.[22]

For medical devices, harmonization of approval-related matters, good manufacturing practices (or quality systems requirements), and adverse-event reporting has been the work of the Global Harmonization Task Force (GHTF). The GHTF comprises officials from industry and governments from Europe, North America and Asia-Pacific (Horton, 1998).

The other method for harmonizing regulations between the EU and various non-EU countries, including Australia, Canada, New Zealand, and the United States, is the use of mutual recognition agreements (MRAs). The EU has ratified all the MRAs it had concluded with these countries, and ratification by these countries is under way. MRAs with other countries such as Japan and Switzerland are currently being negotiated. The MRAs that the EU has concluded cover several industrial sectors, including the pharmaceutical and medical devices sectors. These MRAs harmonize the acceptance of testing and quality inspections for drugs and devices. The annex to the MRAs governing drugs covers pre- and postapproval good-manufacturing-practice inspections, whereas the annex governing medical devices relates to quality control inspections and premarket evaluation reports of certain devices (Horton, 1998).

Other Legal Issues

Several other areas of law affect the manner in which business is conducted by drug and device manufacturers in the EU, including those governing intellectual property (particularly patents) and those governing product liability litigation.

Patents are granted for inventions and are therefore extremely useful tools for protecting the pharmaceutical and medical devices industries that conduct substantial research and development.[23] Patents accord the right, to the exclusion of all others, to exploit an invention for the duration of the patent or to authorize its exploitation (that is, to grant a patent license).

In the EU, patent law has been partially harmonized through the Convention on the Grant of European Patents, concluded at Munich in 1973 and subsequently revised.[24] All member states are currently parties to the convention.

The convention does not provide for a unitary system of protection by patents. It only allows any natural or legal person (business entity) to file a single application to the European Patent Office (EPO) or a national patent office that forwards it to the EPO. The EPO processes the application, and the resulting grant is a bundle of national patents (a European patent), which (subject to certain national formalities) confers the same rights in each country designated in that application as national patents granted by that country, unless otherwise provided in the convention. A patent is in effect for twenty years from the date of filing of the application. Despite the harmonization achieved by the convention, each national legislature may determine the conditions and rules regarding the protection conferred by the European patent, subject to the need to comply with community law.

The EU has attempted on several occasions to revise the current community patent system that is generally regarded as costly and uncertain.[25] In February 1999, the European Commission announced its intention to adopt during 1999 a proposal to create a new unitary and affordable system of community patents. In the meantime, the EU has been successful in creating a mechanism for extending the duration of existing national patent rights on inventions related to medicinal[26] and plant protection products.[27]

Product Liability

The EU recognized that the great divergence of product liability law among member states would impede the free movement of goods within the EU; therefore it began studying proposals for a unified approach in the 1970s (Davis, 1998). After many years of debate, the EU adopted in 1985 Directive 85/374/EEC, which attempted to harmonize liability standards for claims arising from defective products.[28]

The directive embodies a standard of strict liability, which means it requires that the injured person only prove the damage, the defect, and a causal connection between the two. The injured person is not required to show fault on the part of the manufacturers, and privity of contract is no longer required to file a product liability claim. Indeed, liability could extend to all persons involved in the manufacturing process, including importers of medicinal products and medical devices into the community (Davis, 1998).

Several defenses are recognized by Directive 85/374/EEC, including one known as the state-of-the-art defense, which excuses the manufacturer if, based on the state of the scientific and technical knowledge at the time the product was put into circulation, it was impossible to discover the existence of the defect. Finally, EU product liability law does not include the concept of punitive damages nor does Directive 85/374/EEC permit damages for pain and suffering. On balance, product liability awards tend to be considerably lower in the EU than in the United States (Davis, 1998).

Despite Directive 85/374/EEC, member states still have considerable latitude in implementing aspects of the directive, and there are variations among their judicial systems (for example, access to a jury trial).

Conclusion

As highlighted in the discussion, the EU has adopted a comprehensive set of harmonized rules that govern entry to the European market for pharmaceutical and medical device manufacturers. However, many important aspects have not yet been harmonized and therefore depend on the requirements imposed by the individual member states. This is especially the case with respect to the pricing and reimbursement of medicinal products and the standards applicable to medical devices. It is also true for important aspects of the manufacture of medicinal products: the marketing of active ingredients and excipients, the sale of medicinal products in outlets other than pharmacies, the requirements for the advertising of such products, and the intellectual property law and product liability issues. As a result, pharmaceutical and medical device manufacturers will continue to live with the obligation to monitor carefully national legislative and regulatory practices before placing their products on the market in any member state.

Notes

1. See "Communication of the European Commission on the Single Market in Pharmaceuticals," COM (98) 588 final.
2. See Council Directive 65/65/EEC of Jan. 25, 1965, on the approximation of the laws, regulations, and administrative action relating to medicinal products, OJ L 16 of July 12, 1965. This directive was last amended by Directive 93/39/EC, OJ L 214 of Aug. 24, 1993.
3. Council Directive 81/851/EEC of Sept. 28, 1981, on the approximation of the laws of the member states relating to veterinary medicinal products, OJ L 317 of Nov. 6,1981.
4. Council Directive 84/539/EEC on electromedical equipment used in human or veterinary medicine, OJ L 300 of Nov. 19, 1984.
5. Council Directive 90/385/EEC on active implantable medical devices, OJ L 189 of June 20, 1990.
6. Council Directive 93/42/EEC concerning medical devices (hereafter referred to as the Medical Devices Directive), OJ L 169 of June 12, 1993.
7. Directive 98/79/EC of the European Parliament and of the Council of Oct. 27, 1998, on in vitro diagnostic medical devices, OJ No. L 331 of Dec. 7, 1998.
8. Council Directive 87/19/EEC has also created the Committee on the Adaptation to Technical Progress of the Directives on the Removal of Technical Barriers to Trade in the Proprietary Medicinal Products Sector, made up of representatives of the member states and of the commission, which gives its opinion on proposed changes to the particulars and documents that must be submitted in support of applications for marketing authorizations for medicinal products. See also Council Directive 87/19/EEC of Dec. 22, 1986, amending Directive 75/318/EEC on the approximation of the laws of the member states relating to analytical, pharmacotoxicological, and clinical standards and protocols in respect of the testing of proprietary medicinal products, OJ L 15 of Jan. 17, 1987. Council Directive

93/39/EEC changed the name of this committee to the Standing Committee on Medicinal Products for Human Use. See Council Directive 93/39/EEC.

9. See Council Directive 81/851/EEC. The Committee for Veterinary Medicinal Products (CVMP) was set up in 1981, with similar tasks with respect to medicinal products for veterinary use.

10. This committee was set up by Council Directive 83/189/EEC of Mar. 28, 1983, laying down a procedure for the provision of 83/189/EE information in the field of technical standards, OJ L 109 of Apr. 26, 1983.

11. This committee was set up by Directive 90/385/EEC.

12. See Council Regulation (EEC) 2309/93 of July 22, 1993, laying down community procedures for the authorization and supervision of medicinal products for human and veterinary use and establishing the European Agency for the Evaluation of Medicinal Products, OJ L 214 of Aug. 24, 1993.

13. Proprietary and confidential information on active ingredients could be provided directly to the regulatory authorities under the European Drug Master File (EDMF) procedure. In contrast with the situation in the United States, the EDMF procedure is currently not available for excipients and packaging materials.

14. See point 1.1 of the Annex to Council Directive 75/318/EEC of May 20, 1975, on the approximation of the laws of member states relating to analytical, pharmacotoxicological, and clinical standards and protocols in respect of the testing of proprietary medicinal products, OJ L 147 of June 9, 1975. This directive was last amended by Directive 93/39/EC.

15. This procedure is not available for medicinal products that must be authorized under the centralized procedure and those whose marketing has already been refused at the community level.

16. See Article 11 of Directive 65/65/EEC (as amended).

17. There is a recent trend toward a more flexible approach, especially in countries such as Finland, the Netherlands, and the United Kingdom.

18. *Manufacturer* is defined as the natural or legal person with responsibility for the design, manufacture, packaging, or labeling related to a device before it is placed on the market under the person's own name. From a practical point of view, any distributor that undertakes activities such as the repackaging of in vitro diagnostic products, the drafting of instruction leaflets, or the placing of such products on the market under its own name (and without mentioning the name of the manufacturer) may be considered as a "manufacturer" for the purposes of the directives.

19. The Medical Devices Directive defines placing on the market as "the first making available in return for payment or free of charge of a device with a view to distribution and/or use on the Community market, regardless of whether it is new or fully refurbished." "Making available" means either the transfer of the device, that is, the transfer of ownership, or the physical hand-over of the device to the distributor or the passing of the device to the final consumer or user in a commercial transaction or the offer of transfer, in cases where the device is made available in the manufacturer's own commercial distribution chain with a view to direct transfer to the final consumer or user.

20. See the Amended Proposal for a European Parliament and Council Directive on the approximation of the laws, regulations, and administrative provisions of the member states relating to the implementation of good clinical practice in the conduct of clinical trials on medicinal products for human use, OJ C 161 of June 8, 1999; and draft Proposal for a European Parliament and Council Directive on GMP for starting materials and inspection

of manufacturers of both medicinal products and their starting materials (unpublished). A conservative estimation is that the EU legislation imposing a manufacturing authorization for investigational medicinal products will be finally adopted by the end of 2000 and will be binding at national level around mid-2001.

21. References to harmonized standards may also include the EP monographs in certain cases.
22. See http://www.pharmweb.net/pwmirror/pwg/ifpma/ich1.html.
23. *Inventions* could be defined as technological improvements, great or small, which contain at least some scintilla of inventiveness over what is previously known; see Cornish (1996), p. 6.
24. The convention was amended by the act revising its Article 63 of Dec. 17, 1991, and by decisions of the Administrative Council of the European Patent Organization of Dec. 21, 1978; Dec. 13, 1994; Oct. 20, 1995; Dec. 5, 1996; and Dec. 10, 1998.
25. See the Community Patent Convention signed at Luxembourg on Dec. 15, 1975, and the Community Patent Convention annexed to the agreement signed at Luxembourg on Dec. 15, 1989, which have not entered into force and are unlikely to do so.
26. See Council Regulation (EEC) 1768/92 of June 18, 1992, concerning the creation of a supplementary protection certificate for medicinal products, OJ L 182 of July 2, 1992.
27. See Council Regulation (EC) 1610/96 of the European Parliament and of the Council of July 23, 1996, concerning the creation of a supplementary protection certificate for plant protection products, OJ L 198 of Aug. 8, 1996.
28. Council Directive 85/374/EEC of July 25, 1985, on the approximation of the laws, regulations, and administrative provisions of the member states concerning liability for defective products, OJ L 210 of Aug. 7, 1985. Directive 85/374/EEC was amended by Directive 1999/34/EC in order to extend its scope of application to unprocessed agricultural products, OJ L 141 of June 4, 1999.

References

Cornish, W. R. *Intellectual Property.* (3rd ed.) London: Sweet & Maxwell, 1996.

Davis, K. "An International Drug Administration: Curing Uncertainty in International Pharmaceutical Product Liability." *Northwestern Journal of International Law and Business,* 1998, *18,* 693.

Domingues-Urban, I. "Harmonization in the Regulation of Pharmaceutical Research and Human Rights: The Need to Think Globally." *Cornell International Law Journal,* 1997, *30,* 246.

Horton, L. "Mutual Recognition Agreements and Harmonization." *Seton Hall Law Review,* 1998, *29,* 717.

Kidd, D. "The European Medicines Evaluation Agency, and the FDA: Who's Zooming Who?" Paper presented at the International Conference on the Harmonization of Pharmaceutical Regulations, n.d. [http://www.law.indiana.edu/glsj/vol4/no1/kidpgp.html].

PART TWO

EUROPE

Part Two covers health care in nations of the European Union (the Netherlands, Germany, Spain, France, and the United Kingdom), as well as in the non-EU nations of Israel, Poland, and Russia. Contributors analyze these countries in terms of the basic underlying values of the region—universal access, equity in funding, and quality of care—and examine national reform efforts.

The European Union

Chapter Nine reviews health policies and health care reforms in the Netherlands. Kieke G. H. Okma discusses planning and regulation, current health policies, efforts to control expenditures, and the partially implemented reform efforts of the 1980s and 1990s. She then analyzes the changing arena of Dutch social and health care policies.

Germany, with a system that has evolved in a stepwise manner over the past 120 years, presents an interesting case for studying today's challenges. In Chapter Ten, Reinhard Busse discusses the struggle to overcome some of Germany's main health system weaknesses, such as the strict separation between ambulatory and inpatient sectors. He lays out the basic framework of the system, explores health care financing and delivery, and gives an account of major reforms and their objectives over the past decade.

Spain has met the European standard of universal coverage and, primarily with tax-generated resources, financial equity in health care. In Chapter Eleven, Alicia Granados and Pedro Gallo describe the main features of Spain's system in terms of management and organization, prevailing values, and health care priorities and tools. They explore future developments, including the expansion of decentralization, possible pharmaceutical policy changes, and increased resources for research and development.

A branch of France's social security system universally covers the population of that country. In Chapter Twelve, Pierre-Jean Lancry and Simone Sandier discuss France's health care system and the reforms occurring since the mid-1970s. They then look at economic, social, and political reasons for the difficulty encountered in implementing changes over the past thirty years.

The United Kingdom—the last EU country reviewed here—is an industrialized nation with a centralized statutory universal health care financing system, a niche market for private insurers, a mixed public-private delivery system, and a national policy of explicit government rationing of care through control of funding. In Chapter Thirteen, Donald A. Duffy discusses the reengineering of the U.K.'s National Health Service under two different reform strategies, first under Prime Minister Margaret Thatcher and later under Prime Minister Tony Blair.

Non-EU Countries

Israel is a comparatively young state with universal health insurance coverage, a relatively long average life span, low infant mortality, and a comprehensive system of managed health care competition. In Chapter Fourteen, Albert Lowey-Ball summarizes Israel's historical and social context, describes the country's current health care delivery system, looks into the near future in light of Israel's adoption of the National Health Insurance and Managed Competition Law of 1995, and concludes with some lessons learned.

In Chapter Fifteen, Renata Bushko focuses on the potential impact of sociotechnological transformation for the health care system of Poland. Bushko argues that technology-driven reform, coupled with Poland's 1999 market-driven reform, could improve the quality and accessibility of health care in that country. Improvements to the system are measured using the Universal Quality Framework, which is based on quality, cost, outcomes, and patient satisfaction.

Finally, Chapter Sixteen covers health care in the Russian Federation. Youri Lavinski and Steven Vasilev trace the development of Russian health care from the turn of the twentieth century, when the system was based on the concept of social justice, all the way through the Mandatory Insurance Law of 1992 and the Voluntary Insurance Law of 1994. The authors then discuss reform outcomes and the potential for new business opportunities.

EUROPEAN UNION

CHAPTER NINE

THE NETHERLANDS

Kieke G. H. Okma

The Netherlands' health care system shares basic underlying values and principles with other European countries: universal access to health care and health insurance, equity in funding, and good quality of services. In addition, because health care expenditure is one of the main categories of public spending, cost control has become an overriding concern of the Netherlands and other governments (OECD, 1992, 1994, 1996). There is also similarity in the policy problems and dilemmas as well as in the range of policy options and measures considered.

This chapter defines the unique differences of Dutch health care, health policies, and reforms. After an overview of services, the funding and allocation of available resources among institutions are described and contracting models and payment structures defined. Planning and regulation, current health policies, efforts to control expenditures, and the partially implemented reform efforts of the 1980s and 1990s are discussed. Finally, the changing policy arena of Dutch social and health care policies is analyzed.

The author thanks Hans Arnold and Peter Drummond for reviewing this chapter.

Distinguishing Characteristics

Three distinct characteristics of the Dutch system are (1) the mix of public and private funding, (2) the predominantly private provision of care, and (3) the typical Dutch neocorporatist policy arena.

Public-Private Funding Mix

The first characteristic is the mix of public and private funding, with a relatively high share of voluntary, private health insurance. For acute medical care by general physicians and hospitals, about two-thirds of the Dutch population is covered under the mandatory sickness fund insurance (Ministry of Health, 1998a). One-third of the population may opt for private insurance. There is a separate mandatory social insurance for long-term care. Government contributes less than 10 percent out of general taxation; direct payments in the form of deductibles, copayments, coinsurance, and services not covered by social or private insurance amount to another 7 percent. Public funding (social insurance, mandatory private insurance, and tax subsidies) contributes over 85 percent of health care funding. By combining mandatory, employment-related health insurance with populationwide coverage of the costs of long-term care, the Dutch system has become a hybrid—a cross between the Bismarckian and the Beveridge models of health care funding.

Private Provision Dominance

The second important feature of Dutch health care is the dominance of the private provision of services. Most of the Dutch hospitals and other health care institutions are owned and run by religious orders, charities, or nonprofit foundations. State intervention remained modest until after World War II, when government started to intervene in health care by introducing mandatory sickness fund membership, regulating access to private health insurance for certain high-risk groups, and regulating the allocation of resources and planning of facilities. As a logical consequence, this also led to increased interest in controlling health care expenditure. However, the ownership and management of health facilities remained largely nongovernmental, and most general providers are self-employed.

Neocorporatism Policy

Third, the social policy arena in the Netherlands has its own tradition of neocorporatism in which government shares responsibilities for the shaping and outcomes of social policies with a wide variety of organized interests (Lijphart, 1968; Hill, 1993). In the postwar decades, the Dutch health care system expanded by the creation of a wide array of advisory bodies with formal representation of almost all interest groups. Based on the advice of several expert committees inside and outside Parliament in the 1980s and 1990s, governments started to reduce the size and scope of these neocorporatist structures.

Health Care Services

Recent studies confirm that the vast majority of the Dutch population enjoys good health (Ministry of Health, 1997b, 1997c). However, ill health and disability are problems for certain population groups, which are related to social and economic factors, employment status, unhealthy lifestyles, and immigration (Ministry of Health, 1999b, 1995a). In some cases, inequalities in access to health services have increased; specific policy measures seek to redress some of these problems. The main policy goals of universal and equitable access to health insurance and good quality health care have translated into comprehensive health insurance and a wide range of health care services accessible to the entire population.

Mid-1990s Shift

In the second half of the 1990s, there was a shift from separate hospital budgets and payments for self-employed specialists toward lump-sum payments and employment contracts for specialists with hospitals. Most other health professionals are employed by hospitals or other health care facilities and organizations.

Encouraged by changing market conditions, government policies, and modern management models, providers of primary care sought collaboration and forms of horizontal and vertical integration with secondary and tertiary care. They extended their activities far beyond their traditional borders (Okma, 1997). Institutions and organizations for ambulatory care set up collaboration in providing consumer-oriented and efficient services. Hospitals, nursing homes, and home care organizations created formal and informal alliances and regional networks. This also blurred the traditional lines between the different subsectors or "echelons" in health care and related social services. Consequently, traditional definitions of health care services no longer easily apply, and it has become difficult to assess exact distinctions between primary, secondary, and tertiary care.

Health Professionals

Health care is one of the largest service sectors in the Dutch economy. It employs more than 750,000 persons—over 10 percent of all employment. The majority of workers are women, many of whom work part-time.

Together with the Minister of Education, the Minister of Health bears responsibility for the education of health professionals. There are legal restrictions to the number of entrants to medical schools and other education institutions, based on estimates of future needs. In the last decade, several reports predicted dramatic labor shortages, but at the end of the 1990s these had failed to materialize. A recent study suggests possible future shortages in specialized areas (Vermeulen and others, 1998). After the first stage of medical education, physicians have to take further training to become medical specialists; the medical profession itself controls this second stage of education. In December 1998, the health minister announced that she would set up a special institute for regulating the influx of specialist training called the Jan Poorter-Institute.

Freedom of Choice

Dutch patients have free choice of provider. Those insured by the sickness fund are limited to health care providers contracted by their fund. But as most funds have contracted almost all providers in their working area, this rule does not restrict consumer choice. Private patients are usually free to choose a provider. General practitioners have a gatekeeper role in referring patients to hospital and specialist care, but patients still can choose their hospital.

Public Health by Local Authorities

Local authorities bear responsibility for some of the core public health services, including the monitoring of health and contagious disease. The Collective Prevention Act—*Wet Collectieve Preventie* (WCPV)—passed in 1989. A special study of the results of the new legislation found that local authorities had adopted a wide variety of preventive policies and measures. This resulted in diverging levels of public health services becoming available to the population. In order to redress the ensuing inequalities, the health minister asked an expert committee to advise on policy measures (Lemstra Committee, 1998). The committee recommended that local authorities present an annual review of their preventive and public health activities and suggested that the health ministry define a basic package of such services to be mandatory in the entire country (the *basispakket gezondheidsdiensten*).

Recent Organizational Developments

For over two decades, Dutch governments sought to reduce the rate of institutionalization by shifting inpatient care to ambulatory care. Combined with the effects of technological innovations, this led to a sharp reduction in the number of hospital beds. The increased collaboration between services and processes of horizontal and vertical integration enabled such shifts. Although many health facilities collaborate in regional networks, chains of health facilities, and other informal arrangements, most kept their independent legal status until the mid-1990s. But in the second half of the decade, the number of formal mergers and takeovers increased. The Ministry of Health provides financial support for the introduction of such technologies, for example subsidies to general practitioners for computer practice systems.

Based on the recommendations of the Biesheuvel report of 1994 (a committee assessing the need for better integration of ambulatory and inpatient care), the Minister of Health encouraged experiments with new payment methods for medical specialists, aimed at integrating payments for medical specialists with hospital budgets and strengthening the role of physicians in hospital management. In several cases, lump-sum payments replaced separate hospital budgets and physician fees.

Funding Health Care

Social and private health insurance is the main funding source for Dutch health care services. As can be seen in Table 9.1, insurance covers over 85 percent of all health care funding. There is a modest share of government subsidy from general taxation, and direct patient payments amount to about 7 percent of all expenditures.

TABLE 9.1. HEALTH CARE FUNDING IN THE NETHERLANDS.

Source of Funding	Amount (billions of guilders)	Share of All Funding (percent)
Long-term care insurance (AWBZ)	26,641	37
Sickness fund insurance (ZFW)	25,859	36
Private health insurance	10,488	15
Government	3,360	5
Direct payments	4,778	7
Total	71,126	100

Source: Ministry of Health, 1998a.

Note: In June 1999, one euro equaled 2.20371 Dutch guilders, or US$1.05.

Contribution Rates

In 1998, the contribution rate for the sickness fund insured was 6.8 percent of the first taxable income bracket up to 52,983 Dutch guilders (24,043 euros). The share of employers was 5.6 percent, that of employees 1.2 percent. Apart from income-related contributions, which are levied by employers and channeled through the general taxation system into the central fund administered by the Sick Fund Council, those insured by the sickness fund pay a flat rate premium directly to their funds. In 1998, this premium averaged 216 guilders (98 euros) per person per annum, but each fund may set its own premium. Those who are privately insured pay flat rate premiums, with a limited degree of risk-rated premiums. Specific groups of those private insured have access to the special health insurance schemes under the Health Insurance Access Act (WTZ) and pay government-controlled premiums, with a maximum of 225 guilders (102 euros) per person per month. All others who are private insured participate in the mandatory cost-sharing arrangement to subsidize the excess costs of the WTZ schemes (in 1998 they paid 360 guilders or 163 euros per person per year in addition to their regular premium). Reflecting the high degree of solidarity in Dutch health care, all residents pay an income-related contribution for the mandatory, populationwide, long-term care insurance (AWBZ). In 1998 the contribution rate for the AWBZ scheme was 9.6 percent over the first taxable income bracket up to 47,184 guilders or 21,411 euros. Direct payments include the different forms of user fees by patients, as well as noninsured services and (voluntary) supplementary health insurance. Government subsidies out of general taxation mainly support research and education and public health services provided by local authorities.

Allocation of Funding to Subsectors

Government budgeting is the main instrument for allocating funding over subsectors and institutions of Dutch health care. This budgeting takes place on different levels. The first step is the determination of the annual global ceiling (as a quasi-budget) for health care as part of macroeconomic and fiscal policies. Once the cabinet has agreed on the overall budget, the Minister of Health decides the allocation to the specific subsectors. This allocation can be seen as global sectoral budgets. Within this "cascading" budget model, health insurers and health care providers negotiate about the volume, price, and quality of services.

The annual budget document (*Jaaroverzicht Zorg*, JOZ) provides an overview of the sectoral allocation, as presented in Table 9.2.

TABLE 9.2. DUTCH HEALTH CARE FUNDING BY SUBSECTOR.

Subsector	Funding (billions of guilders)	Share of All Funding (percent)
Hospitals, general practitioners, other acute medical care	28,419	40
Nursing homes, retirement homes, home care	15,736	22
Pharmaceuticals and medical aids	7,668	11
Care for handicapped	6,303	9
Mental health care	5,198	7
Public health and prevention	1,219	2
Administration	6,567	9
Total	71,126	100

Source: Ministry of Health, 1998a.

Contracting Models and Payment Structure

The Ministry of Health sets the annual budgets of individual hospitals and other health care facilities, but the institutions receive their payments from the sickness funds and from private health insurers. Representative from organizations of health insurers and providers meet annually to design framework contracts and then negotiate with individual insurance agencies and health care providers. General practitioners receive capitation payments for their sickness fund insured but usually receive fees for services from their privately insured clients. General practitioners receive additional payment for certain types of services, such as flu immunization for elderly patients. Restriction or the delisting of entitlements can cause changes in payment methods. The health care services under supplementary insurance that is offered by the sickness fund or by private insurers are usually provided on a fee-for-service basis.

Planning and Regulation

Even though the majority of health insurers and institutional health care providers are private, not-for-profit organizations, the government plays an important role in regulating them. The Individual Health Care Professionals Act of 1993 (*Wet Beroepen in de Individuele Gezondheidszorg*, WBIG) regulates diploma requirements, certification, and the professional powers of medical and other health professions.

The 1991 Quality of Health Institutions Act (*Kwaliteitswet Zorginstellingen*) of 1991 regulates the quality of service provided by health care institutions. This legislation is based on the principle that health care providers themselves bear primary responsibility for the quality of their services. They have to develop quality systems that include the definition of quality norms and setting procedures, systems of certification, and other rules applicable to all categories of health care institutions. Furthermore, patient rights are safeguarded through several forms of regulation, ranging from consumer protection to new laws regulating the "contract" between doctors and patients (*Wet Geneeskundige Behandelingsovereenkomst*, WGBO).

Health Insurance Schemes

Two types of health insurance schemes will be described—sickness funds and private health insurance.

Sickness Fund Insurance

Sickness fund insurance covers acute medical care provided by general practitioners and medical specialists, related hospital care, medical aids and appliances, obstetrics and maternity care, ambulance and transportation, and some other services (Ministry of Health, 1998a). About 64 percent of the Dutch population belong to a sickness fund. Membership is mandatory for employees with incomes below a certain amount, as well as certain categories of recipients of welfare and unemployment benefits. In 1998, the Dutch Cabinet announced steps to allow self-employed persons with low incomes to join. This not only expanded the fund membership but changed the Bismarckian nature of the sickness fund insurance, as employment status was no longer the crucial eligibility criterion but rather the level of income, regardless of its source.

In 1999, there were thirty independent sickness funds, with an average membership of about 300,000 persons (with a large variation in membership, ranging from fewer than 1,000 to over 1 million). Many funds have sought collaboration with other funds, as well as private health insurance and banking conglomerates, in order to gain strategic market positions exploring new possibilities for offering broader employee benefit packages.

Sickness funds are independent legal entities, with self-appointed boards. They receive their prospective budgets from the Sickness Fund Council, and contract health care services in order to safeguard access to health care for their members. The budgets are based on a number of criteria such as age, gender, region, and disability status. During the first years after the introduction of the prospective sickness fund budgets, they received compensation at the end of the year when the actual expenditures had surpassed the model-based calculations. Gradually this compensation decreased. The funds continue to receive separate payment for capital investments and for excess costs of certain high-risk groups. The funds also administer the long-term care insurance AWBZ on behalf of their members (likewise, private health insurers take care of the AWBZ administration for their insured). The insurers have pooled this administration in regional offices (*verbindingskantoren* or *zorgkantoren*).

The Sickness Fund Council (*Ziekenfondsraad*, ZFR) administers the central funds of the ZFW and AWBZ insurance schemes, sets the budgets of sickness funds, allocates the funding over individual funds and institutions, reimburses health insurance agencies for some of the expenditures not covered by their prospective budgets, administers specific subsidy schemes of the ZFW and AWBZ, and monitors and supervises the administration of sickness funds and private health insurers (the latter only as far as the AWBZ is concerned). Private health insurance is under the supervision and control of the Central Insurance Chamber, *Verzekeringskamer*, which is under the authority of the Minister of Finance. Until 1998, the ZFR also advised the Minister of Health on broader policy issues, but this advisory role has been limited to technical matters only.

Private Health Insurance

Dutch residents who are not eligible for sickness fund insurance may opt to take out private health insurance with one of the fifty or so private health insurance companies. The vast majority of this population segment has done so. Private insurers offer a wide range of insurance policies, with varying coverage, financial conditions, and eligibility criteria. They usually age-relate premiums for elderly people and can exclude preexisting conditions from coverage. In the last decade, in particular during the second half of the 1990s, private health insurers have strengthened their collaboration with the sickness funds for different reasons. In doing so, they gained access to the addresses of those insured by sickness funds to whom they could offer other insurance. In this way, they also benefited from very long experience of the funds with local and regional contracting. Next, they expanded traditional health insurance to a wider range of collective insurance and employee benefits packages, both for the sickness fund insured and the privately insured, under the umbrella of larger conglomerates. Such packages have gained importance in the Dutch market, in particular after recent changes in other social insurance legislation shifted some of the financial risks for sickness and disability from social insurance to the employers, who in turn started seeking insurance coverage for their risks.

Current Health Policies

The main goals of Dutch health policies are solidarity, universal access, equal treatment, and good quality of health care services (*Regeerakkoord*, 1998). Other important principles are professional autonomy and patient satisfaction (Organization For Cooperation And Development, 1992). At the same time, for over twenty years cost control has been an overriding concern, not as a primary goal of health policies but as part of wider macroeconomic and social policies. Health care is one of the major categories of public expenditure (out of taxation and social health insurance). Therefore, reining in the growth of public spending in order to keep labor costs low and strengthen international competitiveness has become one of the main policy goals of Dutch macroeconomic policies. After abandoning the reforms based on the recommendations of the Dekker committee, the 1994 and 1998 coalition cabinets decided to maintain the existing funding structure and to focus on improving the existing system (*Regeerakoord*, 1994). The current coalition chose several measures aimed to improve the quality, flexibility, and user friendliness of both acute and long-term care services; the coalition emphasized the need for better cost control in order to safeguard the future availability of health care for everyone.

Public Health and Quality Assessment

The Inspectorate of Health is responsible for monitoring the quality of health services and health protection measures. In 1997, it published an extensive report on the quality of health care in the Netherlands (Ministry of Health, 1997c). One of the main conclusions of the report is that, compared to other countries the quality and efficiency of Dutch health care is good. Municipal authorities are responsible for the municipal health services and public health measures. In 1998, the Minister of Health announced plans to introduce a standardized minimum package of public health services to be provided by the local authorities.

Acute Medical Care

In acute care, similar to other areas, regionalization of care has become one of the leading themes of health policy. In its governing manifesto of 1998, the government stresses the need for close collaboration within and between intramural and ambulatory services on the regional level (*Regeerakkoord*, 1998).

Changes in Social Security

Changes in the broader area of social policy have also affected health care. For example, reductions in the scope and level of sick leave benefits in social insurance shifted financial risks to employers who realized that they now have a financial stake in a rapid recovery and rehabilitation of their sick and disabled employees. This prompted health insurers to expand their business and combine traditional health insurance with other employee benefits, including rehabilitation, special treatment for labor-related diseases, and waiting list management. Some of these activities raised public concern about the preferential access for employees to health services. In reaction, the Minister of Health felt obliged to take steps to prevent such preferential treatment, but late in 1999 the Cabinet agreed that it would allow employers under certain restrictions to set up special contracts with providers for the treatment of labor-related conditions.

Pharmaceuticals, Medical Aids, and Appliances

The last decades have seen important advances in pharmaceutical science but also rapid cost increases. Compared to other European countries, Dutch patients are moderate consumers of pharmaceuticals. Traditionally, the level of consumption has been low but average prices high in comparison with neighboring countries. The pharmaceutical policies of the Health Ministry reveal a wide range of measures focused on consumers, physicians, and industry. They seek to influence consumption levels, prescription patterns, and wholesale and retail prices, as well as the distribution system of pharmaceuticals. In 1996, the Pharmaceutical Prices Act (*Wet Geneesmiddelenprijzen*) forced the pharmaceutical wholesale industry to lower its prices by an average of 20 percent. In the same year, the Ministry of Health introduced a list of pharmaceuticals reimbursed by the social health insurance. In 1999 over-the-counter drugs were delisted.

There is a special procedure for admitting new drugs to the list, which has slowed the introduction of new pharmaceuticals in the Netherlands. In 1991 the Health Ministry set up the reference price system (GVS) modeled on the German system. Patients can obtain the drugs at or under the reference price without co-payment, but if they insist on receiving higher-priced drugs, they have to pay the price difference themselves.

The report of an expert committee, the Koopmans Committee, contained recommendations for improving cost control. Several measures have been implemented (Koopmans Committee, 1997). In 1999 the ministry reduced the reference price level for many drugs. Other measures focus on influencing the prescription behavior of physicians. For example, every year, the Sickness Fund Council publishes the *Pharmaceutical Compass* for all physicians. Regional groups of general physicians meet regularly to discuss the merits and cost-effectiveness of new drugs and possibilities for substituting brand-name drugs for generic drugs. In 1998 the Health Ministry announced that it would set up similar regional meetings for hospital specialists.

Another change is that pharmacists are now encouraged to sell generic drugs. In recent years, the Ministry of Health has tried to reduce the profit margins of the pharmaceutical producers and wholesale industry. In particular, the system of large sales bonuses and rebates offered to pharmacists came under attack. In order to encourage competition in the distribution system, hospital apothecaries will be allowed to dispense outpatient prescriptions. Sickness funds can now operate pharmacies. The Ministry of Health acknowledges the importance of pharmaceutical innovation, but the new drugs offered are often very expensive.

Cost-Control Policies

At the Cabinet level, there are different, sometimes conflicting policy goals such as improving employment, education, infrastructure, social security, health care and, more recently, meeting the Maastricht criteria for joining the European monetary system. At this level, the main issue is not so much the health of the population but the health of the nation's budget. Macroeconomic policy considerations are often the driving forces of health care policies and health care reform. One of the main policy goals of the Dutch government is to reduce unemployment. One way of doing so is by restraining labor costs, which directly affects health spending, as it is one of the main categories of public spending. In health care, Dutch governments have explored a variety of cost-containment measures: developing budgetary mechanisms at different levels, delisting services from social health insurance, and using policy measures aimed at restraining consumption. Budget mechanisms include the agreement on the annual overall spending limit for health expenditures, the allocation of this amount over different (sub)sectors and regions, the budgeting of individual hospitals and institutions, and the budgeting of individual sickness funds (Ministry of Health, 1994; London School of Economics and others, 1998).

In particular, proposals to delist services and to introduce or increase user charges have proven to be very contentious. Paul Pierson observes that, politically speaking, it is easier to expand entitlements than to contract (Pierson, 1994). Welfare programs often entail direct benefits and diffuse and indirect costs. The expansion of benefits usually implies a very small burden to many (for example, a small rise in contribution rate), with great benefits concentrated on specific groups, whereas contraction implies concentrated costs to certain groups, with small and dispersed benefits for many. Dutch health policies are no exception to this pattern.

Copayments in health care have a mix of purposes: they seek to shift funding from public to private sources, to enhance the cost awareness of consumers, and to increase consumer influence. A specific form of cost containment is the delisting of entitlements from the mandatory coverage of the social insurance schemes. In fact, delisting may be seen as a 100 percent copayment (Okma, 1998).

Health Reform in the 1980s and 1990s

After lengthy debate in 1998, the government decided to accept proposals to reform the Dutch health care system (Ministry of Health, 1988b). It developed a four-year implementation plan. In the period 1989–1992, several steps were taken. Some services shifted from the sickness fund and private health insurance to the AWBZ scheme, which was to become the new populationwide, mandatory health insurance. Rules for planning and setting fees were deregulated. Other steps included the abolishment of regional boundaries of sickness funds, abolition of mandatory contracting of self-employed health care professionals by the sickness funds (with the announcement that mandatory contracting of institutions would end later), removal of local authority control over practices of family doctors, and replacement of fixed tariffs by tariff ceilings. These measures allowed insurers to selectively contract with providers and to negotiate volume, prices, and quality of services.

But during implementation, opposition resurfaced, political support became increasingly hesitant, and public support eroded (Okma, 1997; Willems Committee, 1994). Faced with mounting opposition, the Cabinet began to explore alternative routes, increasingly emphasizing the importance of cost control (Ministry of Health, 1992b). After accepting the legislation for the second phase of reform, Parliament decided to shelve debate over the next steps. Ultimately, this also led to the demise of the Dekker reforms. After general elections in 1994, a new governing coalition stepped into office and announced that it would no longer continue the reforms but opted to shift toward incremental changes of the existing system instead. The new coalition government of 1998 continued this incremental approach. It kept the existing funding model (the mix of public and private insurance, tax subsidies, and direct patient payments) and proposed other measures to improve the quality and efficiency of health care services.

Transformation of the Neocorporatist Policy

In recent years, the landscape of Dutch health politics and policies has undergone major changes. The traditional neocorporatist policy arena came under siege (Okma and de Roo, 1998). Critics felt that the existing structures had become too cumbersome, time consuming, and procedural. Different committees advocated a drastic restructuring of this policy arena, emphasizing the need for strengthening the so-called primacy of politics. This entailed a shift in decision-making power from traditional neocorporatist organizations to Parliament and Cabinet (and ultimately although not intentionally to civil servants). The proposals were inspired by broader changes in society such as changing economic conditions and demographic changes and by the erosion of authority of church, state, and traditional intermediary organizations (Lijphart, 1968).

In 1993, a special parliamentary committee advocated a clear distinction between, and separate organizational forms for, functions such as policy advice, administrative responsibilities, management and control functions, and representation of partial interests (De Jong Committee, 1993). The committee found that there were over 100 different governmental advisory bodies, with a total membership of over 2,200. In the ranking of numbers, the Health Ministry scored the highest, with thirty-six different advisory bodies on health care and related social services. In 1991 they presented more than 500 reports.

Following the recommendations of its own committee, the Dutch Parliament decided to reduce the size and number of advisory bodies and to end the mandatory round of consultations with advisory bodies on each and every piece of legislation. Parliament itself set an example by reducing the number of its own standing committees. For the Health Ministry, this meant an even larger reduction of the advisory structure. Several specialized committees were terminated; some merged with others. The Sickness Fund Council and the Central Tariff Agency are now limiting their advisory activities to specific technical fields and administration. Their advisory role on health policies shifted to the newly established Council for Health Care (*Raad voor de Volksgezondheid en Zorg*, RVZ) that now serves as the major advisory body to the Health Ministry. The Health Council (*Gezondheidsraad*) and the Council for Health Research (*Raad voor Gezondheidszorgonderzoek*, RGO) escaped elimination; they act as nonpolitical, purely scientific bodies advising on scientific developments and research priorities.

Another advisory council under the prime responsibility of the Ministry of Health—the Advisory Council on Social Development (*Raad voor Maatschappelijke Ontwikkeling*, RMO)—focuses on major social and welfare developments. According to the advice of the Committee De Jong, membership in the advisory bodies is to consist of independent experts only, eliminating direct interest group representation, with a relatively small secretariat (De Jong Committee, 1993). Further, it recommended termination of the legal obligation for government to consult with the advisory bodies on each policy proposal and new legislation. In the new set-up, ministries and advisory agencies agree on annual working programs as a guideline for the activities. In one respect, the work of the advisory groups expanded: Parliament itself claimed the right to ask for advice directly rather than via ministerial channels.

The changes in the advisory structure thus have affected the traditional Dutch model of consensual policymaking based on systematic consultation and formalized representation of all major interest groups. The groups now have less opportunity to bring issues to the political agenda via the advisory bodies and to directly influence the shaping and outcome of health care policies by using votes and veto power. A more professional model is replacing the postwar model of consensual policymaking. In some cases, informal arrangements have replaced the formal institutions, such as policy networks that serve as important meeting grounds of different parties, with or without government. Such informal networks are playing an increasingly important role in the shaping of health care policies, but it is not yet clear to what extent they fully substitute for the now-abandoned formalized consultations (Van der Grinten, 1996; Okma, 1997). The 1998 governing manifesto announced a plan to set up consultations with major interest groups in health care about long-term planning of allocation of funding linked to measures to improve the system. To some extent, these consultations have replaced the former formalized advisory structures.

It is ironic that at the time the Dutch are dismantling some of their neocorporatist institutions, other countries show growing interest in the Dutch "polder model" of consensual decision making (Swandson, 1997; Lubbers, 1998; Laetz and Okma, forthcoming). The reduction of certain advisory bodies is not aimed at eliminating the involvement of major interest groups altogether. Rather, government is now searching to find new procedures (also labeled "structural entrance" (*gestructureerd entrée*) to create new meeting grounds without being bogged down by lengthy and ineffective formalized procedures. In order to be effective, policies regarding collective arrangements must have some degree of acceptance in society. This is certainly the case in health care, where the policy decisions so much affect the everyday life of patients and involve so many different actors. But it is also important because we are now, after decades of relative expansion, facing a period of relative constraint. It is easier to find a common ground between different interest groups when the financial situation allows for additional funding for everyone than to agree on limited growth or contraction. When macro-economic policies set limits on the available funding and require hard policy decisions, friendly relations may become strained.

References

Biesheuvel Committee. *Gedeelde zorg, betere zorg* [Shared care, better care].

Report of the Curative Care Modernization Committee. Rijswijk: Ministry of Health, Welfare, and Culture, 1994.

De Jong Committee. *Raad op maat* [Customized counsel.] Report of the Special Parliamentary Committee on the Role of Advisory Bodies in Government Policies in the Netherlands. Parliamentary Documents II, 1992–1993, 21427. The Hague: SDU, 1993.

Dekker Committee. *Bereidheid tot verandering* [Willingness to change]. Report of the Committee on Health Care Reform. The Hague: Government Publication Distribution Center, 1987.

De Swaan, A. *In Care of the State. Health Care, Education and Welfare in Europe and the USA in the Modern Era*. Oxford: Polity Press, 1988.

Dunning Committee. *Kiezen en delen* [Take it or leave it]. Report of the Committee on Choices in Health Care. Rijswijk: Ministry of Health, Welfare, and Culture, 1991.

Hill, M. *New Agendas in the Study of the Policy Process*. New York: Harvester Wheatsheaf, 1993.

Hoekstra Committee. *Report on Inefficiencies in Ambulatory Care*. Rijswijk: Ministry of Health, Welfare, and Culture, 1998.

Koopmans Committee. *Report on Controlling Pharmaceutical Expenditures*. Rijswijk: Ministry of Health, Welfare, and Culture, 1997.

Laetz, T., and Okma, K.G.H. *The Rise and Demise and Resurrection of Dutch Health Care Reforms, 1988–1998,* forthcoming.

Lemstra Committee. *Report on Public Health by Local Authorities*. Rijswijk: Ministry of Health, Welfare, and Culture, 1998.

Lijphart, A. *Verzuiling, pacificatie en kentering in de Nederlandse politiek* [Compartmentalization, pacification, and change in Dutch policy]. Amsterdam: De Bussy, 1968.

London School of Economics and Political Science, van het Loo, M., Kahan, J. P., and Lubbers, R. "In Seeking a Third Way, the Dutch Model Is Worth a Look." *International Herald Tribune*, Sept. 16, 1998.

Marmor, T. R., Mashaw, J. L., and Harvey, P. L. (eds). *America's Misunderstood Welfare State. Persisting Myths, Enduring Realities*. New York: Basic Books, 1990.

Ministry of Health. *Structuurnota gezondheidszorg* [Regional plan for health care]. Leidschendam: Ministry of Health and the Environment, 1974.

Ministry of Health. *Financieel overzicht gezondheidszorg* [Financial summary of health care]. Rijswijk: Ministry of Health, Welfare, and Sport, 1988a.

Ministry of Health. *Verandering verzekerd* [Change assured]. Parliamentary Documents, 1987–1988, 19945. The Hague: SDU, 1988b.

Ministry of Health. *Financieel overzicht zorg 1993* [Financial survey of health care, 1993]. Parliamentary Documents II, 1992–1993, 22808, nos. 1–2. The Hague: Ministry of Health, Welfare, and Sport, 1992a.

Ministry of Health. *Modernisering gezondheidszorg* [Modernizing health care]. Rijswijk: Ministry of Health, Welfare, and Sport, 1992b.

Ministry of Health. *Kostenbeheersing in de zorgsector* [Controlling health care expenditures]. Parliamentary Documents II, 1994–1995, 24124. The Hague: SDU, 1994.

Ministry of Health. *Gezond en wel* [Safe and sound]. Rijswijk: Ministry of Health, Welfare, and Sport, 1995a.

Ministry of Health. *De perken te buiten* [Overstepping the bounds]. The Hague: Ministry of Health, Welfare, and Sport, 1995b.

Ministry of Health. *Financieel overzicht zorg 1997* [Financial survey of health care, 1997]. Parliamentary Documents II, 1996–1997, 25004. The Hague: SDU, 1996a.

Ministry of Health. *Modernisering ouderenzorg* [Modernizing care for the elderly]. The Hague: Ministry of Health, Welfare, and Sport, 1996b.

Ministry of Health. *Financieel overzicht zorg 1998* [Financial survey of health care, 1998]. Parliamentary Documents II, 1997–1998, 25604. The Hague: SDU, 1997a.

Ministry of Health. *Volksgezondheid toekomst verkenningen 1997* [Exploration of the future of public health, 1997]. Rijswijk: Ministry of Health, Welfare, and Sport, 1997b.

Ministry of Health. *Staat van de gezondheidszorg 1997* [State of health care, 1997]. Rijswijk: Ministry of Health, Welfare, and Sport, 1997c.

Ministry of Health. *Jaaroverzicht zorg* [Annual survey of health care]. Parliamentary Documents II, 1998–1999, 26204, nos. 1–3. Rijswijk: Ministry of Health, Welfare, and Sport, 1998a.

Ministry of Health. *Health Insurance in the Netherlands*. Rijswijk: Ministry of Health, Welfare, and Sport, 1998b.

Ministry of Health. *Brief sectorvisie GGZ* [White paper on the health care sector]. The Hague: Ministry of Health, Welfare, and Sport, 1999a.

Ministry of Health. *Nota public health* [Public health memorandum]. The Hague: Ministry of Health, Welfare, and Sport, 1999b.

Okma, K.G.H. "Studies in Dutch Health Politics, Policies, and Law." Doctoral dissertation, University of Utrecht, 1997.

Okma, K.G.H. "Why, When and How Should Patients Be Charged?" (editorial). *Journal of Health Service Research Policy*, 1998, *3*(3).

Okma, K.G.H. "Recent Developments in Health Care Cost Containment in the Netherlands." In E. Mossialos and J. Le Grand (eds.), *Health Care and Cost Containment in the European Union*. Aldershot, England: Ashgate, 1999.

Okma, K.G.H., and de Roo, A. "From Polder Model to Modern Management in Dutch Health Care." Paper presented at the Fourth Four-Country Conference on Health Policies and Health Care Reforms, New Haven, Conn., 1998.

Organization for Economic Cooperation and Development. *The Reform of Health Care: A Comparative Analysis of Seven OECD Countries*. Health Reform Studies, no. 2. Paris: Organization for Economic Cooperation and Development, 1992.

Organization for Economic Cooperation and Development. *The Reform of Health Care: A Review of Seventeen OECD Countries*. Health Reform Studies, no. 5. Paris: Organization for Economic Cooperation and Development, 1994.

Organization for Economic Cooperation and Development. *OECD Economic Studies*. Paris: Organization for Economic Cooperation and Development, 1996.

Pierson, P. *Dismantling the Welfare State? Reagan, Thatcher and the Politics of Retrenchment*. New York: Cambridge University Press, 1994.

Ranade, W. (ed.). *Markets and Health Care: A Comparative Analysis*. Reading, Mass.: Addison-Wesley, 1998.

Regeerakkoord 1994 [Governing manifesto, 1994]. Parliamentary Documents II. 1994–1995, 23715. The Hague: SDU, 1994.

Regeerakkoord 1998 [Governing manifesto, 1998]. Parliamentary Documents II, 1997–1998, 26024, no. 10. The Hague: SDU, 1998.

Swandson, A. "A Model of Economy." *Washington Post,* July 17, 1997, pp. A21–A22.

Van der Grinten. "Scope for Policy: Essence, Operation and Reform of the Policy of Dutch Health Care." In L. J. Gunning-Schepers, G. J. Kronjee, and R. A. Spasoff (eds.), *Fundamental Questions About the Future of Health Care.* The Hague: Netherlands Scientific Council for Government Policy, 1996.

Vermeulen, H.J.J.M., and others. *Prognoses van knelpunten op de arbeidsmarkt van de zorgsector* [Forecasts of bottlenecks in the health care labor market]. Tilburg: IVA, 1998.

Welschen Committee. *Ouderenzorg met toekomst* [The future of elder care]. Recommendations of the Committee for Modernizing Care for the Elderly. Rijswijk: Ministry of Health, Welfare, and Culture, 1994.

Willems Committee. *Onderzoek besluitvorming volksgezondheid* [Investigating decision making in health policies]. Parliamentary Documents II, 1993–1994, 23666. The Hague: SDU, 1994.

CHAPTER TEN

GERMANY

Reinhard Busse

The most important aspect of the German health care system is its major component, the 117-year-old statutory health insurance (SHI; *Gesetzliche Kranken-
versicherung*) that now covers almost 90 percent of the population. The SHI initially
included only blue-collar workers; however, over the last 100 years, more and
more of the population came to be included and the benefit package became more
comprehensive.

Germany presents an interesting case for studying today's challenges because
the system has evolved in a stepwise manner over the last 120 years. It has strug-
gled to overcome some of its main weaknesses, which, for example, include the
strict separation between the ambulatory and the inpatient sectors.

This chapter will first lay out the basic framework of the system and identify
the major actors. Then health care financing and delivery in the major sectors
is explored. The chapter continues with an account of the major reforms and

This article is based in part on the European Observatory on Health Care Systems' "Health Care
Systems in Transition—Germany" (1999), which was written by the same author. That report provides more detailed information on the historical development, the organizational structure and
management, health care benefits and rationing, health care finance and expenditure, health care
delivery, financial resource allocation, and health care reforms. A shorter overview is given in Altenstetter (1999).

their objectives in the last decade and an evaluation of emerging issues; it ends with a description of current developments.

Structural Framework and Major Actors

As for the organization of the system, three main groups of actors can be identified: (1) the federal Parliament and government, (2) the state governments, and (3) the corporatist bodies.

Federal Level

The structural framework of the German SHI system is regulated by the federal Parliament through the Social Code Book V (SGB V), usually upon a proposal by the nine-year-old Ministry of Health. The major sections of the SGB V regulate mandatory and voluntary membership in sickness funds, the sickness funds' benefit packages, goals and scope of negotiations between the sickness funds and providers of health care, the organizational structure of sickness funds and their associations, and financing mechanisms, including the risk compensation scheme between funds.

In 1977, Concerted Action in Health Care was created as an advisory body; its main task is advising the government on how to improve the effectiveness and efficiency of health care. Since 1985, an advisory council consisting of seven medical and economic experts in health care assists the advisory group.

State Level

The states *(Länder)* are responsible for maintaining the hospital infrastructure and for public health programs. Since the 1970s, most preventive measures, such as screening programs and health check-ups for both children and adults, have been included in the SHI benefits package and thus are carried out by office-based physicians. The future role of the public health services is under debate (Busse, 1998).

Other responsibilities of the states include undergraduate medical, dental, and pharmaceutical education, as well as supervision of regional physician chambers, sickness funds operating in the state and regional associations of sickness-fund-affiliated physicians, and dentists.

Corporatist Level

Corporatism has several important aspects. First, it allows for the delegation of certain state rights to corporatist self-governed institutions as defined by law. Second, corporatist institutions have mandatory membership and the right to raise their own financial resources under the auspices of and regulation by the state. Third, the corporatist institutions have the right and obligation to negotiate and sign contracts with other corporatist institutions and to finance or deliver services to their members.

In SHI, legally sanctioned corporatist bodies make up the associations of sickness funds, SHI-accredited physicians, and SHI-accredited dentists. The sickness funds are the payers or purchasers in SHI. In mid-1999, there were 453 statutory sickness funds, with about 72 million insured persons, and 52 private health insurance companies, covering about 7 million fully insured persons.

Sickness fund membership is compulsory for employees whose gross income is below US$40,000 in the West and less in the East and voluntary for those above that level. Currently, 88 percent of the population is covered by the SHI: 9 percent by private health insurance and 2 percent by free governmental health care (for example, police officers and soldiers). Only 0.1 percent of Germans are uninsured.

The legal framework includes the following benefits: prevention of disease, screening for disease, diagnostic procedures, necessary ambulatory medical and hospital care, dental care, drugs, nonphysician care, medical devices, nursing care at home, and rehabilitation. The details of the benefits catalogue are mostly negotiated between the sickness funds and the providers. Hospitals, communities, sickness funds, and others do not have the legal right to offer ambulatory medical care. The absence of corporatist institutions in the hospital sector and the medical profession's monopoly on ambulatory care are largely responsible for the almost complete separation between the ambulatory and the inpatient sectors.

Financing and Delivery

In 1997 (the latest figures available), the total expenditure for health was approximately 517 billion deutsche marks (264 billion euros). These expenditures can be grouped by major payers, such as SHI (46.5 percent), employers (12.7 percent), public finances (10.8 percent), private households (8.8 percent), statutory retirement insurance (6.9 percent), statutory long-term care insurance (5.8 percent), private health insurance (5.6 percent), and statutory accident insurance (2.9 percent), or by type of health care expenditure (see Table 10.1). For the sickness funds, as the most important payers in the health care system, the most recent expenditures are presented in Table 10.2.

The relevant issues in health care delivery are summarized; they focus on the situation in 1999 but include important changes that were introduced through the reform acts of the 1990s.

TABLE 10.1. GERMAN HEALTH CARE EXPENDITURES, 1997.

Type of Expenditure	Total Spending (billions of deutsche marks)	Share of Total Spending (percent)
Treatment	310	59
Hospital care	120	23
Ambulatory medical and dental care	91	17
Pharmaceuticals, medical aids, nonphysician care, dentures	11	2
Spa treatment		
Sickness benefits, rehabilitation and invalidity pensions	137	26
Prevention, maternity, and long-term care	44	8
Education and research	9	2
Not distributable	25	5
Total	526	100

Source: German Federal Statistical Office.

TABLE 10.2. GERMAN STATUTORY HEALTH INSURANCE EXPENDITURES, 1998.

Type of Expenditure	Total Spending (billions of deutsche marks)	Share of Total Spending (percent)
Ambulatory medical care	40.8	16.4
Dental care, including dentures	21.2	8.5
Pharmaceuticals	33.4	13.4
Medical aids, nonphysician care (for example, physiotherapy), dialysis	17.4	7.0
Hospital (inpatient) treatment	85.1	34.3
Sick pay and other benefits	37.2	15.0
Administrative costs	13.1	5.3
Total	248.2	100

Source: German Federal Ministry of Health.

Ambulatory Care Sector

SHI-accredited physicians' organizations have the full obligation for provision of services in their regions. The main elements of the corporatist mission include accepting a total predetermined budget from the sickness funds for providing all covered medical services, which the physicians' associations distribute among their members. This is the "secret" that explains Germany's successful cost containment in the ambulatory care sector.

The sickness funds render total payments for the remuneration of the affiliated doctors to the physicians' associations, which releases them from the duty of paying doctors directly. The physicians' associations have to distribute the sickness funds' lump-sum payments to individual physicians, according to the "unified value scale" and additional regulations among the doctors.

Germany has no gatekeeping system, and patients are free to select a sickness-fund-affiliated doctor of their choice. Legally, sickness fund members select a family practitioner that cannot be changed during the fiscal quarter. Because there is no mechanism to control or reinforce this self-selected gatekeeping, patients frequently choose office-based specialists directly. Even though the number of office-based physicians who treat ambulatory patients has doubled since 1970, a disproportionate share of new physicians have been specialists, who now constitute more than 60 percent of all office-based physicians, despite official statements that 60 percent should be family practitioners.

Hospital Sector

There are around 2,260 hospitals with approximately 572,000 beds (69.7 beds per 10,000 population in 1998) and an average occupancy rate of around 80 percent. Of the 2,030 general hospitals, around 790 hospitals are in public ownership, 820 have private nonprofit status, and 420 are private for-profit hospitals, with bed shares of 55 percent, 38 percent, and 7 percent, respectively. In addition, around 1,400 institutions with 190,000 beds are dedicated to spa and rehabilitative care. More than 1 million persons work in the hospital sector, of which roughly one-tenth are salaried physicians. The number of hospital physicians has tripled since 1970.

Hospitals contract individually with the sickness funds. The negotiated conditions, especially the per diem rates, are then valid for all sickness funds. Regulation of the hospital sector follows a "dual planning" approach: the number of hospitals and hospital beds is planned at the state level. Staff planning and the number of hospital days to be provided are negotiated between hospital owners and sickness funds within the framework of negotiating per diem charges. This also explains why cost-containment policies have been ineffective in the hospital sector.

Pharmaceuticals

The pharmaceutical industry in Germany is among the most powerful in developed countries and contributes significantly to the export market. About 1,200 pharmaceutical companies with around 120,000 workers are operating in Germany. The market segments in Germany comprise pharmacies (including prescription drugs, prescription drugs that could also be sold over the counter, and self-prescribed over-the-counter [OTC] drugs) and hospital pharmacies.

Until the 1970s, the pharmaceutical sector was relatively unregulated; companies could set prices, and all available drugs could be prescribed. Drug licensing for new drugs became mandatory only in 1976. The first real cost-containment measures were the development of reference prices (limits for reimbursement) for certain drugs and the introduction of a "negative list" through the 1989 Health Care Reform Act. Because the resulting effects were very moderate, a price cut, higher copayments, and a global prescribing expenditure cap were issued as part of the 1993 Health Care Structure Act. In the case of overspending, physicians were liable for the debt. Initially, sickness funds' pharmaceutical expenditures dropped by 19 percent. Approximately one-third of this drop was attributable to higher copayments and more over-the-counter sales; one-fifth was attributable to the price cut, and one-half to fewer prescriptions. However, the necessary shift in the practitioners' prescribing behavior from unproved or ineffective pharmaceuticals to the "standard therapy" was not achieved. Also, the effects on prescribing habits were not lasting, and expenditure soon rose again. The only lasting effect was the rise in patient cost sharing. Alternative concepts in both improving prescription quality and containing costs, such as a "positive list," were recalled through a change in legislation proposed by the Federal Minister of Health (Busse and Howorth, 1996).

Reforms and Cost Containment

The era of cost containment in the German statutory health insurance sector started in 1977 with the introduction of the Health Insurance Cost-Containment Act. The act ended a period of rapid growth in health care expenditure, especially in the hospital sector. This growth was intended as a way of overcoming infrastructural deficits and shortcomings. Since 1977 the sickness funds and providers of health care have been required to pursue a goal of contribution stability, defined as holding increases in contributions level with the rate of rise in contributory income. Compliance with this legislation is a main task of Concerted Action in Health Care. However, health politicians also felt the need to intervene at increasingly shorter intervals in order to achieve the objective.

Stable contribution rates are viewed as an important objective. Employers and employees jointly pay contributions. For many employees, rises in contribution rate come about because of international competitiveness. A series of cost-containment acts led to a moderation of health care cost increases and stabilized sickness funds' expenditures as proportion of GDP per capita (between 6 and 7 percent since 1975; see Busse and Howorth, 1999), at least until reunification. This was achieved almost without the explicit rationing of services. The following factors were employed in these acts (Busse and Howorth, 1999):

- Budgets for sectors or individual providers
- Restriction of high-cost technology equipment and number of ambulatory care physicians per geographical planning region
- Increased copayments (both in terms of size and number of services)
- From 1997 to 1998, an exclusion of certain dental benefits for persons born after 1978

Reform Acts in 1989 and 1993

The Health Care Reform Act introduced health promotion into the benefit package and increased preventive services. However, the Health Insurance Contribution Rate Exoneration Act cut the former in 1996. Other elements included the introduction of reference prices for pharmaceuticals and medical aids, new benefits for long-term care, introduction of quality assurance measures, and increased scope of the medical review boards of the sickness funds.

Key elements of the Health Care Structure Act were as follows:

- The introduction of legally fixed budgets or spending caps for the major sectors of health care (Busse and Howorth, 1996; Busse, Howorth, and Schwartz, 1997; European Observatory on Health Care Systems, 1999; Schwartz and Busse, 1996)
- A partial introduction of a prospective payment system in the hospital sector (Busse and Schwartz, 1997)
- A lessening of the strict separation of the ambulatory and hospital sector (for example, ambulatory surgery in hospitals became possible)
- The introduction of a positive list of pharmaceuticals (later abolished)
- Increased copayments
- Restrictions in the number of ambulatory care physicians

- The introduction of a "risk compensation scheme" to redistribute contributions among sickness funds
- The freedom to choose a sickness fund for most insured (Busse and Richard, forthcoming)

Reform and Re-Reform, 1996 to 1998

The Health Insurance Contribution Rate Exoneration Act and, even more explicitly, the first and second SHI Restructuring Acts represented a shift from strict cost containment to a policy of restricting employers' contributions on the one side and an expansion of private payments on the other. Copayments were presented as a way to put new money into the system.

In effect, the 1996–1997 acts broke several traditional rules of the system:

- Uniform availability of benefits
- Contributions shared equally between employers and employees
- Financing depending only on income and not on risk or service utilization
- Provision of services as benefits-in-kind

The abolishment of these changes, as well as the reversal of the tendency to shift costs onto patients while easing the financial pressure on providers, became the most important part of the health policy program of the opposition parties. In the expectation of reversals after the elections, the sickness funds undermined the implementation of the de jure end of forcing providers to limit their income for the sake of cost containment. They refused to sign contracts to that end but acknowledged they would reconsider this standpoint after the election, that is, if the former government remained in power.

Change of Government

After the change of government in the fall of 1998, the Act to Strengthen Solidarity in SHI reversed the changes that were not in line with traditional approaches. In addition, copayment rates for pharmaceuticals were lowered, and budgets or spending limits reintroduced; the relevant sectors of health care were defined more strictly than ever. The renewed introduction of budgets and spending caps gave prominence to these instruments again which, over the years, have been of varying forms and efficacy but have been generally more successful in containing costs than any of the other supply- or demand-side measures, which have largely failed. Table 10.3 provides an overview of the rise, fall, and resurrection of budgets and spending caps.

TABLE 10.3. COST CONTAINMENT THROUGH BUDGETS AND SPENDING CAPS SINCE 1989.

Year	Ambulatory Care	Hospitals	Pharmaceuticals
1989 to 1992	Regional negotiated fixed budgets	Individual negotiated target budgets	No budget or spending cap
1993			National legally set spending cap
1994	Regional legally fixed budgets	Individual legally fixed budgets	
1995			Regional negotiated spending caps
1996			
1997	Regional negotiated fixed budgets	Individual negotiated target budgets	
1998	Target volumes for individual practice		Target volumes for individual practice
1999	Regional legally fixed budget		Regional legally set spending cap
2000	Regional negotiated fixed budget with legal maximum	Individual target budget with legal maximum	Regional negotiated spending caps

Source: German Federal Ministry of Health.

Emerging Issues

The German system puts more emphasis on free access and high numbers of providers and technological equipment than on cost-effectiveness or cost containment per se. The public is supporting these priorities; using them as criteria, the system works well. Waiting lists, as well as open rationing decisions such as not providing care to certain patients, are virtually unknown. Currently, however, a shift toward evidence-based medicine and health technology assessment, as well as the will to cut benefits accordingly, can be observed.

In the past, public opinion did not support many changes in the health care system. The new red-green government was aware of this and reversed the most unpopular decisions—exclusion of persons from certain benefits, increased co-payments, and private health insurance mechanisms—through one of their first new laws, programmatically termed the SHI Solidarity Strengthening Act. However, it explicitly took the risk of opening a public debate on priorities, steering mechanisms, and financial incentives when it reintroduced budgets for ambulatory care and spending limits for pharmaceuticals, both of which are extremely unpopular with physicians.

Four "hot" topics are emerging: (1) financing, (2) health technology assessment, (3) the fragmentation of health care between sectors and payers, and (4) collectivism versus competition.

Financing

A major controversy is centered on the financial situation of the SHI. There is now growing recognition of the fact that the perceived "cost explosion" in German health care never happened. This perception led to efforts to contain costs and to the policy of income-oriented expenditures in health care, with the aim of stabilizing contribution rates. Although the absolute amount of health care expenditures had increased five-fold or so since 1970, the percentage of health care expenditures of the GNP remained relatively stable, at least until reunification. This is even more remarkable, as a number of new services had been introduced in health care, such as prevention measures and health promotion. It is now perceived that there is a financing crisis rather than an expenditure crisis or cost explosion. Two facts are especially relevant to this: (1) the high number of unemployed persons narrows the financial basis of the social insurance system, and (2) labor is responsible for an ever-decreasing share of the national income, whereas the share of capital is increasing in tandem. This results in a relative reduction of the financial flow to the social insurance system because contributions are based only on labor.

However, due to reunification, health care expenditure as a percentage of GDP has risen substantially (and now remains at that high level) because health care costs per capita are almost the same in the East as in the West, whereas the GDP is not. Cost containment will, therefore, remain high on the political agenda, and budgets are here to stay for the near future.

Health Technology Assessment

There are considerable inconsistencies in health care sectors. In general, the ambulatory sector appears to be much more regulated than the in-hospital sector in terms of coverage decisions and steering of diffusion and usage of technologies.

Licensing, as a prerequisite for providing SHI-funded services, applies to pharmaceuticals and medical devices (independently of the health care sector in which they are used). Although most licensed pharmaceuticals are covered by the SHI, coverage decisions for medical and surgical procedures in the ambulatory care sector are made explicitly through the Federal Committee of Physicians and Sickness Funds. Explicit coverage decisions are currently nonexistent for the in-hospital sector.

The future direction is to both extend existing health technology assessment mechanisms to other sectors, especially the hospital sector, and to ensure that assessments and coverage decisions are co-coordinated between sectors.

Separation Between Sectors

One weakness is the fragmentation of the German system, especially between ambulatory care and inpatient care. Related to the separation issue are the weak role of primary care and the absence of gatekeepers to steer the patient through the system. The sickness funds are apparently ambiguous about this issue: on the one hand, they claim to support gatekeeping by family practitioners; on the other hand, many of their "disease management" and other models may be intended to increase their own role in gatekeeping.

Collectivism Versus Competition

Throughout the history of the German SHI, regulations have become much more uniform. The Reform Act of 1988 was an attempt to strengthen the purchasers' side by standardizing and centralizing all negotiating procedures, which also standardized the benefits catalogue (Busse, Howorth, and Schwartz, 1997). By introducing a risk compensation mechanism, the Structure Act of 1992 led to a narrowing of difference in contribution rates. The act also introduced free choice of funds for members and therefore competition between funds (Busse, Howorth, and Schwartz, 1997). True market-like competition is not possible, however, as the sickness funds have to offer (almost) the same benefits for a very similar contribution rate; in addition, the range of providers is the same because they are contracted collectively (Brown and Amelung, 1999). In this situation, it is no wonder that funds, particularly the more successful ones in terms of gaining new members, are demanding greater flexibilities for selective contracting. Recent preliminary court verdicts have supported the move toward selective contracting, with the reasoning that joint decisions of sickness funds constitute monopoly power. The issue will remain a case for debate for the future.

Year 2000 Reforms

After the short-term Act to Strengthen Solidarity in SHI, the current government introduced a new medium- to long-term reform into Parliament in June 1999, which was passed in a modified form in December 1999. This Reform Act of SHI 2000 has been effective since January 2000. This reform tries to address three of the system's weaknesses.

1. *Removal of ineffective or disputed technologies and pharmaceuticals from the sickness funds benefits catalogue.* Although these measures are undisputed (or rather unnoticed and undiscussed by the public), the third measure, that is, the introduction of a "positive list" of reimbursable drugs, was opposed by the pharmaceutical industry, especially the smaller companies with a high percentage of "disputed" products.

2. *Improvement of the cooperation of family practitioners, ambulatory specialists, and hospitals.* The new act allows contracts between sickness funds and providers that cross the line between the ambulatory and the inpatient sectors, that is, a group of providers could contract with funds to provide both kinds of care. To promote a (voluntary) gatekeeping function of family practitioners, the act allows sickness funds to give their insured a bonus if they access specialists via their family practitioner only.

3. *Introduction of "global" budgets for sickness funds.* The proposal had called for the introduction of global budgets for sickness funds through which they would have been legally obliged to spend only as much money as they receive through contributions. Additionally, it had called for a change in hospital financing from the "dual" approach to a "monistic" way in which the sickness funds would have to cover all costs, including capital costs. Another piece of the reform relating to financing is the introduction of a budget for family practitioners, that is, separate from the ambulatory specialists.

These pieces of the reform received by far the largest public attention. Although most actors said they agreed in principle with the aim of these measures, they were opposed to different parts of the way to achieve it. The physicians presented the fiercest opposition to the global budget. They openly threatened to ration benefits by setting patients on waiting lists for drugs and procedures; with certain exceptions such as for transplantations, that had been unknown. The physicians' camp, however, was divided about the issue of separate budgets for family practitioners. Both physicians and hospitals were afraid that they might be the losers if certain parts of "their" budgets were used for trans-sectoral contracts. The employees of physicians' practices and hospitals staged demonstrations because they were afraid that jobs would be cut because of the global budget. The sickness funds welcomed global budgets and, in principle, also monistic financing of hospitals. But they insisted on getting the power to plan hospital capacities as well. The *Länder*, although happy to leave capital financing to the sickness funds, wanted to retain their power to determine hospital capacities.

Conclusion

In the end, the act that finally passed did not contain the requirement for global budgets but retained sectoral budgets that will be reduced by the expenditure necessary to finance care delivered under trans-sectoral contracts. The proposal to change hospital financing to a monistic approach also failed. As far as the reimbursement of the running costs is concerned, from 2003, a new payment system based on uniform case fees will replace the current mixed system, with per diems varying between hospitals but with uniform case and procedure fees.

The debate over the current reform act once again demonstrated that changes to Germany's system are slow and stepwise or, to put it positively, carefully debated and thought through. Germany has not done badly this way. Countries that have tried to radically restructure their systems in a short time would do well to consider that fact.

References

Altenstetter, C. "From Solidarity to Market Competition? Values, Structure, and Strategy in German Health Policy, 1883–1997." In F. D. Powell and A. Wessen (eds.), *Health Care Systems in Transition*. Thousand Oaks, Calif.: Sage, 1999.

Brown, L. D., and Amelung, V. E. "Manacled Competition: Market Reforms in German Health Care." *Health Affairs*, 1999, *18*(3), 76–91.

Busse, R. "The German *Länder:* Health Care and Public Health." *Eurohealth,* 1998, *4*(1), 20–22.

Busse, R., and Howorth, C. "Fixed Budgets in the Pharmaceutical Sector in Germany: Effects on Cost and Quality." In F. W. Schwartz, H. Glennerster, and R. B. Saltman (eds.), *Fixing Health Budgets: Experience from Europe and North America.* New York: Wiley, 1996.

Busse, R., and Howorth, C. "Cost Containment in Germany: Twenty Years' Experience." In E. Mossialos and J. Le Grand (eds.), *Health Care and Cost Containment in the European Union.* Aldershot, England: Ashgate, 1999.

Busse, R., Howorth, C., and Schwartz, F. W. "The Future Development of a Rights-Based Approach to Health Care in Germany: More Rights or Fewer?" In J. Lenaghan (ed.), *Hard Choices in Health Care: Rights and Rationing in Europe.* London: BMJ, 1997.

Busse, R., and Richard, S. "Open Enrolment and Risk Structure Compensation in Germany's Statutory Health Insurance: Mechanisms and Effects." *European Journal of Public Health,* forthcoming.

Busse, R., and Schwartz, F. W. "Financing Reforms in the German Hospital Sector: From Full Cost Cover Principle to Prospective Case Fees." *Medical Care,* 1997, *35*(10), OS40-OS49.

European Observatory on Health Care Systems. *Health Care Systems in Transition—Germany.* Copenhagen: World Health Organization, 1999.

Schwartz, F. W., and Busse, R. "Fixed Budgets in the Ambulatory Care Sector: The German Experience." In F. W. Schwartz, H. Glennerster, and R. B. Saltman (eds.), *Fixing Health Budgets: Experience from Europe and North America.* New York: Wiley, 1996.

CHAPTER ELEVEN

SPAIN

Alicia Granados, Pedro Gallo

Spain is one of the European countries where health outcome indicators are good; health expenditures are well within European standards, even though there is increasing pressure on costs. The system has achieved universal coverage, and resources are mainly generated by taxes; the system has provided overall financial equity (De Miguel, 1994). Health services are mainly provided by the public sector, through the hospital network, although the role of the private sector is important and the public-private relationship is complementary. Despite minor improvements, primary care is still lagging behind as a service network in most Spanish regions.

This chapter describes the main features of the system in terms of management and organization, prevailing values, and health care priorities and tools. Future developments, including the extension of decentralization, possible pharmaceutical policy changes, and increased resources for research and development are explored.

Overview

Spain's GDP per capita is $15,162 (purchasing power parity in 1996) and has a population of over 39 million. Despite spending only 7.4 percent of GDP (1997) on health care, it performs remarkably well in morbidity and mortality indicators: 674.5

mortality rate for all causes (per 100,000 population), 6.0 infant mortality rate (per 1,000 live births), life expectancy of 81.0 years (for females) and 73.3 (for males; 1994), and 9 percent of the population made use of a hospital (Rodríguez, Gallo, and Jovell, 1999). The system covers 99.8 percent of the population and is mainly publicly funded (75 percent), largely through taxes. Almost 90 percent of the private funding (25 percent of the total) is in the form of direct payments. Private insurance premiums only account for 2 to 3 percent of the total expenditures, although there are significant differences across regions. Most of the available hospital beds are publicly owned, although this also varies greatly between regions.

The organizational structure is decentralized across seventeen regions but, to date, only seven of them are invested with full competencies. The allocation of resources to the regions is mainly allocated on the basis of the population in the territory. Ten regions are directly controlled by central Madrid-INSALUD (National Health Institute) and seven highly autonomous regional health services. The whole of the INSALUD and the regional health services shape the Spanish National Health System.

Management and Organization

Major objectives of the system include the protection of health, the promotion of health, and the prevention of illness, with a special emphasis placed on public health, primary care, and maternity and infant care. Protection of health is recognized by the ruling 1978 Spanish Constitution and further reinforced by developments such as the 1986 General Health Act (GHA) and the regional legal arrangements.

Universal Coverage and Equity

Universal coverage and equity are two highly valued policy objectives. The GHA claimed that public health care should be extended to cover all of the population and provide equal access to services. This demonstrates a clear commitment of public authorities to universality and equity.

The extension of coverage has been remarkable and, today, almost the entire population (99.8 percent) enjoys public coverage in health care. A public provision network largely guarantees coverage. However, this varies from region to region, partly for historical reasons and partly because of development and investment trends in public facilities. In this respect regions like Catalonia are characterized by a large, nonpublic sector. The nonpublic sector has created universal contracts with public health authorities for the provision of services.

Public-Private Mix

The four main sources of finance are taxes and social contributions on the public side, and out-of-pocket payments and private insurance premiums on the private side. Despite this, public and private financing have historically followed different paths, and the balance has changed since the 1960s and 1970s.

During the 1960–1987 period, public expenditure grew at a real annual rate of 9 percent, well above all other OECD countries. Today, it represents approximately 5.8 percent of the GDP, that is, three-fourths of total expenditure in health care.

Public finance, however, has undergone substantial changes in time, particularly in the balance of public sources that is made up of taxes and social contributions. During the 1960s and 1970s, tax contributions to the health system were less than 5 percent of total public expenditure in health. By 1980 they represented 10 percent; since 1982 there was a rapid increase to 30 percent in 1988, 80 percent in 1993, and 99 percent in 1998. Social contributions to health care expenditures today are almost nonexistent.

As mentioned, private finance represents approximately 25 percent of the total expenditure in health. Out of this 25 percent, more than 90 percent are out-of-pocket payments on pharmaceuticals and on private providers. In respect to the latter, it should be noted that private insurance in Spain accounts for approximately 3 percent of total expenditure on health care.

Patient Payments

Patients receive free care at the point of use at any public institution or private hospital whose contracting status has been previously negotiated. There is no copayment for medical services, physiotherapy, transportation for medical emergencies, or basic dental care.

Pharmaceuticals are free of charge when administered while receiving inpatient care; however, for most drugs prescribed during outpatient and primary care, the patient pays 40 percent of the total amount. The remaining 60 percent is directly refunded to the pharmacist by central authorities within the Ministry of Health, except for pensioners, who are exempted from any form of copayment. The Ministry of Health regulates the price of drugs; over 1,600 pharmaceutical products are excluded from public coverage and are only available on an out-of-pocket payment basis.

The consumption of pharmaceutical products has increased considerably; today Spain is among the top European countries in pharmaceutical expenditures (Rodríguez, Gallo, and Jovell, 1999).

Hospital and Primary Care

A number of factors should be noted regarding hospital and primary care services. The size and staffing of hospitals in Spain varies according to ownership. In general, publicly owned hospitals have better staffing ratios per beds and the most sophisticated high-technology equipment. Reimbursement for hospital services is largely prospective by budgeting. Payment to private hospitals contracting with public authorities is based on a formula that takes into account the type of institution and the type of patients. Hospitals are generally paid for days of stay at a fixed price that is renegotiated every year.

Unlike hospital care, primary care services under the National Health System are almost exclusively provided in public facilities and increasingly by full-time primary teams, including general practitioners, pediatricians, and nurses serving a well-defined geographical area (Rodríguez, Gallo, and Jovell, 1999). The payment of physicians who provide ambulatory services is made partly on a capitation basis and partly on a salary basis. Hospital doctors are largely paid in the form of salaries, with an incentive scheme that takes into account experience and full-time status. Private medical practices are paid on a fee-for-service basis.

Utilization

The number of consultations and visits per capita is lower than the OECD average, but recent survey data indicate that the reported average number of physician visits was 5.9 in 1991. The lowest rates of utilization correspond to the highest income group (3.7 visits a year on average), and the highest utilization rates to the lowest income group (9.1 visits), which is also the group that reports a higher number of health problems. These facts, together with results coming from similar studies on equity, point to a reasonable utilization of services according to need (Blendon and others, 1991; Navarro, 1997).

Further, other studies of the utilization of health care services at regional levels have shown that the provision of such services is largely equitable, that is, based on the different needs of the population, with particular emphasis on lower-income groups and on limiting chronic health indicators (Gallo, Serra-Prat, and Granados, 1999).

Physician Freedom

An important consideration in understanding the delivery of services is the status of physicians as a professional class, who enjoy a great degree of medical practice freedom. In the seventies Spain doubled its number of practicing physicians; the number of physicians per 1,000 inhabitants today is considerably above the average of OECD countries. Although half of these professionals have at least two jobs, the number of unemployed physicians remains very high: 10 percent in 1983 and 20 percent in 1987 (Rodriguez, Gallo, and Jovell, 1999; Rodríguez and De Miguel, 1990). Active physicians work as full- or part-time employees of public or private health care organizations, and about 40 percent also have a private practice (Rodríguez and De Miguel, 1990). For 76 percent, their main position is salaried and is hospital-based (Rodríguez, Gallo, and Jovell, 1999).

Critical Regional Issues

The decentralization of health services to the seventeen Autonomous Communities in the form of devolution and the creation of their respective regions is an omnipresent issue in the organization of Spanish health care (Mills and others, 1990; Rico, 1998). The country's legal frame in this regard is shaped by three elements: the 1978 Spanish Constitution, the regions' Estatutes, and the General Health Authority. The GHA is part of a much wider, comprehensive and constitutional process of decentralization and state redefinition known as the State of the Autonomies.

Regional Authority

The regions are the administration level in charge of health management and control through their regional health services (RHS). Each region uses its competencies and, according to the Estatute (*Estatutos de Autonomía*), elaborates on the GHA through development and complementary laws, creates regional health plans, and distributes resources.

The resulting seventeen health plans are essential in the shaping of the National Integrated Health Plan (*Plan Integrado de Salud*). This plan is developed from the combination of four sources: (1) the regional health plans, (2) plans of a national scope, (3) common plans of the regions and the state, and (4) other particulars related to financial and resource allocation arrangements. To date however, no national integrated health plan has been developed.

Decentralization Difficulties

The decentralization process has experienced difficulties. The transfer of authority in the area from central government to the regions has been accomplished differently and has resulted in diverse levels of autonomy. Accordingly, only seven of the seventeen Spanish regions, accounting for 60 percent of the population, live in a fully decentralized region and enjoy a thorough body of competencies (Catalonia, 1981; Andalucia, 1984; Basque Country and Valencia, 1987; Navarre and Galicia, 1990; and the Canary Islands, 1994).

The other ten regions (40 percent of the population in Spain), although with some degree of autonomy, are still under the central and direct management of the National Health Institute-INSALUD in Madrid (De Miguel, 1994). Much of the debate regarding decentralization, however, is centered in the regional allocation of resources and, hence, in the most equitable ways to account for regional differences in demography, morbidity, mortality, patients' movement, and tourism.

Territorial Equity

Despite some GHA articles encouraging equity, there remain geographical differences among regions regarding the number of total beds per 1,000 inhabitants, doctors per bed, and doctor-to-nurse ratios. In reference to those disparities, two significant issues should be noted. First, North-East regions and Madrid prevail as the best-equipped regions in terms of beds per 1,000 inhabitants and personnel per 100 beds, whereas the South-West areas in Spain remain undersupplied (De Miguel, 1994). Second, *conciertos* (pay agreements) correct to some degree the existing public sector differences among regions. Indeed, private-public agreements in regions such as Catalonia and the Basque Country are the solution to a lack of beds provided by the public system. This has defined a mutual dependency relationship between both sectors because the private sector sees *conciertos* as the means to survive in the health care market. The private sector remains dependent on the public sector because the latter has become the most important client in terms of resources.

The NHS not only has to deal with an unbalanced distribution of resources in terms of geographical location but also in terms of the types of facilities available. The NHS is taking deficiencies into consideration, and 80 percent of INSALUD hospitals are currently undergoing partial (50 percent) or total (30 percent) renovations so they can be more responsive to sociodemographic changes, spontaneous increases in demand for services, and technological changes (Rodríguez, Gallo, and Jovell, 1999).

Regional Reforms

Particular emphasis should be given to reform initiatives at the regional level. For example, the Health Care Organization Law (*Liei d'Orden Sanitara de Catalunya*, or LOSC), enacted by the Catalan Parliament in 1990, has shaped health care in

Catalonia and reflected the socioeconomic development and health care characteristics. In developing the LOSC, the Catalan government considered the unique characteristics of the market, including the fact that over 60 percent of the beds are privately owned. A purchaser-provider split was implemented as a means to rationalize the organization of a mixed health care system that includes services supplied by the public and private sectors under the general direction and organization of the Catalan government (Rodríguez, Gallo, and Jovell, 1999). The market in Catalonia today could be better defined as a relational market rather than as a *stricto sensu* internal market, as is implemented in other European countries (Gallego-Calderón, 1998).

Key Challenges

Spain faces the dilemma of maintaining health care coverage, developing primary care services, providing support systems for long-term care patients, and encouraging investment in the least privileged regions, while simultaneously controlling costs. An additional challenge is to implement full decentralization of services without endangering the equity principle and maintaining or improving health outcomes of the population.

Rising Costs

Policymakers are concerned with rising costs because of the increased health needs of an aging population. In addition to increased demand and use of services, additional cost pressures are driven by the adoption and introduction of new health care technologies.

New Policies

Continuing concerns in policy include primary care reform, rationalization of hospital care, integration of services (particularly for the elderly and for those needing mental health services), cost-containment measures, the well-known purchaser-provider split, and the increasing role of HTA in research and education initiatives.

Research Initiatives

Different approaches regarding research strategies coexist in Spain. The main public source for financing and supporting research is placed in the central Ministry of

Health through the National Health Research Fund (*Fondo de Investigación Sanitaria,* or FIS). This initiative is investigator-led. In 1996, 140 HTA-related projects were funded at over US$2 million. Other research initiatives may be found at the regional level.

In Catalonia, a 1996 an agreement between CAHTA and the Catalan Health Service led to the design and implementation of a health services research strategy linked to the process of HTA, taking into account the priorities identified in the Catalan Health Plan (Granados and others, forthcoming).

Health Technology Assessment Role

HTA has a long history in Spain, beginning with the advisory board on high technology in the Catalan Department of Health in 1984. This board evolved into the Catalan Agency for Health Technology Assessment (CAHTA) in 1994. The Basque Country established an HTA unit in 1992 (OSTEBA), and the Andalusian government did so in 1996 (AETSA). A national agency for health technology assessment (AETS) was also created in 1994.

These different organizations coordinate their work, in part through the Working Group on HTA, which is an advisory committee in the Interregional Council of the Spanish NHS. HTA is firmly established as a sound tool to inform the health care decision-making processes as regards the safety, efficacy, and efficiency of existing and new technologies (Granados and others, forthcoming).

Opportunities and Limitations

When pinpointing market opportunities in Spain, one has to consider the context or setting of implementation, its historical development as regards the health care market, the role of the various providers (public and private), the legal framework, and the social values and preferences that prevail.

New Planning Opportunities

The first to consider is the increasing heterogeneity of health care policies because of devolution to the regional level. This has translated not only in the different planning and organization strategies of health care services but in contracting and incentive arrangements. New approaches or initiatives may well be easier to implement in some regions than in others. Further, the policymaker is not just one central authority in Madrid but also many at both the national and regional level. The increasing concern about health expenditures and rising costs in health care, together with the need to control the public sector deficit according to the EU standards, could also be seen as an opportunity for the implementation of such approaches.

Managed Care Limitations

Any new initiative such as that for managed care would face a series of opportunities and limitations to its implementation in the Spanish health care market. As regards limitations, we would like to highlight the possible conflict facing existing and prevailing values in the Spanish health care system. We refer particularly to solidarity, equity, participation, costs, quality concerns, physician freedom, and the standardization of clinical practice.

Further, managed care initiates will probably encounter a set of internal competitors in the Spanish setting, not only coming from public institutions but also from the well-known private interests, both at the purchaser and provider levels. It should be acknowledged that private providers might be seen as competitors only in some regions in Spain and not in others. Finally, accountability should be mentioned. Certainly, the Spanish system works under a clear definition of responsibilities, particularly in reference to public sector performance. Control over the private sector is also present in areas such as accreditation and authorization of new centers and services.

Future Policy Developments

A number of policy developments can be foreseen.

Completing Decentralization

First, the decentralization of public health services is still to be completed in Spain, not only regarding the number of regions presently benefiting from full competencies but also regarding the need to correct existing inequities in the finance and delivery of services among regions.

The effective integration of these regional health services is a basic condition to achieve the right to health protection of all citizens, the coordination of public policies, the uniform levels of functioning of public services, and an effective health plan that would result in the improvement of service-related issues.

Pharmaceutical Policy

Second, a new pharmaceutical policy regarding generic drugs is need. The pressure of pharmaceutical expenditures on the health budget and the need to control costs would foster a greater use of these drugs. On the management side, there is bound to be a greater differentiation between purchaser and provider responsibilities, allowing for the introduction of more flexible schemes in the way public health care institutions are managed. This would also mean a major role to be played by health technology assessment in informing decision making.

Increased Research

Third, a major implication of public resources to research and development is foreseen, particularly in areas of great health concern such as cancer, leading to the strengthening of a National Institute for Cancer Research. Similarly, regional governments such as Catalonia, in the use of its competencies, will continue to emphasize research-oriented initiatives in their own territory.

Conclusion

Spain is one of the European countries where health outcome indicators are good, keeping health expenditures well within the European standards but with an increasing pressure on costs. Further, the system has achieved universal coverage, and resources are mainly generated by taxes; overall financial equity has resulted (De Miguel, 1994). Health services are mainly provided by the public sector, through the hospital network, although the role of the private sector should be acknowledged. A public-private relationship may be understood as complementary. Despite minor improvements, primary care is still lagging behind as a service network in most in Spanish regions.

References

Blendon, R. J., Donelan, K., Jovell, A. J., Pellisé, L., and Costas-Lombardía, E. "Spain's Citizens Assess Their Health Care System." *DataWatch/Health Affairs*, Fall 1991, pp. 216–228.

De Miguel, J. M. "Salud y Sanidad" [Health and Ministry of Health]. In *Informe sociológico sobre la situación social de España* [Sociological information and the situation in Spain] (Vol. 1). Fundación FOESSA, Madrid, 1994.

Gallego-Calderón, R. "New Public Management Reforms in the Catalan Public Health Sector, 1985–1995: Institutional Choices, Transaction Costs, and Policy Change." Doctoral thesis, London School of Economics and Political Science, 1998.

Gallo, P., Serra-Prat, M., and Granados, A. *Equitat en la provisió de serveis sanitaris a Catalunya* [Equality in the provision of services in Catalunya]. Barcelona: Agencia d'Avaluació de Tecnologia Médica, 1999.

Granados, A., Sampietro-Colom, L., Asua, J., Conde, J., and Vázquez-Albertino, R. "The Role of Health Technology Assessment in Spain." *International Journal of Technology Assessment in Health Care,* forthcoming.

Mills, A., and others. *Health System Decentralization: Concepts, Issues, and Country Experience.* Geneva: World Health Organization, 1990.

Navarro, V. "Topics for Our Times: The 'Black Report' of Spain—the Commission on Social Inequalities in Health." *American Journal of Public Health,* 1997, *87*(3), 334–335.

Rico, A. "La descentralización sanitaria en España" [Decentralization in Spain]. *Papeles de Economía Española,* 1998 [Spanish Economic Papers, 1998]. *76,* 49–66.

Rodríguez, E., Gallo, P., and Jovell, A. J. "Sharing Lessons with Newly Industrialized Countries: The Experience of the Spanish Health Care System." *Health Policy and Planning,* 1999, *14,* 2–3.

Rodríguez, J. A., and De Miguel, J. M. "The Case of Spain." *Health Policy,* 1990, *15,* 119–142.

CHAPTER TWELVE

FRANCE

Pierre-Jean Lancry, Simone Sandier

On the whole, the French declare themselves satisfied with their health care system. The population is now universally covered by the *assurance-maladie,* a branch of the social security system that lifts the financial barriers to access to medical care provided by health professionals and the health care industry.

Affiliation with the *assurance-maladie* is through different schemes, according to the individual's socioprofessional category. The main scheme, the *régime général,* covers employees and pensioners from trade and industry sectors, as well as their families—more than 80 percent of the population. The *régime général* is financed mainly by payroll contributions of employers (around 13 percent of gross salaries) and a special contribution levied on total income (around 5 percent).

Within the provisions of the *assurance-maladie,* patients are free to choose among health care services, but they contribute a significant proportion of the cost of care. Patients pay the provider directly and are reimbursed later, but in most cases only partially. The difference is expressed through a patient cost-sharing scheme (the *ticket modérateur*), in which the patient is charged different amounts depending on the type of care and treatment necessary. There are exceptions to

The authors based this chapter on an earlier work of theirs, "Twenty Years of Cures for the French Health Care System." In E. Mossialos and J. Le Grand (eds.), *Health Care and Cost Containment in the European Union.* Aldershot, England: Ashgate, 1999.

these general rules for certain patient groups or types of diseases and treatments, however. Of the population, 87 percent are affiliated with voluntary, supplementary sickness funds *(mutuelles)* or purchase private insurance, both of which supplement compulsory insurance and cover to varying degrees the charges that the *assurance-maladie* does not. Because of the combined effects of the compulsory and the complementary coverage, different payers contribute differently to financing health care expenditure, according to the extent of coverage and type of services provided. If a patient pays directly for only 13.9 percent of overall expenditure, for example, the amount rises to 22 percent in the case of physician services, 20 percent for pharmaceutical products, and 40 percent for dental treatment—but is only 6 percent for hospital charges.

Services and goods covered by the *assurance-maladie* that are listed as professional acts and reimbursable medicines must come from registered health providers. Moreover, a doctor must prescribe these services and goods. In certain cases, such as for eyeglasses and physiotherapy, prior approval is needed for reimbursement. Under these circumstances, the number of services covered is unlimited.

Services provided vary widely. With respect to ambulatory care, health professionals and health care facilities are mainly in the private sector. In contrast, the public sector dominates hospital care and owns 75 percent of all beds.

The relationship between private doctors, their patients, and the *assurance-maladie* is regulated by contracts *(conventions)*, the last of which was signed by only one doctors' trade union in 1997. Patients may consult a specialist without a referral from their general practitioner (GP). Private doctors can prescribe any treatments or diagnostic tests for their patients. They are paid on a fee-for-service basis, according to a negotiated fee schedule. About 25 percent of doctors, mainly specialists *(Secteur 2)*, are allowed to exceed these fees.

At the regional level, public bodies *(Agence Régionale d'Hospitalisation)* regulate planning, as well as the allocation of hospital beds and big-ticket technology. Changes in numbers of beds or in hospital equipment must abide by the *carte sanitaire*, within the framework of a national planning procedure. Public hospitals receive funding through global budgeting, whereas private hospitals are paid on a per diem basis, with set expenditure targets.

Reimbursable drugs—about 90 percent of the pharmaceutical market—are listed by category, price, and reimbursement rate as set at the ministerial level. Expenses covered by the *assurance-maladie* range from 35 percent for nonessential drugs to 100 percent for essential medications such as anticancer drugs.

According to comparative statistics from the Organization for Economic Cooperation and Development (OECD), in 1997 France ranked fifth among OECD countries in terms of health expenditure per capita ($2,100 in purchasing power parity) and fourth in terms of health care expenditures as a share of GDP (9.9

percent). In 1997, according to the French National Health Accounts Commission, total health care expenditure amounted to 781.4 billion francs, or 10.2 percent of GDP. Expenditure for medical goods and services represents 87.2 percent of that total. This amounts to an average of 11,728 francs per person, with an average growth of 3.2 percent per year, at a constant 95 francs, between 1980 and 1995.

In the long run, the growth rate of health expenditure per person at constant francs has decreased. Over the five years between 1990 and 1995, the rate of growth was more than 2.4 percent per year. Since 1980, modification of the reimbursement scheme has meant an overall decrease in the contribution of compulsory health insurance toward health care expenditure, from 76.5 percent in 1980 to 73.9 percent in 1995. In 1995, the National Health Insurance (NHI) still contributed up to 90 percent of the hospital expenditure but only about 60 percent of doctors' fees. An equal percentage was attributed to pharmaceutical expenditure and less than one-third to dental care expenditure. Supplemental health insurance (*mutuelles* and private insurers) and patients have come to play a more important role in financing ambulatory care and pharmaceutical consumption.

The Period 1975–1995

Since the mid-1970s, the slowed rate of growth in economic activity and increasing unemployment have led to a decline in social security revenues, particularly for the *assurance-maladie*. Faced by new financing challenges and a recurrent deficit in the public accounts, the government and the *assurance-maladie* took reform measures that went beyond ordinary management of the *assurance-maladie*, which had evolved according to social, economic, and technological change.

The measures are discussed in the sections that follow.

Adding Resources

During this twenty-year period, government policy focused on *increasing the amount of resources* available to the *assurance-maladie* in order to limit its deficits in the short term. This strategy, politically less risky than reducing benefits, involves raising the salary base of payroll contributions as well as progressively increasing contribution rates from both employees and employers. To complement payroll contributions, new resources from taxes and other levies on revenues have been allocated to the *sécurité sociale*. These new revenues, initially conceived as temporary provisions, have been gradually adopted on a wider scale as ordinary sources of financing. Salary contributions rose from 1.5 percent to 6.8 percent between 1975 and 1995. During the same period, employers' contributions increased from 2.5 percent to 12.8 percent.

Increasing Copayments

Public opinion often opposes measures that affect the degree of public financing of health care expenditure. An overall increase in copayment rates in 1967 had to be reviewed the following year, after public demonstrations of social discontent. After this experience, the government waited twenty-five years before proceeding with another measure of this kind, establishing a general increase in patients' financial contribution to their health expenses in the summer of 1993. Prior to this reform, the *assurance-maladie* reduced its obligations to finance certain expenses through partial measures with direct or indirect effects. Those having a direct effect included the limitation of exemptions from copayment (*Plan Seguin*, 1986), the introduction of patient charges to cover hospital hotel costs (*Plan Bérégovoy*, 1983), and successive adjustments of pharmaceutical reimbursement rates to a level as low as zero, varying by type of drug. One measure having an indirect effect on the share of health care expenditure financed by the *assurance-maladie* is the creation in 1980 of a sector of physicians with unregulated fees.

Beyond their short-term effects, the restrictive measures have led to a reduction in the participation of the *sécurité sociale* in financing health expenses. As a result, a growing number of people have resorted to supplemental insurance. Between 1980 and 1995, for instance, the component of health expenditure financed by the *mutuelles* increased from 5.0 percent to 6.8 percent of overall health care expenditure and from 8.5 percent to 12.4 percent of pharmaceutical expenditure.

The declining role of the *sécurité sociale* has certainly affected the equity of access to health care. When compulsory social welfare benefits decrease and complementary benefits do not cover the difference, inequalities in the use of health care tend to increase.

Regulating Care Providers

In the early 1970s, measures regulating the relationships between the state and the *assurance-maladie* on one side and private providers of care on the other were generally concerned with the supply of health care. First, a *numerus clausus* was introduced in medical schools to reduce the number of doctors in the medium and long terms. Second, a fixed number of training posts for specialists was set for hospitals, a move that was expected to influence the distribution of doctors between general practice and specialist care. Finally, the *carte sanitaire* was introduced to ensure that the demand for health care was met with appropriate hospital services, as well as to control the diffusion of big-ticket technology.

During the 1980s, new measures were introduced, initially targeting the methods of payment for providers of care, either directly or through more general cost-containment measures. Subsequent steps have focused on professional practices.

Reforms After 1995

After the general election of 1995, the new government took a different approach to measures concerned mostly with budgetary matters, which did not really deal with the various factors governing changes in the health care system and its costs. On November 15, Prime Minister Alain Juppé presented to Parliament a comprehensive program of reforms of the whole welfare system in France, publicized as the *Plan Juppé*. On the one hand, the plan called for emergency short-term financial measures; on the other, it set forth guidelines for a major revision in the medium term of the functioning of the health system.

The *Plan Juppé* is, in fact, a synthesis of various proposals, many of them suggested in earlier technical reports and political programs or even already planned by former administrations. As such, it drew approval and blame from both the left and the right of the political arena. Despite great social turmoil at the end of 1995 and various other protests, however, the main measures of the plan were maintained. Although a new left-wing government was called in during June 1997, the different provisions in the *Plan Juppé* are currently being implemented.

To analyze the extent to which implementation of the *Plan Juppé* has changed or will change the functioning of the health care system in France, we will first provide a glimpse at its short-term measures and then discuss some of the structural measures in the field of general management of the system and of physicians' services.

Short-Term Measures of the *Plan Juppé*

Implementation of short-term measures was started within a month of the announcement of the plan. These measures are somewhat standard; they were designed, for example, to increase social security revenues or contain costs. An increase of contributions from pensioners and the unemployed was determined; hospital care reimbursement rates dropped as deductible amounts per diem increased (from 55 to 70 francs); the pharmaceutical industry was required to pay an exceptional taxation of 2.5 billion francs (around 3 percent of its turnover). A target growth rate for both hospital and ambulatory care expenditure was set for 1996–1997 that was equal to the general inflation rate (greater than 2.1 percent), with the prospect of reinforced control mechanisms.

The plan also introduced an exceptional annual tax of 0.5 percent of total incomes effective for thirteen years starting from 1996, aimed at paying the past and current debt of the *sécurité sociale* (250 billion francs). At the end of 1997, considering that the deficit will be higher than foreseen, the period of application of this measure was extended by five years. Theoretically, the tax should end by the year 2014.

Structural Prescriptions of the *Plan Juppé*

Other provisions of the plan are more innovative but require more time for implementation. They could well alter in the long term the respective roles, responsibilities, and behaviors of the different actors in the system: the state, the insurers and other payers, the providers, and the population. Thus, some of the main features characteristic of the French health care system might well be phased out gradually—for example, monopolistic national health insurance linked to occupation, free access to and free choice of provider for the patient, absence of the gatekeeper role of the primary physician, freedom of prescription enjoyed by physicians, and lack of control over the volumes of services provided.

The *Plan Juppé* was intended to improve financial access to health care services through implementation of universal health insurance based on residence rather than on occupation. This measure is important not only because 0.5 percent of the population was still not insured at the time but also because this would legitimize other measures, including the following:

1. National health insurance is now levied on the total income of persons instead of on salaries alone.
2. The state's role in overseeing sickness funds managed by employees and employers' unions has increased.
3. Parliament now has overall control of financing and the orientations of the health care system.

Universal health insurance has proved to be more difficult and more costly to implement than anticipated but finally will be in effect as of January 1, 2000.

Current Regulations

New regulations concerning the financing and monitoring of health care are moving forward in the following ways:

- *Controls over functioning of the health care system have been enhanced.* Now the government controls directly both public and private hospitals instead of only public hospitals. Moreover, the government now appoints chairpersons and directors of various new agencies created at the national or regional level to monitor and supervise the development of the hospital sector.

- *National Health Insurance organizations have lost some of their autonomy.* They continue to negotiate with private health professionals, but the results of their decisions have to fit within the preexisting framework decided by the Parliament. Moreover, National Health Insurance has to abide by the objectives of management defined every third year in a contract with the government *(Contrat d'Objectifs et de Gestion).*

- *A target expense growth rate was set.* In December 1999, for the fourth time, the Parliament voted a *Loi de Financement de la Sécurité Sociale,* based on the proposal of the government and after the analysis of the report of the *Conférence Nationale de Santé* created by the *Plan Juppé.* According to this law, a target growth rate of more than 1.5 percent is set for 1999–2000 in overall health expenses covered by the health insurance.

The fact that prospectively set target budgets constrain the rise of health expenditures from now on, not only as a whole but also by regions and for each type of care, will be remembered as a tribute to cost containment and as one of the major changes introduced or considered by the *Plan Juppé.* As if those financial measures were not reckoned to warrant a lower rate of growth for health care expenses without harming equity in access to care and quality of services provided, however, the *Plan Juppé* has designed a series of measures concerning the delivery of medical services. We will focus hereafter on physician services.

Until now, no major changes in the regulations concerning access to care and fee-for-service payments have been mandated. In the future, however, the *Plan Juppé* might be viewed as a milestone that paved the way for restricting the rights of both patients and providers.

The plan adopts a soft approach by introducing new optional mechanisms that patients, doctors, and others may comply with or not, according to their will. Such a method prevents possible conflicts with opponents and allows, before full-scale implementation, a test of the popularity of the devices, their cost, their efficacy, their efficiency, and their limitations and failures. Three of the mechanisms are as follows:

- Each person receives a *carnet de santé,* a type of booklet in which doctors record patients' medical records. The patient is invited (but not legally required) to produce that booklet at each contact with a health professional or hospital. The idea is to ensure continuity of care and also to limit the number of visits as well as unnecessary prescriptions. For the time being, this experiment seems to be failing. Three years after the introduction of the *carnet de santé*, very few use it regularly. Only incentives such as a higher reimbursement rate could be a boost to such a measure.

- For the first time, in early 1997, the sickness funds signed agreements (conventions) separately with private generalists and specialists. The targets set in 1996–1997 in those agreements for growth of expenses (income and prescriptions) were higher for general practitioners (more than 1.5 percent) than for specialists (more than 1.1 percent). Targets were met by the GPs and slightly exceeded by the specialists. Targets were higher for 1998 and 1999 than for previous years but should be the same for year 2000.

- In October 1997, GPs were given the possibility of becoming, on a voluntary basis for both physicians and patients, a *médecin référent* (a kind of gatekeeper). This new design opens the door to the possible alteration of the free choice of physician by the patient, because the registered patient has a "moral commitment" not to directly visit a specialist without being referred. The GP has to keep a detailed record for his patients, and 10 percent of his prescriptions must be for cheaper drugs, including 3 percent for generic drugs. As financial incentives, patients of *médecins référents* do not have to pay directly out of pocket the full cost of the visit but only the *ticket modérateur* (30 percent), whereas doctors receive an extra annual payment of 150 francs per registered patient (the price of an office visit is 110 francs). Up until now, only 12.5 percent of GPs and around 100,000 patients have chosen this option. Although it is too soon to fully appreciate the success or the failure of *médecin référent* contracts, most GPs appear to have been more influenced by warnings concerning a potential danger of an increased control by the sickness funds than by the prospects of immediate financial benefits.

After three years, should the *médecin référent* experiment be widely accepted by physicians and patients and generate significant savings, it would be politically wise to extend it.

Conclusions

During the last twenty years, cost-containment and regulation measures have mainly targeted *sécurité sociale* expenditures rather than considering health expenditures as a whole. The growth of total health expenditures has slowed markedly, and the share of expenses met by sickness funds has decreased. It seems, however, that inequity is increasing.

Despite the deceleration of health care expenditures, there are still concerns about its financing. Thus, policymakers will continue to consider regulatory measures as a lever to ensure the balance between resources and expenses. The trend over the last thirty years shows that changes are very difficult to implement for economic, social, and political reasons.

Perhaps in the years ahead, as in many European countries, French GPs will be gatekeepers; that could logically lead to a shift, partial if not total, from fee-for-service compensation to capitation-based payment. That in turn could reduce consumption of specialty care.

The policymakers should take into account a few conclusions that emerge from a recent Eurobarometer opinion survey: people regard health policy as a priority, and people do believe in their doctor's judgment and decisions. The idea of constraining health care costs faces hostile reaction, and agreement by the medical profession seems to be prerequisite for the success of any measure of rationalization of health care provision.

CHAPTER THIRTEEN

UNITED KINGDOM

Donald A. Duffy

The United Kingdom is an example of an industrialized country with a centralized statutory universal health care financing system, a niche market for private insurers, a mixed public-private delivery system, and a national policy of rationing care through government control of funding for the public delivery system. The United Kingdom may be unique among countries with a statutory universal system in that its National Health Service (NHS) underwent one significant reengineering under a reform strategy that never was fully implemented and now is undergoing a second reengineering under a second and different reform strategy (see Table 13.1).

The National Health Service

When the National Health Service was established in 1948, it was centrally controlled. The British Medical Association quickly declared war on this "socialized medicine scheme." Physicians had a choice of becoming full-time salaried employees of the NHS and its publicly owned hospitals and clinics, practicing part-time for the NHS as consultants, or remaining in the shrinking, private fee-for-service sector. According to anecdotal reports, creation of the NHS led to a brain drain, as many British physicians wedded to private practice fled the country to reestablish clinical practices elsewhere. Many who remained in the United

TABLE 13.1. STATISTICAL PROFILE OF THE UNITED KINGDOM.

Population:	58.6 million
Health care expenditures as a percentage of GDP:	7.3% (low range among OECD countries)
Government share of total health care expenditures:	84%
Health care expenditures per capita:	US$1,366
Life expectancy at birth:	74 years, males; 79 years, females
Infant mortality rate:	7 per 1,000 live births
Physicians:	1.6 per 1,000 population
Hospital beds:	2.9 per 1,000 population

Kingdom finally but reluctantly participated in the NHS as a means of economic survival.

The feud between organized medicine and the NHS continued almost unabated for nearly half a century. In recent years, the NHS and British policymakers have gained praise from medical ethicists elsewhere on two counts. First, U.K. politicians explicitly adopted a policy of rationing access to costly elective and high-technology-based procedures. A widely publicized longitudinal health services research study supported this policy decision in its finding that NHS cardiac patients treated on a regimen of medications and medical management did as well as those who received bypass surgery.

Second, the NHS was among the pioneers in supporting the concept of hospice care under which terminally ill patients agree to forgo heroic interventions that only prolong the process of dying. With their informed consent, they opt instead for palliative treatment, pain management, and counseling under a combination of home care and inpatient care when necessary for pain management and intermittent relief for family caregivers.

In 1985, internationally renowned American health care economist Alain Enthoven developed an "internal markets" concept, described in a white paper issued by the National Health Service. Prime Minister Margaret Thatcher began the first reengineering of the NHS under a strategy of decentralizing management and creating internal markets involving annual contracts between "fund holders" or payers and individual hospitals or groups of hospitals administered by regional hospital trusts. The Thatcher concept continued under her successor, Conservative Prime Minister John Majors, but then was abandoned by his successor, Laborite Tony Blair.

Blair singled out the NHS as an example of his "third way" political ideology for redefining the central government's role. The "first way" refers to the traditional ideology of liberals and social democrats. The "second way" refers to the market-oriented ideology of conservatives such as Thatcher. Blair's "third way" refers to a new and more pragmatic ideology shared by German Chancellor Gerhard Schroeder, U.S. President Bill Clinton, and others on the world's political stage.

Blair's Labor government articulated its paradigm shift for the NHS in a white paper, published in 1997. "I want the NHS to take a big step forward," Blair wrote in his foreword to this document, "and become a modern and dependable service that is once more the envy of the world."

To advocates of market competition in health care, the Blair initiative represents not a big step forward but one in the reverse direction. It focuses on reversing the trend toward decentralization in favor of more centralized controls, while retaining some aspects of market reforms.

Even though the pace of reform may be demanding, some analysts who have peeled away the political rhetoric see the NHS reengineering now under way as primarily incremental, with some structural reforms, rather than a wholesale overhaul.

The Blair white paper set a number of ambitious goals for the NHS, including the following:

- Guaranteeing to establish in the year 2000 a nationwide, twenty-four-hour telephone advice service staffed by trained nurses, similar to the U.S. concept of advice nurses. (The NHS demonstrated its global outlook by contracting with a U.S. company as its prime consultant in designing this system.)
- Guaranteeing that by the second quarter of 1999, all patients diagnosed with suspected breast cancer will gain access to specialists within two weeks after referral by their "gatekeeper" primary care physicians.
- Guaranteeing that in the year 2000, all patients with other suspected types of cancer will also gain access to specialists within two weeks of referral by their primary care physicians.
- Guaranteeing to reduce waiting times substantially for patients awaiting specialists' care in hospitals and ambulatory surgery clinics. (Estimates are that as many as 1 million patients are on waiting lists for access to hospitals for all types of elective, nonemergency procedures.)
- Establishing national clinical practice guidelines that will "help establish clear national standards for services to improve quality and reduce unacceptable variations in standards of care and treatment." (Guidelines for heart disease and mental health services were targeted for publication in 1999, those for the elderly in 2000, and those for diabetes in 2001).
- Establishing a national institute to evaluate new technologies and pharmaceuticals and provide advice to providers on the cost-effectiveness of alternatives for treatments.

From a restructuring standpoint, the "third way" of NHS reengineering focuses on empowering regional groups of primary care physicians as gatekeepers, decision makers, and allocators of funding. Under this concept, so-called primary care groups (PCGs) are the successors to the Thatcher concept of "general practitioners' fund holders."

The NHS envisions establishing hundreds of PCGs. Each will be allocated fixed budgets for providing and arranging for a wide range of health care services for defined population groups.

This concept of fixed budgets is similar to that applied by many U.S. HMOs such as the Kaiser Permanente Medical Care Program, in which the HMO (the entity functioning as the insurer) contracts with independent groups of physicians to provide all covered medical services on a capitation payment basis, with the capitation payment fixed by annual contract.

The NHS application of this principle differs from the Kaiser Permanente application in three major ways. One, the NHS's fixed payment to PCGs is adjusted to reflect variations in demographics and other risk factors for the populations that each PCG serves. Two, the NHS concept extends beyond medical services to include hospital, home health, ambulance, and other services, as well as outpatient prescription drugs. Three, under the NHS application, PCGs are allowed to retain any surplus annual revenues without penalty in succeeding years' funding allocations but are restricted to applying any surpluses only to improving facilities and services.

In contrast, the principle of fixed capitation payments to physician groups, as applied by Kaiser Permanente, provide for the HMO, or insurer, and contracting physician groups to share in any surplus revenues. The physician groups typically distribute their shares of revenue surpluses to individual physicians as bonuses or incentive payments. The amounts of these incentive payments at risk were substantially reduced after critics of HMOs contended the concept provided participating physicians with financial incentives to erect barriers to care or withhold or deny costly care.

HMOs with those financial arrangements argue that, to the contrary, when some portion of individual physicians' income is at risk based on the financial performance of the total HMO enterprise, they have compelling financial incentives to emphasize preventive care, early diagnosis, and prompt intervention through medically appropriate treatment. Delays in diagnosis and appropriate medical treatment, they contend, only lead to costlier care at the expense of the physician group.

The NHS plan for governance and management of the PCGs involves a complex multiyear transition to its final phase. Ultimately, the PCGs will be governed by a body of trustees consisting of a majority of government-appointed laypersons and a minority of up to ten participating providers, including physicians and registered nurses, who will form a "professional executive body." The trustees will be responsible for overseeing the PCG's health care facilities and determining its infrastructure. The professional executive body will determine priorities for professional services, emphasizing preventive care and health education, and for capital investments.

One analyst of the NHS—Julian Le Grand (1999), professor of social policy at the London School of Economics—has written that Thatcher's proposed internal market reforms were predestined to failure because decentralization is inimical to both the legislative and administrative branches of the U.K. government. He characterized both as being strongly oriented to "keeping tight central control" because "it may be that health is too sensitive an issue in Britain for central government ever to let the relevant agents have enough freedom."

"Only time will tell," Le Grand concluded, "whether Labour's new version of the market will dominate the continuing need for the central government to retain control. If the story told here [that is, in his recent article in *Health Affairs*] is correct, however, a shrewd gambler would not bet on the market to win."

The NHS and Organized Medicine

One might assume that the NHS reform policy of the conservative Thatcher government would have attracted the support of private-sector-oriented organized medicine. To the contrary, the British Medical Association (BMA) vigorously opposed the Thatcher "internal market" reform strategy.

At the BMA's annual membership meeting in 1995, it adopted a policy position calling for "the abolition of the NHS internal market," adding that "vast" savings from reducing administrative personnel "would be better spent on direct services to patients." It also contended the Thatcher reforms were based on a "policy of competition rather than co-operation between primary and secondary care and between service providers."

At the same time, the BMA warned that the Thatcher reforms were "leading to increasing tensions and thereby deteriorating patient care."

In contrast, the relieved BMA accepted the Blair government's white paper on NHS reform in principle, including its reliance on the medical profession to regulate itself in terms of individual physicians' adherence to jointly set, evidence-based clinical practice guidelines. It became evident that the BMA and government had established the necessary conditions for a working partnership.

It may have appeared to that historian that the BMA had realigned its thinking to become the NHS's loyal opposition in the literal—not just the gentlemanly rhetorical—sense. The BMA, however, kept its options open. At its 1999 annual meeting, its policymakers proclaimed "the National Health Service remains fundamentally under-resourced" and added that "changes in administrative structure will never correct this problem."

"We welcome the recognition of the crucial importance of professional self-regulation," the BMA announced. "Clear evidence-based standards must be set, and performance against (them) must be monitored."

Like its decentralized statutory system counterparts in its former colony of Canada, the NHS appears to have become a fixture in the United Kingdom's social and political fabric, too. Unlike in Canada, however, where private insurers cannot cover services funded by the provinces' statutory systems, British dissenters have a choice of opting out and enrolling in private plans. Those who elect to do so, however, are not excused from paying their shares of the tax burden earmarked for supporting the NHS.

The Role of Private Insurers

Explicit decisions to rationalize access to elective surgery and other access issues plaguing the NHS have been a small boon to sustaining private insurers. About thirty of them provide coverage to about 11 percent of the United Kingdom's total population. By far the largest private insurer—the nonprofit British United Provident Association (BUPA), which has expanded elsewhere in Europe—accounts for over 40 percent of its industry's annual premiums.

Some large employers offer employee health benefits and contribute to their costs. Group and individual coverage may exclude care for specific chronic diseases, compelling the privately insured to rely on the NHS for some necessary care.

Some insurers have attempted to contain costs by negotiating caps on the fees of specialists. Some have adapted the PPO concept by contracting only with selected private hospitals.

Some private groups of physicians, particularly in London and other major population centers, have been exploring the concept of bypassing insurers and contracting directly with major employers to provide specified medical services for their workforces and dependents.

As long as the NHS remains an integral part of the United Kingdom's cultural and political fabric, private insurers will remain only niche players in the British health care market. Their best bets for more attractive business development opportunities may well be in looking to the Continent as the European Union addresses the issues of a common market for private health insurance, either as supplements or alternatives to member-countries' statutory systems.

The Pharmaceutical Market

In comparison with other OECD-member countries, the United Kingdom spends a high proportion of its national health care monies on drugs. They account for nearly 16 percent of total expenditures, almost double the figure for the United States and substantially more than for Germany and Sweden.

Unlike Japanese physicians, British physicians do not dispense most prescription drugs; therefore, they have no personal financial interest in overprescribing. The situation appears ripe for the application of pharmaceutical benefits management systems. The "third way" of reform for the NHS involves capping funding to PCGs for drugs and assuming that peer pressures within PCGs will compel over-prescribers to cease to be outliers and fall back into the mainstream of prescribing habits.

The government's pharmaceutical price regulation scheme uses a carrot-and-stick approach targeted at controlling the profit margins of manufacturers selling to the NHS, which is the primary source of drugs for nearly 90 percent of the population. Manufacturers that voluntarily comply with controls on their profit margins are reasonably assured of continuing to do business with the NHS. Those who do not run the risk of sacrificing these sales opportunities.

A search of the Website of the Pharmaceutical Research Manufacturers Association (PhRMA), the trade association of U.S., research-based pharmaceutical companies, failed to reveal any PhRMA complaints about U.K. restrictive trade barriers or failure to honor its commitments to protecting the patent rights to branded drugs. In some countries, PhRMA's complaints prodded the U.S. Trade Representative to initiate formal protests to the World Trade Organization (WTO) about failures to honor WTO commitments in the prescription drug area of international trade.

Opportunities

For health services and health policy researchers and analysts, the nonprofit Cochrane Collaboration, based in Oxford, offers an extremely useful opportunity for applying the Internet as a tool in "preparing, maintaining and promoting the accessibility of systematic reviews of the effects of health care." Founded in memory of the noted British epidemiologist Archie Cochrane, the Cochrane Collaboration has affiliated Cochrane Centres in a number of other European, Asian, North and South American countries, and Australia.

The Cochrane Collaboration's Website (www.cochrane.de) maintains general information on health services and health policy research; guidelines, manuals, and software; contact details for Cochrane Groups outside the United Kingdom; links to other Internet resources; and a site index. It also provides for interactive e-mail communications among its users.

From a business development perspective, the "third way" of reform for the NHS already has produced several new business opportunities for foreign holders of intellectual properties. As examples, the NHS contracted with one U.S. firm to be its prime consultant in establishing its twenty-four-hour hot line for health care advice and another to design and conduct its periodic surveys of consumers' attitudes toward the NHS.

As the NHS turns more to health informatics systems as tools for achieving its new goals and objectives, opportunities are likely to arise for holders of other intellectual properties and systems.

Websites

Website for the National Health Service: www.nhs50.nhs.uk/nhs today

Website for the British Medical Association: www.bma.org.uk

References

Dobson, F. "Modernizing Britain's National Health Service." *Health Affairs*, May-June 1999, pp. 40–41.

Le Grand, J. "Competition, Cooperation or Control? Tales from the British National Health Service." *Health Affairs*, May-June 1999, pp. 27–39.

NON–EUROPEAN UNION

CHAPTER FOURTEEN

ISRAEL

Albert Lowey-Ball

In the mid-1990s, a leading Israeli politician—the mayor of Jerusalem and a prominent member of the conservative Likud Party, Ehud Olmert—casually mentioned that "health care can't be run entirely as a free market system, because you can't allow too much cost-cutting, and because people don't buy health care like other services" (Meyer, 1997, p. 63). This statement probably reflects a near-consensus among leading Israeli politicians, academics, industrialists, entrepreneurs, and soldiers that

- Everyone should have equal access to a basic set of health care benefits and services.
- There should be limits on the extent to which income and prices can be used to allocate health services to the population.
- Quality of and access to health care services should be maintained and improved.
- Health care spending should not be more than about 9 percent of the GNP.

The author would like to thank Yaakov Nevo, a senior health care analyst with the Israel Health Ministry in Jerusalem and a longtime colleague, for his insights and support.

Israel is still a comparatively young state, with slightly fewer than 6 million people, about 81 percent Jewish and 19 percent Israeli Arab (Government of Israel, 1999). Both the Jewish and Arab populations are ethnically and religiously diverse. Israel's existence has usually been imperiled by war, and the country's defense expenditure as a share of the GDP is among the highest in the world.

Conversely, its health care spending as a proportion of GNP (about 8.5 percent) is *less* than that of many other countries (Rosen and Shamai, 1998). Yet Israel has universal health insurance coverage (except for small groups with special legal status), a relatively long average life span (78.2 years), a relatively low infant mortality rate (8.3 deaths per 1,000 births), and a comprehensive system of managed health care competition.

This chapter gives a brief summary of Israel's historical and social context, including a review of the country's managed health care organizations known as *sick funds*. Following is a description of the country's current health care delivery system. Next is a brief look into the near future in light of Israel's adoption of the National Health Insurance (NHI) and Managed Competition Law of 1995. We project that health expenditures in Israel will rise significantly between 2001 and 2005 (with inflation in the health care sector greater than in other sectors) and that opportunities for foreign direct investment in health-related high-tech industry and health services will expand. Finally, we conclude by summarizing some of the lessons learned through Israel's health care system.

Historical and Social Context

The State of Israel was founded in May 1948 amid invasion and turmoil but with a solid basis in the *Yishuv* of the Palestinian Mandate. The early settlers (mostly European), both before and after World War I, developed strong social, political, and economic institutions. In the late 1940s and early 1950s, the country was inundated with waves of Jewish immigrants, mostly from Europe, the Middle East, and North Africa. Since the 1970s large numbers of immigrants have come mostly from Russia.

Israel's population is diverse, with major cultural and ethnic differences between and among Arabs and Jews. Income variations, educational levels, levels of welfare dependence, and incidence of crime vary substantially among different population groups. The diversity is reportedly reflected in widely different cultural styles with respect to health care (Barg, 1998). So far, though, a strong sense of social cohesion and community has accompanied this diversity, at least among the Jewish population (Elon, 1971). Israel's Arabs also participate relatively well in the health care system, in terms of access and coverage, especially since 1995.[1]

In spite of its high immigration rate and the attendant massive social and budgetary costs, along with ongoing security issues with its neighbors and consequent high defense budgets, Israel has accepted a goal of universal health care coverage at a relatively low percentage of the GNP. To a large extent, it has achieved this goal.

Even before 1948, sick funds had been established in Israel based on voluntary associations of workers making small contributions for their health care. The first and long-dominant sick fund, the Kupat Holim (later the Kupat Holim Clalit, KHC or Clalit), started in the early 1920s and was until 1995 closely linked to the powerful Labor Federation—the Histadrut—and the Mapai Party and its successors. KHC and other sick funds covered about 53 percent of the population in 1948 and about 85 to 95 percent of the population from the early 1970s to 1995. KHC has served for a long time as the insurer of most of the country's population; it owns many general acute hospitals and primary care clinics. After the government itself, KHC is the country's largest employer of physicians.

As a major oligopoly on the insurer and payer sides, a significant player on the provider side, and a strong force inside government itself, KHC by the 1970s and 1980s seemed to have lost its sense of accountability to consumers and the government. It faced no strong competition, and the expectation was that the government or the Histadrut would largely cover its budgeting deficits. By the early 1980s, its hospitals and clinics were losing large amounts of money, and KHC had become ever more dependent on continuing "emergency" government payments. Benefits packages became unclear; resources were partly allocated on political grounds; and service queues at hospitals and clinics became ever longer (Meyer, 1997). Many people thought Clalit had become "bureaucratically calcified."

Increasingly, sick funds competed for the younger, healthier portions of the populace. Allegations were that these smaller sick funds "target marketed" and denied membership status to some higher-risk members of the populace (Rosen, 1998). They developed supplemental benefits packages to target the well off. By the late 1980s, dissatisfaction with the semi-socialist KHC and the health system as a whole had dramatically increased. KHC's market share began to decline. Many people thought that quality of care and access was declining. KHC's membership had become noticeably older than the membership of its competitors. The government was deeply concerned over the mounting losses at Clalit and some of the other sick funds (personal communication, Yaakov Nevo, senior official with the Israel Ministry of Health, 1999). Public dissatisfaction and criticism had reached high levels and could no longer be ignored (Rosen, Gross, and Barg, 1996).

National Health Insurance and Managed Competition

During the late 1980s, Israel's parliament, the Knesset, appointed a judicial committee to develop recommendations on the structure and financing of the health care system to increase the degree of consumer accountability, expand coverage, improve quality, and increase competition.

The resulting National Health Insurance (NHI) law passed the Knesset in late 1994. This law contained a number of principles that embody "managed competition." It sought to foster fair competition among the sick funds, turn them into "real" HMOs, and split the provider from the HMO side and the HMOs from the payer. The law sought to make the sick funds more independent of government and more accountable to health care consumers. It mandated a separate financing mechanism, the National Insurance Institute (NII), which would collect health taxes from employees and employers and negotiate rates with the sick funds. The NHI law, effective January 1, 1995, guaranteed universal health insurance coverage and ushered in a more rigorous approach to managed competition. The law mandated that there would be

- No discrimination by sick funds in terms of enrollment, access, and service with respect to potential enrollees
- A defined benefits package applicable to all sick funds and enrollees
- Risk-adjusted payment to the sick funds by the government
- Divestiture of hospitals and clinics from the government to new nonprofit trusts
- A government health premium and tax collection mechanism, through the National Insurance Institute
- A progressive premium structure based on employee income and a payroll tax on employers
- Equal "governmental budgetary" status of the sick funds and freedom of choice to consumers among them

The law did not specifically mandate risk-adjusted payment to clinics and hospitals (Rosen and Shamai, 1998).

A number of the concepts included in the NHI Law are similar to those that govern health policy in some other advanced countries: universal coverage, premium risk adjustment, competition among sick funds, and some freedom of choice among plans. The Israeli approach also outlawed adverse selection and did not allow for such entities as Regional Health (purchasing) Alliances. It did not permit direct employer purchasing of standard health benefits or involvement in selection of health plans—features of health systems in some other countries.

Israel's 1995 law mandates the following benefits: medical diagnosis and treatment, preventive medicine, hospitalization (general acute, maternity, psychiatric, and chronic), surgery and transplants (including some coverage for such services abroad), preventive dental care, first aid and medical transportation, medical services at the workplace, medical services for drug abuse and alcoholism, medical equipment and appliances, obstetric and fertility treatment, treatment of injuries caused by violence, medications, chronic disease treatment, long-term care, physical therapy, speech therapy, and occupational therapy (Rosen and Shamai, 1998). This package, monitored and enforced by the Ministry of Health, is universal.

The Israeli approach does not eliminate private insurance or fee-for-service medicine. Prior to 1995, Israelis had the right to purchase private health insurance from local or foreign firms. They continue to have this right and typically exercise it by purchasing supplemental health insurance (Government of Israel, 1999).

Current Health Care Delivery System

The effort to strengthen managed competition occurred within a framework of a health system thoroughly dominated by the government, including the Ministry of Health, the Ministry of Finance, and the NII, and by KHC. Largely, the national government, municipalities, the KHC, other sick funds, and religious organizations own hospitals. The central government is a strong regulator of health services, the principal owner of hospitals and primary clinics, and a key investor in health services. And NHI has made the government virtually the exclusive payer. Most physicians work on salary in primary care and other clinics owned by the Health Ministry, municipalities, or Clalit.

Sick Fund Coverage

All of Israel's population is covered by at least one of the country's four sick funds. In 1997, according to the JDC-Brookdale Institute, sick fund enrollment was distributed as follows: Clalit (3.77 million, or 64 percent of the population), Maccabi (1.12 million, or 19 percent), Meuhedet (530,000, or 9 percent), and Leumit (530,000, or 9 percent). Competition exists among the sick funds for enrollees, among hospitals for admissions, and between hospitals and sick funds for primary care clinic services and for hospital beds and quality physicians (Rosen, 1996).

Sick funds are HMOs in the sense that they provide defined benefits packages to enrolled populations for fixed prospective payments. Some sick funds own some hospitals and clinics, and all are involved with provider networks.

The NII establishes age-adjusted premium rates for each sick fund and pays in periodic monthly amounts. The funds allocate the monies among their member hospitals and clinics, based on enrollee linkages to physicians in clinics (mostly primary care) and hospitals (mostly specialists). Clinics typically are paid on an age-adjusted capitation basis as well, whereas hospitals are paid on a per diem basis. Both provider types may, if they run deficits, seek periodic settlement payments either from the sick funds, who in turn seek payments from the NII, or, if government-owned, from the Ministry of Health.

The main sick fund—KHC—owns fifteen general and specialty hospitals, or about 32 percent of all hospitals in the country. It has over 6,000 physicians on salary, or about 22 percent of all physicians in the country, and owns 1,250 primary care clinics—62.5 percent of all such clinics (Kupat Holim Clalit, personal communication, 1997). It may be viewed as a dominant purchasing oligopoly. KHC is heavily involved in medical research and specialty services such as care for the elderly and occupational health care. KHC's fiduciary connection to the Histadrut has largely been severed since 1995.

Financing

Following the adoption of NHI in 1995 and continuing until 1998, all employers and employees in Israel paid a health tax based on payroll and income earned. The tax averaged about 5 percent of payroll paid by employers; employees paid up to 4.8 percent of their income, the amount depending on their income level. Individuals who were unemployed, low-income, self-employed, or retired paid a set fee of about $22 per month (Rosen and Shamai, 1998). No one was denied coverage if they could not pay. Health tax payments were made to the NII, a semi-independent public entity operating under the joint authority of the Ministry of Labor and Social Affairs. It negotiated age-adjusted capitated rates with four sick funds. (Eventually, other factors such as service mix and outcomes may be considered in the risk-adjustment mechanism.) Capitation payments were supplemented to varying degrees by government subsidies through periodic adjustments. In 1998 the employer tax was abolished and replaced with direct government payment to the sick funds for the standard benefits package. The Ministry of Finance is interested in reducing the subsidies by authorizing the sick funds to charge higher out-of-pocket payments to consumers and for supplemental insurance coverage premiums (Rosen, Ivenkovsky, and Nevo, 1997). The Finance Ministry is trying to make the sick funds more competitive, more private, and less dependent on government subsidies. It is also seeking to turn the sick funds into tougher negotiators with their contracted providers. Some hospitals currently negotiate forms of global capitation with the sick funds on behalf of themselves and their affiliated clinics (interview with an Israeli, 1999).

The Ministry of Health

This ministry has overall responsibility for health services in Israel. Its responsibilities include

- Establishing and maintaining health access and quality standards and enforcing them
- Licensing medical personnel
- Owning and operating about 50 percent of the nation's hospital beds, about 75 percent of the primary care clinics, and 40 percent of the mother and child centers
- Promoting medical research
- Maintaining and enforcing drug, environmental, and public health standards
- Preparing and carrying out health care legislation (Government of Israel, 1999).

The ministry employs about 14,000 physicians (52 percent of all physicians in the country), mostly through its clinics and hospitals. The relationships between the Health Ministry and the sick funds are tortuous, but somewhat less so since 1995, when the NII took over the payer role. The Health Ministry is currently involved in a major effort to spin off its hospitals to nonprofit trust companies; so far those attempts have failed. The government wants hospitals to compete more effectively for scarce HMO admissions and revenue and believes that this will be more achievable if its hospitals are in the private sector and operate on better business principles.

Physicians

About 27,000 physicians are active in the country—a serious oversupply. This high number is partly a consequence of historical, cultural, and educational factors and partly a consequence of substantial immigration of Russian physicians over the past thirty years. Close to 55 percent of Israeli physicians are foreign-born; most from Russia were also trained there (Shvarts, de Leeuw, Granit, and Benbassat, 1999).

About 80 percent of Israel's doctors are salaried, and 20 percent are exclusively private, fee-for-service providers (Government of Israel, 1999). The substantial oversupply of physicians results in relatively low physician incomes, with strong downward pressures continuing on these incomes. Some physicians are reportedly underemployed or unemployed.

Many physicians are employed by over 2,000 primary care clinics and 850 mother-and-child care clinics owned by the central government, municipalities, or the sick funds, especially Clalit (Shvarts, de Leeuw, Granit, and Benbassat, 1999). Hospital positions are prized by physicians and difficult to obtain. Hospital and clinic physicians do not have much to do with one another. Clinic physicians rarely have hospital privileges and do not follow their patients into hospitals (Meyer, 1997). Physicians with largely private, developed fee-for-service practices reportedly increased rapidly in numbers in the 1980s and early 1990s. They tend to focus on the relatively healthy, young, and well-off and on those who are otherwise dissatisfied by the services of the sick funds.

Hospitals

There are forty-eight hospitals in Israel, with about 13,000 general acute care beds. The country also has about 14,000 chronic and long-term care and 7,000 psychiatric beds. Israel's rate for acute care and psychiatric beds (3.39 per 1,000) is slightly higher than that of the United States (3.19 per 1,000) (Government of Israel, 1999). Of the hospital beds, 45 percent are owned by the Health Ministry, 30 percent by KHC, 6 percent by the Hadassah Medical Organization; the remaining 19 percent are owned by other nonprofit, for-profit, or religious entities. Israel's hospital use rate is not markedly different from that of other advanced nations. Beds are full, with occupancy rates averaging about 95 percent in recent years (Shvarts, de Leeuw, Granit, and Benbassat, 1999). Israel's hospitals have a fine international reputation, especially for computerized services and high-tech health services related to military casualties (Government of Israel, 1999). Hospitals remain under the domination of their senior medical staff physicians. Mostly prestigious specialists, these senior staff influence physician, nursing staff, capital equipment, and expenditure allocation within hospitals. As elsewhere, senior hospital physicians tend to regard hospitals as their own rent-free workshops (personal communication with anonymous source, 1995).

The Model and the Near Future

Israel's commitment to equitable and universal access to health care benefits on a cost-effective basis is firm. Since 1995, insurance coverage levels have increased from 95 percent to almost 100 percent of the population for a basic set of health care benefits. In fact, Israeli residents living abroad occasionally return to Israel for health care coverage and services when they get older.

Also since 1995, Israel's health care marketplace has more fully exemplified a number of features of managed competition than before. Coverage of the population is universal, based on prescriptive right. The single governmental payer, the NII, is technically independent of the regulator and public health entity, the Health Ministry, and serves as the health care premium collector. Coverage has been delinked from employment status. The four competing health plans act to optimize economic net revenue, with premiums determined by enrollee age and eventually condition or outcome.

Israel's managed competition and national health insurance experiment, if it works over time, could serve as an interesting guidepost for other countries. The low cost of health care as a percentage of the GNP may be an underestimate, however, partly because some health care expenditures are "off the books"—that is, fee-for-service expenditures in the gray or black markets are not always reported for legal and tax reasons. The magnitude of this underestimate is unknown. The low percentage is also due in large part to the government's exercise of its monopoly purchasing power. We forecast that the added sense of entitlement will result in health care inflation greater than in other sectors over the next five years, thereby adding to the fiscal pressures on the national budget and taxpayers.

Possible Changes

Since NHI took effect in 1995, government hospitals are to be devolved to independent, nonprofit trusts, enabling them to act in a more businesslike fashion—more oriented toward the bottom line. Geriatric, chronic disease and long-term care, and psychiatric services will eventually become the responsibility of the sick funds and no longer the direct responsibility of the government. These reforms are strongly opposed by nurse and physician unions, the medical community in general, and elements within the Ministry of Health. Hence, they have not yet been implemented (Government of Israel, 1999).

Israel's health system expenditures will probably increase to over 9 percent and possibly reach 10 percent of GNP between 2001 and 2005. Out-of-pocket enrollee payment requirements will increase significantly, as will pressures on sick funds to "target market" certain population groups through further supplementary insurance product variation. Health taxes will increase more than will other taxes. The Finance Ministry may take a larger role than the NII in rate negotiations with sick funds. Emigration of Israeli physicians may increase. Some hospitals may close.

Opportunities

Given Israel's history, its social and institutional relationships, and its commitment to universal coverage, can firms outside the country contribute to the health care system and find opportunities to build valuable business relationships? Possibly. Opportunities in the health care arena probably lie in the following areas:

- Capital, technology transfer, and administrative infrastructure for further development of advanced computerized diagnostic, medical, and surgical techniques and equipment.
- Sale of state-of-the-art pharmaceuticals, by pharmaceutical firms, especially to the Health Ministry, sick funds, and hospitals. KHC is one of the world's largest purchasers of pharmaceuticals, mostly from European firms.
- Technical assistance with further development of advanced risk-adjustment paradigms, especially as they approach outcome measures and are applied to hospital and clinic payment. The Ministry of Health and the sick funds are interested in more sophisticated measures.
- Joint ventures with Israeli hospitals and hospital systems for selected foreign hospital-health systems. Officials believe that Israel's hospitals need considerably more professional management. The services could include network development and management, rate negotiations, and technology transfer. The Israeli government is interested in exploring full or partial sales of its hospitals.
- Joint ventures of successful foreign health plans and insurers with Israeli sick funds, whereby the outside organizations could potentially serve as sources of capital and management expertise, particularly in network management and provider negotiations.
- Sale of selected fee-for-service products, including supplemental health insurance products targeted to well-to-do and well-traveled Israelis.

Lessons Learned

The Israeli health system provides the following lessons:

- *Universal coverage and access can be achieved without breaking the bank.*
- *Managed competition, though imperfect in some ways, can work.*
- *Managed competition can maintain equity simultaneously with competition.* Israel's implementation of the 1995 NHI statute mandating managed competition serves as a test case of whether 100 percent population coverage and elimination of adverse selection is consistent with competition among more or less private organi-

zations. The NHI law sought to privatize the nonprofit sick funds and nationalize payment.

- *Adequate risk-adjustment methods can be devised and implemented, and age-adjusted HMO premiums significantly reduce adverse selection.* The NII is fiscally constrained by the tax and premium moneys it collects and the willingness of the government to provide subsidies. Preliminary evidence suggests that age-adjusted rates have indeed reduced adverse selection and improved the financial status of health plans with older enrollee profiles and worsened that of plans with younger profiles.

Note

1. Confidential interview, Ministry of Health, Israel, Aug. 1999. 12 percent of Israeli Arabs were uncovered in the early 1990s; by 1998, this figure had dropped to about 3 percent.

References

Barg, J. "Comparing U.S. and Israeli Health Care Systems." *Physician's News Digest,* June 1998.

Elon, A. *The Israelis: Founders and Sons,* New York: Bantam Books, 1971.

Government of Israel. "The Health Care System in Israel: A Historical Perspective" In *Israel at Fifty, 1948–1998.* Jerusalem: Ministry of Foreign Affairs, 1999.

Meyer, H. "Out of Israel: Israel's Nationalized Health Care System." *Hospitals and Health Networks,* 1997, *71*(7), 63.

Rosen, B. *Price Competition and the 1998 Budget Arrangement Law.* Jerusalem: JDC-Brookdale Institute, 1998.

Rosen, B., Ivenkovsky, M., and Nevo, Y. *Changes in the Sick Fund Economy: Sick Fund Revenues and Expenses Before and After the Introduction of National Health Insurance.* Jerusalem: JDC-Brookdale Institute, 1997.

Rosen, B., Revital, G., and Barg, A. *National Health Insurance: The First Year.* Jerusalem: JDC-Brookdale Institute, 1996.

Rosen, B., and Shamai, N. *Financing and Resource Allocation in Israeli Health Care.* Jerusalem: JDC-Brookdale Institute, 1998.

Shvarts, S., de Leeuw, D.L.A., Granit, S., and Benbassat, J. "Public Health Then and Now: From Socialist Principles to Motorcycle Maintenance: The Origin and Development of the Salaried Physician Model in the Israeli Public Health Services, 1918 to 1998." *American Journal of Public Health,* 1999, *89*(2), 248.

CHAPTER FIFTEEN

POLAND

Renata Bushko

Poland has a unique opportunity to improve the quality and accessibility of health care by introducing technology-driven health care reform in addition to its 1999 market-driven reform. This study focuses on the current Polish health care system and its potential for accelerated sociotechnological transformation. If technology-driven health care reform is implemented, significant improvement will occur by 2005 without unnecessary administrative overhead.

In this analysis, we measure improvement using the universal quality framework (Bushko, 1995), which consists of four components: (1) organizational quality, as measured by compliance; (2) process quality, as measured by cost; (3) clinical quality, as measured by outcomes; and (4) service quality, as measured by patient satisfaction.

Political Structure and Economic Outlook

Under the 1997 constitution, Poland is a democratic parliamentary republic, with a directly elected president holding some veto powers. In 1989, Poland went through a major political change when it shifted from communism to democracy.

The quotations in this chapter were obtained in personal communications unless otherwise indicated.

According to Jeffrey Sachs (1993), author of *Poland's Jump to the Market Economy*, "the reforms in Poland, introduced on January 1, 1990, have been especially far reaching, and have been widely recognized as a model for the reforms in other parts of Eastern Europe and the former Soviet Union" (p.1). Since then, Poland's economy has been improving steadily. Its population of 38.7 million (62 percent in cities, 38 percent in rural areas) is served by 120,000 physicians (55 percent women) and 214,000 nurses (more than 80 percent women) in more than 3,000 health care facilities (Ministry of Health, 1998).

Transformation: The 1999 Health Care Reform

In 1999, Polish health care underwent major reform; national budgets were separated from state (*voivodship*) budgets. Until 1999, all institutions had been financed on a historical budget basis (funding based on prior spending), at US$8 billion annually, or US$219 per person (European Observatory, 1999). Beginning in 1999, all providers are supposed to be self-financed, and hospitals belong to local governments.

Employees now pay 7.5 percent of their income to state health insurance, called Sickness Funds; in all, seventeen Sickness Funds exist, including sixteen located in *voivodships* and one that serves the army and the state administration. Sickness Funds buy services from providers, except for highly specialized procedures, which are purchased by the Ministry of Health. Primary care services are purchased on a capitation basis, specialist care on a fee-for-service basis. Hospitals are paid based on the number of admissions. Employers cover occupational medicine; drugs are partially paid for by patients. The primary care physician coordinates care, but a patient can go directly to an oncologist, dermatologist, dentist, or gynecologist. Patients have full choice among hospitals within a given Sickness Fund.

The distribution of modern technologies in health care is not uniform across the country; major use is in central cities. Despite an increase in the use of non-invasive visualization technologies (MRI and CT scans), these procedures are much less common than in the United States.

Organizational Quality, as Measured by Compliance

Making providers responsible for their own financial management, with a possibility of going bankrupt, affects organizational quality by creating pressure to comply with cost and quality expectations of the market. Because of the current lack of competition, health care providers and payers are now monopolists on their respective territories, dictating prices and rules. The 1999 reform aims to spin off health care organizations into autonomous units, each competing for patients based on service—with the best competitors winning a larger share of the insurance funds and patients. The wave of innovation and change has just begun, and providers will need to improve organizational quality in order to survive.

Process Quality, as Measured by Cost

Medical work is based on dynamic, cross-functional, interdepartmental, interorganizational collaboration that requires constant communication and effective sharing of professional knowledge. It takes place in health care institutions that are constantly restructuring themselves in order to survive in a turbulent, competitive environment. With self-financed providers and *voivodships* as designated coordinators, multiorganizational TQM techniques will be useful in the management and evaluation of health care delivery networks. Building consensus among loosely affiliated institutions delivering health care for one community is complex, challenging, time consuming, and expensive, but it is critical to success. The implementation and use of an information infrastructure can accelerate development of communitywide leadership and coordination processes toward a common mission, vision, and values. With utilization management, case management, or disease management, average length of hospital stay, for example, might be reduced from twelve to five or six days. Investment in the national, state, and organizational process redesign and Internet/EDI-enabled health information infrastructure will improve health care processes, reduce costs, and make possible implementation of performance measures, such as an automatic accreditation system, as opposed to an administrative, inspection-based system.

Technology-driven reform will ensure that medical reporting becomes instantaneous. Reports can be generated on a system monitor as the doctor dictates. They can be instantly transmitted with electronic data interchange (EDIFACT and HL7 standard) to the information system, thus becoming available to accreditation centers, statistical bureaus, other specialists, and the patient (for example, via Web-based personal medical records) (Sutherland, 1999). This assures continuity of care and puts less administrative burden on the patient. It also enables physicians to generate real-time, patient-specific instructions, which increase patient compliance with treatment plans. Enforcing compliance is a big issue for achieving good clinical outcomes, which is the basis for overall process efficiency and patient satisfaction.

Clinical Quality, as Measured by Outcomes

Steady progress is being made in clinical outcomes due to public health programs, as measured by morbidity, infant morbidity, and life expectancy since 1990. Poland does not have clinical guidelines in place, so the choice of drugs or clinical treatment is based on the individual experience of a given physician. Evidence-based medicine has not been introduced. Although tools exist to transfer medical knowledge (Internet use is steadily growing), there are no requirements or incentives to use them. Technology-driven reform could help without introducing major guidelines or regulation through a sociotechnological-learning loop (Bushko, 1998), not a bureaucratic process:

- Clinical guidelines, best practice knowledge, and reporting requirements are embedded in templates and in the knowledge-base-driven prompting system used by physicians in medical reporting.
- Physicians internalize guidelines and new medical knowledge while doing medical reporting with the knowledge-based system on a daily basis. The intuitive, voice-enabled interface makes using this system easy. Repetition encodes knowledge in memory.
- Physicians are more prone to follow guidelines and collect pieces of clinical information needed for future outcomes studies, so there are better clinical data for analysis.
- This leads to the improved pool of information available for the creation of physician guidelines, eliminating a potential false learning phenomenon that occurs when research is based on poor-quality or incomplete data sets.
- New guidelines get embedded in knowledge-based systems, and the sociotechnological medical learning loop closes and repeats itself continuously, improving diagnostic quality.

Service Quality, as Measured by Patient Satisfaction

With a growing economy, highly educated, well-paid, knowledge workers seek good-quality health care and demand better service and improved access. According to Dr. Adam Kruszewski, medical director of Warsaw-based MediCover, "They like to participate in decisions about their own health, and they are willing to pay extra for that. They start to realize that it would be useful to compare doctors and make treatment choices based on the objective criteria."

Technology-driven reform would encourage self-care and disease prevention through medical education and behavioral modifications. For example, cellular phones that can be used to search the Internet for health-related topics and to send preprogrammed e-mail reminders (for example, reminders to exercise or take medication, no-smoking messages, or healthy behavior hints) will have a significant impact on life and health satisfaction levels in the near future.

Future Health Services and Technologies Market

Given current reforms and growing demands from consumers, Poland is a major market for knowledge-intensive health care services in the form of consulting or software that embeds medical knowledge and guidelines for cost-effective care. Because the health care informatics business requires customized user interfaces, major players in health care information systems have not yet delivered integrated solutions ready to serve Poland's rapidly changing health care needs.

The hardware and medical devices market is also substantial. Historically, major suppliers of electronics to Poland have been Germany, Japan, the Netherlands, France, and the United States. Poland's historically low health care spending by the government as compared with other countries (that is, 4.2 percent of GNP in 1997 compared to an average of 11.2 percent in other countries) will be outbalanced by new privatization efforts giving purchasing decision power to health care organizations.

Policy Changes

Future policy changes will continue to be directed at the health care market-driven reform, with emphasis on self-financing of health care organizations and autonomy of states. Because the reform process is highly political and involves social discourse among many professional interest groups, the public, and the government, we concentrate here on the predictions of technology-driven developments.

Technological Acceleration

Poland requires health care products that can demonstrate the improved quality of care while reducing costs.

Electronic Data Interchange (EDI)

Hardware allowing implementation of electronic data interchange, or EDII, is essential for the 727 major Polish general hospitals (232,856 beds) and for all 3,000-plus health care facilities (US$50 million market potential in EDI software) ("Kto ma w domo komputer," 1999). This technology will dramatically improve processes in both clinical and administrative areas and thereby produce savings that can be used to finance new equipment in the clinical area and to finance point-of-care devices including telemedicine. This will ensure the ability to pay health care professionals higher salaries and thus will accelerate technology acceptance.

Speech Recognition as a Key Technology

The second important aspect is to invest in the speech-recognition model for Poland's physicians of various specialties and to implement a nationwide strategy of clinical data that are captured via mobile, voice-enabled devices. This will help reduce the health care cost of administrative information processing and prepare the ground for population-based health care management and evidence-based medicine. According to Dr. Michael Fitzmaurice of the Agency for Health Care Policy and Research, U.S. Department of Health and Human Services, "Speech to data conversion and wireless technologies are keys to improving health care quality by enabling health professionals to capture vital clinical data in a non-intrusive and intuitive way at the point of care." Some vendors (for example, Lernout and Hauspie Speech Products, or L&H) have already developed adaptive learning technologies that use speech to create documents or control applications but also recognize, locate, and access critical patient data stored within documents. As described by Jo Lernout, leader of the speech and language industry and founder of L&H, at the 1999 Future of Health Technology Summit, "A new breed of clinical documentation solutions is emerging that combines voice and knowledge-based systems to provide immediate benefits to both the clinician and the healthcare organization."

Personalization and the Internet

With new developments in bioinformatics, genetic profiling, and individualized drug design, it is critical to develop technology-mediated patient-physician communication via the Internet that would maintain a high-level personalization of service. With aggressive planning for the National Information Infrastructure and investment in "Community Internet Access Stations" for everybody, the Polish population can start participating in its own health care. There is no reason to wait for consumer empowerment; such participation should be encouraged via technology-driven health care reform to make it truly successful. It should be a cornerstone of the reform, not a by-product.

Currently, about 4 million people in Poland have access to the Internet through home and workplace computers. Of these, 15 percent access the Internet every day, 17 percent a couple of times a week, 32 percent a couple of times a month (European Observatory, 1999). The "no service fee" Internet access model that originated in the United Kingdom has not yet reached Poland, but with tighter links to the European Union, it is inevitable. According to a survey conducted by Find/SVP (1999), two-thirds of the people on-line sought health information at least once; one-third regularly use the Internet for health care problems; and the AOL (America Online) health care site has more than 2 million users. In the United States, the Internet reached 50 million people over the last five years. Worldwide traffic on the Internet is doubling approximately every 100 days. Seniors over fifty-five represent a growing segment of Internet users, thus increasing the possibility of dissemination of health knowledge through that medium.

If the infrastructure is in place, the Polish market for health care, knowledge-based, on-line services will grow from 20 million (2 million users paying $10 a year) in 1999 to approximately 500 million in 2005. With rapid progress in machine translations, all health-related information currently being developed in English can be quickly translated and easily adapted to the Polish market. Considering that it is possible now to browse the Internet via cellular phone, this is a good opportunity for content-driven Internet service providers.

Conclusion

Poland can move toward mobile, user-friendly health technology and patient empowerment without experiencing administrative slow-down if the vendor community invests in products that are well suited for the Polish medical market. The size of the country justifies that investment. If technology-driven health care reform is implemented, dramatic improvement will occur by 2005, as measured by (1) compliance with best practice standards, (2) cost, (3) clinical outcomes, and (4) patient satisfaction. Technology will enable the introduction of real-time performance measures based on quality data, automatically collected, without any administrative burden; those data will be immediately transferred into useful guidelines and behavioral changes, without costly inspection methods. It is a historic opportunity to ensure that Poland's 1999 health care reform, like its 1990 market reform, will be recognized as a model for reforms in other parts of the world, with health care organization not only self-financed but self-accredited.

References

Bushko, R. "Leadership Challenges in the Twenty-First Century: Seven Strategies to Leadership." Workshop conducted at the IMIA'95 conference, Healthcare Executives' Challenges in the Twenty-First Century: Leadership, Quality, Technology, and Innovation-Driven Process Management, Vancouver, Canada, 1995.

Bushko, R. "From Transcription to Total Transformation: National Impact of Voice-Enabled Clinical Dictation and Reporting." [www.fhti.org]. Hopkinson, Mass.: Future of Health Technology Institute, 1998.

European Observatory on Health Care Systems. *Health Care Systems in Transition: Poland.* Geneva: World Health Organization, 1999.

Find/SVP Research Publications, Inc. Survey cited at [www.intel.com]. 1999.

"Kto ma w domo komputer" [The computer]. *Rzeczpospolita,* Sept. 29, 1999, p. A2.

Lernout, J. "Future of Voice, Speech, and Language Technologies." *Future of Health Technology Summit, 1999* (CD-ROM). Hopkinson, Mass.: Future of Health Technology Institute, 1999.

Ministry of Health. *Biuletyn Statystyczny: Ministerstwo Zdrowia I Opieki Spolecznej, Centrum Organizacji I Ekonomiki Ochrony Zdrowia.* Warsaw: Ministry of Health, 1998.

Sachs, J. *Poland's Jump to the Market Economy.* Cambridge, Mass.: MIT Press, 1993.

Sutherland, J. "Future of Medical Computing." *Future of Health Technology Summit, 1999* (CD-ROM). Hopkinson, Mass.: Future of Health Technology Institute, 1999.

CHAPTER SIXTEEN

RUSSIA

Youri Lavinski, Steven Vasilev

The health care system in Russia has been developing over the last three centuries very much in line with the rest of the world. The great social changes that affected Russia at the turn of the twentieth century made the concept of social justice a cornerstone of official policies. The Semashko system, named after one of the first commissars (ministers) of health, was adopted in the Soviet Union.

The characteristics of this system were, and largely remain, as follows:

- *Eligibility:* The entire population is eligible for services.
- *Benefits:* The state provides all necessary health services at no charge.
- *Financing:* The public system is financed from the general state budget (for example, national general revenues), enterprise budgets, and extra budgetary funds. Private payments in the past were limited to a few nonessential services and some unofficial payments to public providers for preferential treatment.
- *Payment of medical care providers:* Virtually all facilities were owned by the state, and all health care personnel were state employees. Polyclinics and hospitals were reimbursed, based on eighteen-category line-item budgets. Physicians and other health personnel were salaried employees. Provision and financing were combined (that is, the public financing authority owned, budgeted, and managed facilities).
- *Service delivery system:* The system was conceptually a well-integrated hierarchical structure of primary care stations; health posts; polyclinics; and local, re-

gional, and national-level hospitals. The human and physical capital infrastructure of the system was based on planning norms used to allocate facilities and personnel across geographical areas. Quality of care was enforced through a hierarchical review process based on reprimanding inappropriate behavior. Public health programs were targeted to maternal and child health and communicable diseases (Klugman, Schieber, Heleniak, and Hon, 1998).

The system achieved dramatic improvements in public health. The ability to participate in private practice was limited to physicians of certain specialties that were considered less important to public health, like plastic surgery.

The missing market influence and chronic underfunding slowed progress and eventually caused the crash of public health care institutions. By the end of the socialistic period, state funding was dramatically depleted; physicians and entire organizations were forced to struggle for their very survival. Both state and newly born private systems started looking for a panacea, often instead of scrupulous learning and planning, which led to further disappointments.

Transition to Capitalism

Health care entrepreneurship became not only possible but was a widespread phenomenon in Russia from the late 1980s to the early 1990s. There were several positive and negative factors influencing this process. The positive factors were as follows:

- A popular demand for better services
- A population accustomed to direct payments to physicians and other medical personnel (under the table)
- A dramatic growth in the numbers of people ready to pay, no matter what (middle- and upper-class people)
- An openness and readiness of the society to accepting a Western example
- An ability to use state-funded clinics and hospitals, often well equipped and well staffed, to provide private or "paid" services
- The weakness of the state, including its inability to regulate and tax new businesses—essentially a tax-free environment for entrepreneurs

Unfortunately, negative factors played a significant role and in many cases prevailed over positive ones. Also many positive factors became negative in the long term:

- An absence of appropriate laws often kept private health care practice at odds with government, tax authorities, and even the criminal code.
- An ability to use state facilities and equipment practically free of charge discouraged investment in long-term maintenance and purchase programs and made the construction of new, independent private clinics and hospitals unreasonable.
- An inability of the state to pay decent salaries encouraged physicians and other personnel to embrace under-the-table schemes and created a gray market, which is very harmful to true entrepreneurs.
- The official policy—free health care for all—and lack of political will to support privatization of health care discouraged both providers and payers from developing new systems and mechanisms.

Finally, the mind-set of the population, including that of officials and physicians, is still changing very slowly and represents a major problem for years to come.

Financing and Delivery

Russia has been conducting pro-market experiments in health care since the late 1980s. These experiments were staged on a municipal or regional level and supported by the Ministry of Health. Three major regions were involved: the City of St. Petersburg, the Samara Region, and the Kemerovo Region. The experiment involved introducing financial self-governance at the facility level within the budget assigned by a local health authority. The physicians became gatekeepers, and monies left after paying for patient treatment in hospitals and other services were distributed to physicians and used to improve facilities. The experiments were highly successful and promoted by federal authorities, but this coincided with a severe economic crisis in the early 1990s, which has aborted most further attempts (Curtis, Petukhova, Sezonova, and Netsenko, 1997).

The Mandatory Insurance Law was adopted in 1992, which outlined mechanisms for providing universal coverage guaranteed by Article 41 of the Russian Constitution. The employers contribute 3.6 percent of their payroll to the federal and regional state insurance funds. The regional funds keep 3.4 percent and distribute monies to independent insurance companies on a per capita basis. The federal fund gets 0.2 percent, which is used to equalize the distribution of benefits throughout the country, fund public health bodies and research, and deal with national epidemics (Field, 1999).

The insurers pay providers for each hospitalization, mostly on a diagnostic-related group basis, and reimburse outpatient facilities on a per capita basis. Global budgeting and fee-for-service mechanisms are also in use. The local administrations pay for the unemployed, children, retirees, and other segments of the nonworking population, usually through state-owned insurers. There is no personal contribution to premiums or copayment (Semenov, 1998).

Although laws permit direct contracting between employers and insurers, the territorial distribution of monies is more common (for example, employers pay into a local mandatory insurance fund, which in turn pays insurers). This model is supported by local governments, to which these funds report; a few large employers have secured legal means of allowing direct contracting with insurers.

Patients have freedom of choice for both physicians and facilities, although free choice is often difficult to implement in practice. Private providers are compensated on the same basis as state hospitals and clinics. Finally, the government finances treatment for such conditions as tuberculosis and AIDS, as well as for services such as psychiatry.

The Voluntary Insurance Law was introduced in 1994, but employer and personal contributions are not tax deductible, which makes its effect limited mostly to introduction of high-end health insurance products that are unaffordable for the majority of the population.

The gray market controls a significant amount of the funds that the population spends on health care. Because this activity is external to official channels, it depletes state coffers even more and discourages investment.

Providers

Providers generally fit in one of three groups: (1) state-controlled agencies, (2) enterprise- or union-controlled agencies, and (3) private institutions.

Many state-controlled facilities are permitted to form quasi-private ventures and may be the best bet for a Western partner. This is because they are relatively stable, despite a lack of state funding. The bureaucracy may be foreboding, but if a decision is made, they are reliable partners.

Enterprise or union-controlled ventures are widespread and represent a heavy mix of state and private components. They are also an attractive and often overlooked choice for entrepreneurs and investors. They may have a wide range in numbers of employees or members, as well as solid support from a parent organization, if such an organization has been successful in the new economy. Distributors of medical equipment, who sold enormous amounts of new equipment and even built new hospitals, successfully exploited this.

Private ventures are mostly small. Some have a few expatriate physicians and minuscule facilities; some use state clinics' personnel and equipment. Those founded or managed by Western entrepreneurs have gained the most acceptance among the expatriate community and foreign travelers. Still, they largely failed to attract a significant number of Russians, mostly due to higher-than-average prices and cultural barriers between expatriate physicians and locals. Most private enterprises are highly specialized and work in such areas as plastic surgery, dentistry, and alternative therapy.

Another group of private ventures are those owned by religious organizations. They emphasize quality and service and have been able to attract many private clients. Although emergency services are provided mostly by the government, there are several examples of successful private initiatives.

Payers

Payers include government, insurers, employers, and individuals. The significance of each payer category differs in different regions of Russia: the government is usually the only payer in rural, remote, poor regions, whereas such cities as Moscow, St. Petersburg, and Nizhni Novgorod boast significant number of individuals willing to pay premium prices for good care.

Government and Legislature

Government forces at the national level are very powerful in Russia despite a lack of financial resources. Unfortunately, they are unwilling, or at least are very slow, to make changes (Chernichovsky, 1999). In contrast, local governments in Russia have been the primary movers and shakers. They have significant freedom from the federal authorities and have been experimenting since the late 1980s.

Reform Outcomes

There are positive and negative outcomes from the recent changes in political structure. On the positive side, one can say that health economics came to life even in the most backward regions. The government, the regional authorities, and the managers of health care facilities were forced to start counting money. This in turn put pressure on physicians, and they started looking for new efficiencies.

The dramatic decrease in length of hospital stays, introduction of new utilization management techniques, and increased attention to patient rights contributed to a changing atmosphere in health care.

Many positive developments have been related to increased information exchange. Physicians and health care administrators now have the ability to travel and learn from the best examples. Such organizations as the U.S. Agency for International Development (USAID), World Bank, and the European Bank for Reconstruction and Development have been distributing grants and providing other types of assistance (Rice, 1995; U.S.-Russia Commission, 1999).

Entrepreneurs also contributed significantly to dramatic changes within the system. It became possible to establish private practice, form a venture, build a hospital, or start an insurance company. This created new jobs and helped retain talent that otherwise would have been looking for a better life in the West or forced into the gray market.

The existence of a private health insurance market is extremely important for further advances in health care market development. Although this is limited to high-end insurance and travel products, it breaks the government monopoly and establishes new incentives for all players.

On the negative side, the continuous underfunding and in most cases a severe decrease in the absolute amount of funds available has undermined both patient care and health care organizations' ability to survive.

Successful organizations were able to embrace changes and tangibly improve their technical base, personnel training, and level of patient care. Others became little more than degrading buildings and demoralized medical staff. Many physicians and nurses quit health care altogether; they started businesses or began working in unrelated fields.

Still, the professionalism of the medical staff, which was largely preserved within hospitals, medical schools, and other institutions, along with rediscovered entrepreneurship, have created a new class of physicians-entrepreneurs and reform-minded administrators.

Critical Success Factors

Three major factors are required for success in Russia. First, the existence of a local partner is necessary for doing business in Russia, even if this is not required by law. The local partner helps jump-start everything from the registration of a venture and opening a bank account to making sure that relationships with authorities proceed smoothly.

The second requirement is local (regional or city) government support. This helps with everything, sometimes even with finding a local partner. Licensing is also a critical issue, which is usually easy to resolve with support from the government.

Third, a respected and efficient manager must be identified. A local partner may not be qualified to run a health care venture. The alternatives are scarce. There is a great lack of competent local managers because physicians with little formal management training occupy most of the administrative and managerial positions. Therefore, an expatriate manager may be the only initial alternative, until a local replacement can be trained (Economist Intelligence Unit, 1999a, 1999b).

Summary of Opportunities

Any entrepreneur or insurance company must be very patient and prepared for protracted bureaucratic and political battles if they want to implement anything statewide. The best option is to conduct an experiment on a regional or local level, with the assistance of federal and local authorities, and then try to make a case in respective parliaments and governments.

Regional opportunities. There is a much greater opportunity for entrepreneurial initiatives on a regional level in Russia, where regions have powers similar to the powers of the American states. Most of the health care budget is held regionally; decision making is also done on this level.

Opportunities with financial groups. This is a valuable option to explore at the level of big industrial and financial groups. They have a great deal of independence from the state and great influence on authorities, as many cities and even regions may depend on their tax contributions.

Opportunities at the private level. There are few barriers to private enterprise. The initial taboos on some types of activities, such as hospital business, maternity, imaging, and cancer care, were removed; aggressive entrepreneurs may be very successful in this area.

References

Chernichovsky, D. "Genuine Federalism in the Russian Health Care System: Changing Roles of Government." *Journal of Health Politics, Policy and Law,* 1999, *24*(1).

Curtis, S., Petukhova, N., Sezonova, G., and Netsenko, N. "Caught in the Traps of Managed Competition? Examples of Russian Health Care Reforms from St. Petersburg and the Leningrad Region." *International Journal of Health Services,* 1997, *27*(4).

Economist Intelligence Unit. *Business Russia.* Chicago: Russian-American Publications, 1999a.

Economist Intelligence Unit. *Russia Market Atlas: An Exhaustive Guide to One of the World's Biggest Emerging Markets.* London: Economist Intelligence Unit, 1999b.

Field, M. G. "Reflections on a Painful Transition: From Socialized to Insurance Medicine in Russia." *Croatian Medical Journal,* 1999, *40*(2).

Klugman, J., Schieber, G., Heleniak, T., and Hon, V. "Health Reform in Russia and Central Asia." In J. M. Nelson, C. Tilly, and L. Walker (ed.), *Transforming Post-Communist Political Economies: Task Force on Economies in Transition.* Washington, D.C.: National Research Council, 1998.

Rice, T. "Cross-National Trends in Health Sector Reform: Thinking Revolutionary, Acting Evolutionary." Paper presented to Duma. Zdrav Reform Project (USAID), May 15, 1995.

Semenov, V. "Contracting Methods: Reimbursement and Incentives: Case Study of Russia: Federal Mandatory Insurance Fund." Paper presented at the Third Annual Summit on International Managed Care Trends, Miami, 1998.

U.S.-Russia Commission on Economic and Technological Cooperation. "Joint Report of the 8th Health Committee Meeting." Washington, D.C., Mar. 23, 1999.

PART THREE

LATIN AMERICA

Contributors to Part Three analyze health care in Brazil, Argentina, Chile, and Mexico and present a case study from Mexico. They look at the traditional Latin American model of centralized health care, often with great inequality of care for poor and for upper-middle-class populations.

In Chapter Seventeen, Daniel Whitaker and Bianca Camac analyze Brazil's shift away from the traditional Latin American model. Like other Latin American countries, Brazil has a health care system segmented into a struggling publicly funded sector for the poor and a high-quality private sector for the upper-middle classes. Brazil is unique, however, in its degree of decentralization and in the symbiosis between its public and private sectors. They discuss the potential for growth in the private sector to address serious inequalities within the Brazilian health care system.

As in Brazil, every Argentine theoretically has access to some form of health care. But the quality of care in that country has deteriorated, according to Paul Doulton, while the cost has increased. And poor and rural populations often lack access altogether. In Chapter Eighteen, Doulton discusses reform initiatives of the 1990s designed to improve quality, efficiency, and access, and he identifies future anticipated developments.

Chapter Nineteen covers health care in Chile—a system considered progressive twenty years ago but now facing a better-informed, democratic society.

Pat Vitacolonna and Franz Schenkel discuss the attributes of the Chilean system, what should be retained, and what cracks have appeared, given the country's changing demographics and position in the world economy. The chapter concludes with an in-depth discussion of one company's effort to help insurance companies in Chile deliver a high-quality managed care product.

The first of two chapters on Mexico, Chapter Twenty reviews that country's health care system and the potential for investment there. The Mexican Constitution explicitly recognizes the right of all persons to health protection, Neelam Sekhri points out, but as in the South American countries reviewed, services are often limited in accessibility, quality, or scope. Sekhri looks at the economic and political factors that make Mexico particularly rife for investment but also warns of possible protests against privatization.

Finally, valuable lessons can be learned from an international business that failed. In Chapter Twenty-One, Keith F. Batchelder and Laurence Dene McGriff assess how a start-up health plan at one time positioned to become a major managed care company in Mexico ended in failure. They use the case study as a lesson in the clash of cultures and plans gone awry.

CHAPTER SEVENTEEN

BRAZIL

Daniel Whitaker, Bianca Camac

Health care in Brazil is quickly shifting away from the traditional Latin American model. Brazil's health care system, like the systems of its neighbors, is segmented into a struggling, publicly funded health sector (the *Sistema Único de Saúde*, or SUS) for the poor and a high-quality private sector for the upper-middle classes. Brazilian health care is distinguished not only by the fact that a less interventionist government largely assumes the role of purchaser of services rather than provider but also by the municipally decentralized nature of the public health sector. The vigorous growth of the Brazilian private health sector over the past decade, as a contractor to the SUS and as a private provider, has presented new opportunities for the future direction of Brazil's health sector as a whole. The potential of the private sector to assume a majority role as a cost-efficient provider of integral health services offers a powerful public-private symbiotic model for health sector reform and growth in Brazil.

This chapter reviews health care in Brazil and the evolution of the current health service. The public and private sectors are discussed in terms of structure, provision, and finance; new reforms and legislation are also considered. Finally, possible avenues for growth of the Brazilian public and private sectors from 2001 to 2005 are described.

Brazil in Context

Brazil's economic, social, and demographic situation reveals a striking degree of inequality. It is within this setting that the activities of the public and private health sectors can best be understood.

Inequality

Brazil is characterized by significant diversity and inequality, even by Latin American standards. With a population of about 175 million, Brazil is the fifth-largest country in the world, sprawling over half the continent of South America. According to the Human Development Index (HDI)[1], in 1994 Brazil ranked very close to the measure at which countries are considered to have attained a high level of human development. Yet this figure disguises the alarming degree of internal disparity that can be found across the five major regions of Brazil and the social groups therein. For example, the HDI of the highly populated urban south-southeastern regions (for example, São Paulo and Rio de Janeiro) compare to Argentina and Chile, whereas the less populated northeastern states have an HDI equivalent to El Salvador and the Congo. Brazil's Gini index[2] consistently places the country in the ranks of the most unequal societies in the world. In 1995 Brazil's Gini index was 60.1 (World Bank, 1998). Furthermore, the richest quintile of Brazil's population controls over 64 percent of the income, whereas the poorest quintile shares only 2.5 percent (World Bank, 1999).

Demographics

Brazil's population, with a median age of 23.2 years, is younger than other countries of similar size and economic status (Carvalho de Noronha and Ruth da Silva Pereira, 1998). The mean annual population growth for 1990–1998 was 1.6 percent, and total fertility rate (births per woman) in 1997 was 2.3 percent (World Bank, 1999). Thirty percent of the population of Brazil is under the age of fifteen, although this figure has fallen from 42 percent in 1970 (Pan-American Health Organization, 1995). These facts indicate that many of the main epidemiological effects of an aging population are still to come for Brazil.

Epidemiological Shift

Since 1960, Brazil has experienced an epidemiological shift, as the economy has evolved from one that is agricultural-dependent into one that is urban and industrialized. Brazil's disease profile has encountered a sharp decrease in the incidence of mortality from waterborne, infectious, and parasitic diseases and a rise in the magnitude of mortality due to noncommunicable disease (Latufo, 1997). For the period 1990–1994, the major causes of total mortality in Brazil were diseases of the circulatory system (33.9 percent), injuries and poisonings, including homicide (14.8 percent), malignant neoplasms, especially stomach and lung cancer (13.0 percent), and communicable diseases (11 percent; Pan-American Health Organization, 1998a).

Evolution of a System

Brazil's recent economic and political history has created the current public and private health care models.

Formation of the SUS

Before 1987, the *Ministerio da Saúde* (Ministry of Health) provided health care for the poor and uninsured, and the *Instituto Nacional de Assistência Médica da Previdência Social* (INAMPS—National Institute of Medical Assistance for Social Security) covered the formally employed; the private sector catered to the middle and upper classes. In 1988, the federal constitution declared that health care was a public right to be provided as a duty of the State. The result was the *Sistema Único de Saúde* (SUS—the Unified Health System), which merged the INAMPS under the direction of the Ministry of Health, to create a universal public system. As many middle-class Brazilians fled a public sector they felt was overburdened and failing to deliver quality health services, there was an explosion in demand for private health care. The result has been a divided health sector providing relatively good, comprehensive private sector care to about 45 million upper-middle-class Brazilians and uneven and poorer quality care for another 125 million Brazilians, or *carentes*, who are dependent on the SUS.

Health Care Spending and Reform

Brazil's economy is the eighth largest in the world, with a GNP (expressed in U.S. dollar equivalents according to purchasing power parity) of US$1.02 trillion, or US$6,160 per capita in 1998 (World Bank, 1999). As a proportion of GDP, government health care spending made up 2.7 percent, whereas the private sector contributed 4.7 percent, for a total of 7.4 percent of GDP (US$77 billion) spent nationally on health care in Brazil in 1998 (Economist Intelligence Unit, 1999). During the "lost decade" of 1980 to 1990, the pattern of inequality in Brazil became very severe as the Brazilian government, like most in Latin America, chose to focus on macroeconomic adjustment rather than on the deteriorating social situation during this turbulent economic period. The result was a serious cutback on social spending, including health, which prohibited the SUS from providing a health care package consistent with that of other middle-income countries.

By the late 1980s, glaring social inequality was evident, and the government recognized the role of health as a determinant of economic growth. This produced efforts to reform the financing, self-management, and incentives of the public health sector. Emphasis on the decentralization of SUS services, mandated in the Organic Health Laws 8080 and 8142 of 1990, is the most obvious example (see Table 17.1). Despite the SUS's efforts to improve, consumer demand for private sector health services has sharply accelerated since 1988.

The size of Brazil's private sector offers important opportunities to both foreign and domestic investors. But perhaps more interesting from a policy perspective, the symbiotic relationship between public and private health care finance and provision offers great potential benefits (as well as some risks) for Brazil. And it is an example for Latin America as a whole.

TABLE 17.1. MAJOR HEALTH LEGISLATION IN BRAZIL SINCE 1988.

Date	Law	Summary
1988	Constitution	Establishes the legal obligations and decentralized foundation for Unified Health System
9/90	Law 8080	Organic Health Law: Establishes responsibility, obligations, and financial and administrative structure at the federal, state, and municipal levels; delineates the rights and responsibilities of the private sector and prohibits foreign private health care
12/90	Law 8142	Organic Health Law: Details administrative network and function
1/96	NOB	Basic Operational Guidelines: Defines managerial responsibility at each level of government; strengthens the capacity of the municipal governments to deliver services; promotes further decentralization by constructing automatic transfer of federal resources to the state and municipal levels
6/98	Law 9656	Private health insurance regulation: Stipulates a basic package of care that must be offered by private health care plans and requires the private sector to reimburse the public sector for expenses incurred treating privately insured patients

Source: Buss and Gadelha, 1996, p. 290.

Public Health Care: The Unified Health System (SUS)

The SUS is a decentralized, universal, and publicly funded system that provides and purchases integral health care services. The decentralized SUS depends on empowered regional and local initiative to organize appropriate health care. In general, the SUS provides outpatient services and purchases inpatient services. The SUS operates from federal, state, and municipal government funds, and the distribution of federal funds is skewed toward wealthier southeastern states. The SUS pays for inpatient services according to a prospective payment system and for outpatient services by volume.

Structure and Change

The SUS can be characterized as a universal, publicly (under)funded system that purchases the health services it provides. A system that emphasizes decentralization, the SUS has devolved into three relatively autonomous federal, state, and municipal tiers. Each level possesses organized bodies responsible for operations, finance, and social representation (see Table 17.2).

Decentralization

The depth to which the SUS provides a decentralized service depends largely on local initiative. Without required provisions in a city charter, neither a municipality nor technically a state can receive funding or administrative recognition at

TABLE 17.2. STRUCTURE OF THE BRAZILIAN UNIFIED HEALTH SYSTEM (SUS).

Level	Executive Body	Operational Management	Financial Management	Social Control
Federal	Ministry of Health	Tripartite Intermanagerial Commission	National Health Fund	National Health Council
State	State Health Board	Bipartite Intermanagerial Commission	State Health Fund	State Health Council
Municipal	Municipal Health Board	Municipal Health Secretary	Municipal Health Fund	Municipal Health Council

Source: Buss and Gadelha, 1996, p. 290.

the next-highest SUS tier. Neither can it create *Conselhos Municipais de Saúde* (Municipal Health Councils, or CMSs) (Grimes, 1997). The incidence of the CMS, a good gauge of SUS decentralization, varies significantly by region and is best developed in the south-southeast. As a result the picture of health inequality in Brazil becomes one in which locally empowered health services are often absent in the regions where they are most needed. The World Bank estimates that about 11 million Brazilians have no real access to health care because of geographical isolation. The severity of this situation is reinforced by the fact that the south-southeast registers nearly twice as many annual ambulatory consultations per capita (World Bank, 1996).

Effects of Decentralization

At its best, the result of SUS decentralization has been an increase in accountability and responsiveness on the part of local health authorities. Consequently, both the CMS and the local executive branch, which maintains the real legislative authority over local health policy, have recognized that responding to the health needs of the community mines considerable political capital.

SUS-Financed Provision

The public sector, consisting of both SUS-owned and contracted private services, provides health care services to 75 percent of Brazilians. Private providers contracted to the SUS deliver over three-quarters of inpatient care and about half of ambulatory care. In 1995, SUS-funded hospital admissions made up 40 percent of the for-profit private hospital admissions, 33 percent of nonprofit private hospital admissions, 27 and 10 percent, respectively, of public and university hospital admissions (Carvalho de Noronha and Ruth da Silva Pereira, 1998).

Responsibilities

Although the SUS attempts to present itself as an integrated system, generally the federal level (Ministry of Health) assumes responsibility for national sanitation, evaluation of health system performance, and co-coordination of the nationwide Health Information System (SIS). The state level (SES) focuses on chronic care and works with other tiers of the SUS to prevent injuries and communicable diseases. The municipal level (SMS) is officially responsible for organizing local health care services, including primary and acute care, disease surveillance, and sanitation efforts.

Facilities

In 1998, there were 6,358 inpatient facilities under the umbrella of the SUS, of which 33.6 percent belonged to the public sector (DATASUS, 1999). The majority of these are small hospitals with fewer than seventy beds each. As in many countries, the regional distribution of both public and private health facilities strongly favors the highly populated urban areas. In Brazil, the southeast and center-west regions have 3.3 and 3.6 total public and private hospital beds per ten thousand, respectively, although the northern region has only 2.0 (Ministry of Health, 1999). Over two-thirds of SUS hospital beds are in the private sector; 23 percent are in the public sector; 10 percent are in research and teaching university hospitals.[3]

In June 1999, there were about 54,000 outpatient and primary care facilities (public and private) in Brazil. In the public sector, 68.4 percent of these were operated at the municipal level, 4.3 percent by state governments, and 5.8 percent at the federal level. The private sector contributed the remaining 21.5 percent (11,596).

Health Professionals

The distribution of physicians, nurses, and dentists is also concentrated in the southeast and in urban areas. Over the last decade, there has been a real increase in the number of nurses and dentists per capita, although the number of physicians per capita has remained stable (Pan-American Health Organization, 1998b). Any medical professional may hold more than one position in Brazil, as more than 57 percent of physicians have more than two jobs; 17 percent hold only one (Morrissey, 1999). In 1992, the public and private sector accounted for 48 and 51 percent of physician positions held, respectively (Instituto Brasileiro de Geografia e Estatística, 1992).

Finance of the SUS

In 1998, the SUS spent about US$27.5 billion (purchasing power parity) on health care, drawing on tax revenues and social contributions collected at the federal, state, and municipal levels. The public sector does not recover the cost of providing health services through copayments, deductibles, or charges for comfort services. Despite the strain on the SUS's scant resources, according to the Pan-American Health Organization (1998b)—though some observers think this to be an overestimate—the SUS finances 95 percent of primary care, 70 percent of secondary care, and 90 percent of highly complex tertiary care to the whole population.

Federal Finance and Distribution

In 1993, the federal Ministry of Health provided about 72 percent of the financial resources to the public health sector at all tiers, though this figure had fallen from about 85 percent in 1987. According to the Ministry of Health, about 72 percent of federal health resources originate from contributions to social funds and 20 percent from fiscal stabilization funds; the remaining resources stem from national treasury bonds, taxes, and other sources (Pan-American Health Organization, 1998b).

The distribution of financial resources by the Ministry of Health exacerbates Brazilian health inequality. The relatively wealthy and developed southeastern region receives nearly double the amount per capita of total SUS financial resources than the northern region (DATASUS, 1999). Figure 17.1 demonstrates the profound disparity in the spread of federal resources.

Purchasing Services

The SUS finances outpatient services according to volume of services performed, using a fixed payment for aggregate treatments, although there is an increasing shift toward a capitated prospective payment system. The Ministry of Health pays both public and private providers directly, except for services contracted at the municipal level (Carvalho de Noronha and Ruth da Silva Pereira, 1998). The reimbursement of providers by the federal Ministry of Health was about 40 percent of the 1998 Ministry of Health budget—a very low figure, considering that the Ministry of Health has few obligations to provide health care services itself (Ministry of Health, 1998).

The SUS purchases hospital services according to the *Autorização da Internação Hospitalar* (AIH) system. The AIH system links prospective fees and guidelines for a particular diagnosis treatment, such as a normally attended in-hospital birth or an appendectomy. The median value for a SUS-funded hospital admission was $US270 in 1995 (Carvalho de Noronha and Ruth da Silva Pereira, 1998). Because AIH prices do not fully reflect the real cost of care, the World Bank claims that the prices paid to providers do not provide incentives for efficient allocation of resources because they are too low to cover costs, maintenance, depreciation, and innovation. Also, there are perverse incentives for public providers to be inefficient and poor allocators of resources (World Bank, 1996). For example, public hospitals have incentives to turn away patients because they are not interested in expanding capacity. Furthermore, the public sector has an advantage over private hospitals because public hospitals receive extra budgets for salaries and other inputs.

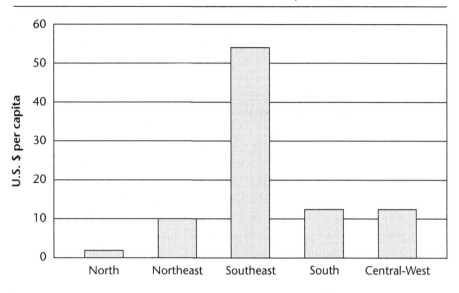

FIGURE 17.1. PER CAPITA DISTRIBUTION OF FEDERAL HEALTH RESOURCES, BY REGION.

Source: DATASUS, 1998.

Purchasing from the Private Sector

There are strong incentives, however, for the private hospital sector to be efficient allocators of the limited resources they receive from government AIH payments. Private hospitals claim to receive only a fraction of the cost of providing care to SUS patients, with one estimate, since they receive only about US$2 per day for treatment (Morrissey, 1999). Moreover, unlike the autonomous private sector, private hospitals under contract depend critically on the SUS for income. An estimated 70 percent of the income of for-profit private hospitals and 85 percent of the income of private philanthropic and nonprofit hospitals is from public funds (Viana, Queiroz, and Ibañez, 1997). Private hospitals have consistently felt undervalued and underpaid by the SUS, and the public-private strain has been exacerbated by frequent delays in payment. Also, despite significant tax breaks that many private hospitals receive by admitting a specified percentage of patients from the SUS, a growing number of such hospitals stopped accepting these patients because of poor and delayed remuneration from the SUS. This situation has intensified at the municipal level, as it is the municipalities who are responsible for organizing and financing local health care services. Fraud control is a serious issue;

the government estimates that 10 percent of inpatient reimbursements are fraudulent, although other sources estimate this figure to be as much as 40 percent (World Bank, 1996). In addition, the relationship between the private and public sectors has recently begun to change as the Ministry of Health has started to play the role of referee by regulating the "rules of play" in a previously unregulated private sector.

Private and Supplemental Health Care

The private health sector is divided into a component consisting of health insurance plans and a private hospital sector, which depends partly on public finance. Private insurance is divided into four main models. Private hospitals tend be organized around a particular social group or issue. The private health sector as a whole has grown rapidly over the last decade. New legislation will force the insurance plans to pay for more comprehensive health care services. The private sector provides most secondary inpatient care, whether directly to its own private patients or as contracted by the SUS.

The private health care sector has grown rapidly in the last two decades and continues to grow, although now the future is more uncertain. It is estimated that roughly 30 percent of the Brazilian population (45 million people) is covered by privately purchased health services (Pan-American Health Organization, 1998b). This figure has more than quadrupled from 11 million in 1988.

Although the private hospital sector can be found in many forms, sometimes organized around a single hospital, geographical area, or ethnic group, the autonomous private sector has four main models:

• *Group medicine (planos de saúde)*, or HMOs, serves roughly 18.3 million people, mostly in the south, especially in the state of São Paulo. The formal representatives of *Planos de Saúde* are the Brazilian Group Medicine Association (ABRAMGE) and the associated National Syndicate of Group Medicine Companies (SINAMGE). Together these groups directly employ 27,000 medical doctors and own more than 225 hospitals, 21,000 beds, and 2,850 diagnostic centers, although most have contracted agreements expanding access to many more facilities and health professionals (ABRAMGE, 1998).

• *Medical cooperatives (cooperativas médicas)* offer private health care to about 11 million Brazilians. Represented by UNIMED, a union of medical doctors, cooperatives contract directly with employers to provide moderately priced, nonprofit health services. Cooperatives own a small network of hospitals and employ over 90,000 medical doctors in Brazil in 366 cooperatives formed by the medical association of a city (Morrissey, 1999).

- *Autonomous plans (autogestão)* cover about 8 million private patients. The *autogestão* are self-managed providers run by state-owned companies or large private companies. The Brazilian Association of Company Services (ABRASPE) represents these plans (Viana, Queiroz, and Ibañez, 1997).

- *Indemnity medical insurance (seguradoras)* serves about 4 million people. Consisting of about eleven organizations, this model offers a wide range of coverage, from extensive and expensive coverage to very restricted and inexpensive coverage. Such coverage takes the form of cash reimbursements rather than the organization of actual health care provision.

Growth and Reform

The first economist to hold the post as minister of health, José Serra introduced the first-ever legislation to regulate the private sector (see Table 17.2). Law 9656 of June 1998 created strict requirements on private health care plans through two main measures directed at managed care (that is, the first three of the private insurance forms discussed earlier). First, plans will be required to offer more comprehensive health plans with a mandatory minimum package of services (*plano de referencia*). In the past, many private sector insurers provided care to the secondary level but forced patients back into the public sector for high-cost, tertiary treatment. Second, the private sector will be required to reimburse the public sector for treating privately insured patients. Formerly, the public sector provided care to private patients without charging their respective private insurers for the cost of their publicly provided care. Restrictions concerning foreign investment in Brazilian companies have also recently been removed, allowing several large U.S. insurers into the Brazilian market (Morrissey, 1999).

Private Sector Reaction to New Regulations

Understandably, the private health sector is unhappy with Serra's new regulations. The industry has protested that the changes will lead to a vicious circle of higher premiums and an even more overburdened public sector. ABRAMGE has stated that managed care premiums will increase dramatically, as private plans not only are forced to pay for a wider and more expensive range of services but to reimburse the public sector for treatment incurred by their own private patients as well. As a result, ABRAMGE predicts that many middle-income consumers will be forced out of the private market, further straining an already struggling SUS. Also, because the new law does not affect indemnity insurers, it is possible that there will be a proliferation of relatively useless, cheap, and limited financial health insurance plans that abandon consumers in cases of serious illness.

Private Provision

In general, the private insurance sector (that is, group medicine and medical co-operatives) focuses on the provision of secondary-level services and has not been particularly concerned with the provision of primary and preventive care. The private hospital sector also provides most secondary- and tertiary-level care, though it has not always been encouraged to be an efficient provider, given its contractual relationship with the SUS. About two-thirds of all facilities with beds in Brazil are private, whereas about 75 percent of all outpatient facilities are owned by the public health sector. Public secondary care (inpatient) facilities serve about 70 percent of the population (Pan-American Health Organization, 1998b). The ratio of total (public and private) inpatient to outpatient facilities is roughly 4 to 1 (World Bank, 1994). Nearly three-quarters of diagnostic support facilities and blood banks are private. Furthermore, the overwhelming majority of clinical laboratories (96.8 percent) are also privately owned and maintained (Pan-American Health Organization, 1998b).

Finance of the Private Sector

The private health care system spent US$16 billion in 1998 in Brazil. Per month, HMOs spent US$17.94 per enrollee, compared to the public sector, which spent just US$4.16 per person (ABRAMGE, 1998). Most private health care plans are maintained by contributions from employers and, to a smaller extent, individuals and businesses. Services are moving away from fee-for-service orientation toward capitated and diagnosis-related fixed remuneration—a move that has provided the private sector with incentives to control costs and be more efficient. Often offered as part of an employment package in large urban areas to attract skilled workers, private health care packages are partially paid by the employee and subsidized by the employer. Many middle-income Brazilians tend to opt for the moderately priced, medical cooperative insurance. Indemnity insurance also offers a spectrum of coverage at a wide range of prices.

As private health care plans have been pushed to control costs, the contracted private hospital sector has been forced to move away from the traditional fee-for-service reimbursement toward the *pacote* system—a flat-rate, cost-per-case system similar to the DRG system in the United States. If Serra's new law damages the whole private sector in the way ABRAMGE predicts, then the law will ultimately shrink the entire hospital business as it places further financial strain on the contracted private hospital industry.

2001–2005: Directions for Growth

The potential growth of the private health sector in Brazil is vast, given the number of underserved health consumers and the current state of the public health system.

The dependent nature of the public-private relationship indicates the magnitude to which the private sector has the possibility to assume an even larger role in Brazilian health care delivery. Although there are many possible directions for private growth, three avenues are as follows:

- To continue to cater to the needs of the privately financed health service community.
- To encourage greater involvement in the supply of publicly funded services, especially for tertiary-level care as a contractor or a private provider. This model would require AIH prices to rise.
- To increase the amount of primary and complex tertiary care offered by managed care in order to make coverage fully integral. This change by the private sector will most likely occur as a necessary measure to control costs.

Whichever route is taken, remuneration systems need to be modified in order to ensure that processes not only improve outcomes but also reduce costs. An appropriate avenue for growth and reform would be the expansion of prepaid, integral plans offering a wide range of health care services.

As the private sector has grown, new legislation has encouraged behavior that is efficient and controls costs. What remains to be seen is whether the private sector will be able to diversify into primary and ambulatory care to the extent necessary in order to significantly contain the cost of the tertiary-level services for which it is now required to pay. Furthermore, the potential of the private sector to take on the role of a cost-efficient provider of tertiary-level services is important, given the current lack of incentives for cost control and efficiency.

Despite the discomfort the private sector might feel because of Serra's new regulations, there must be recognition of the benefits of offering prepaid, integral health plans from which consumers are able to acquire a full package of health services.

Conclusion

Although the consequences of the recent reform of the private health sector are still hard to predict, they are important in that they introduce an agenda of public sector health care costs and consumer concerns in what has been a traditionally unregulated private industry. Closer integration of the public and private sectors is a possibility but is not yet certain.

Unlike most countries with a comprehensive public health service, the Brazilian private sector plays a surprisingly large role—directly through private health care plans and indirectly though contracting—in the provision of health care services. Despite the fact that public health services are supposed to be universal, the public health system has acknowledged that it cannot meet the demand of all consumers. Consequently, the public sector, in essence if not in practice, has encouraged investment in the private sector through contracting and purely private services.

The Brazilian health care system remains like much of the rest of Brazil—striking in its degree of inequality. However, the system is unique in its degree of decentralization and in its symbiosis with the private sector. As a possible model for other countries suffering from problems often inherent in a highly centralized health care system, the Brazilian SUS has provided a structure that empowers communities to create health models according to local health needs. Although the legislative principles governing the SUS are somewhat cloudy in terms of the real power granted to municipal health councils, there does exist both a voice and a legal channel for funding from the federal to the municipal level. Yet significant financial problems persist in a public sector lacking necessary financial resources. The result is that the public sector's role as a provider rather than a contractor of services must be emphasized.

Regardless of the direction of growth, the Brazilian public and private health care market must address the serious nature of inequality within the country if truly comprehensive care is to be provided. In a system already rife with glaring disparities, it is essential that new legislation not oblige the current public system to provide even lower standards of health care to the poor. This could happen if the new private sector regulations force middle-class Brazilians out of the private market and back to the SUS. The possibility that both the public and private sectors in Brazil can work together, in symbiosis, to contract and to provide an integral package of health care services must be recognized, encouraged, and enabled if the entire health system is to grow successfully.

Notes

1. The Human Development Index is a measure of the United Nations Development Program that focuses on three determinants: deprivation of life expectancy, literacy, and income for a decent living standard. The third determinant is an adjusted figure for per capita income based on the purchasing power of GDP figures.
2. The Gini index measures the extent to which the distribution of income among individuals or households in an economy deviates from a perfectly equal distribution (the Lorenz curve). A Gini index of 0 implies perfect equality, whereas an index of 100 implies perfect inequality. Sample Gini indexes for selected countries: Sweden (1992), 25.0; United States (1994), 40.8; Mexico (1992), 50.3; Poland (1992), 27.2; South Africa (1993), 58.4.
3. This implies much higher utilization at university hospitals than other public hospitals (DATASUS, 1999).

References

ABRAMGE [Brazilian Group Medicine Association]. [http://www.abramge.com.br]. 1998.

Buss, P., and Gadelha, P. "Health Care Systems in Transition: Brazil, Part I: An Outline of Brazil's Health Care System Reforms." *Journal of Public Health Medicine*, 1996, *18*(3).

Carvalho de Noronha, J., and Ruth da Silva Pereira, T. "Health Care Reform and Quality Initiatives in Brazil," *Journal on Quality Improvement*, 1998, *24*(5).

DATASUS. *Recursos Federais do SUS: Pagamentos Federais.* Brasilia: Ministry of Health, 1998.

DATASUS. [http://www.datasus.gov.br]. 1999.

Economist Intelligence Unit. "In Focus: Four Countries, Four Health Sectors." *Healthcare Latin America*, 1999, *60*.

Grimes, M. F. *Brazil's Municipal Health Councils: An Experiment in Direct Democracy.* Austin: University of Texas, 1997.

Instituto Brasileiro de Geografia e Estatística [Brazil Institute of Geography and Statistics]. [http://www.ibge.org].1992.

Ministry of Health. *Informaçoes em Saude: Recursos, Acesso e Cobertura.* [http://www.saude.gov.br]. 1999.

Morrissey, J. "Brazilian Healthcare at a Crossroads: Private Sector Flourishes as the Government's Program Buckles Under Heavy Demand, Lack of Funding." *Modern Healthcare*, May 15, 1999, p. 6.

Pan-American Health Organization. *Health Statistics from the Americas.* Washington, D.C.: Pan-American Health Organization, 1995.

Pan-American Health Organization. *Brazil: Health in the Americas.* Washington, D.C.: Pan-American Health Organization, 1998a.

Pan-American Health Organization. *Brazil: Profile of the Health Services System.* Washington, D.C.: Pan-American Health Organization, 1998b.

Viana, A. L., Queiroz, M. S., and Ibañez, N. "Implementation of a Single Health System in Brazil: New Relationships Between Public and Private Sectors in Brazil." In C. Altenstetter and J. W. Björkman (eds.), *Health Policy Reform: National Variations and Globalization.* Hampshire, England: International Political Science Association/Macmillan, 1997.

World Bank. *Brazil: The Organization, Delivery and Financing of Health Care in Brazil: Agenda for the '90s.* Washington, D.C.: World Bank, 1994.

World Bank. *Brazil: The Organization, Delivery and Financing of Health Care in Brazil: Agenda for the '90s.* Washington, D.C.: World Bank, 1996.

World Bank. *World Development Indicators, 1998.* Washington, D.C.: World Bank, 1998.

World Bank. *Entering the 21st Century: The World Development Report, 1999/2000.* Washington, D.C.: World Bank, 1999.

CHAPTER EIGHTEEN

ARGENTINA

Paul Doulton

Argentine health care schemes were created in the 1950s and 1960s out of Peronism, with a heavy union underpinning. The backbone of health care in the country is the *obra social* (OS), to which all employees are required to belong. There are as many OSs as there are trade unions, resulting in fragmentation and inefficiencies.

In theory, every Argentine has access to some form of health care. The quality of care has deteriorated, however, while the cost has increased. Doctors are in oversupply (one for every 370 inhabitants) and are unevenly distributed, with most concentrated in the capital or large provincial cities. Furthermore, most physicians are specialists, with an undersupply of primary care physicians and nurses.

Argentina spent an estimated 9 percent of its GDP on health care in 1998, or $710 per capita—a generous amount by Latin American standards. However, this does not mean that Argentines receive better health care than other Latin Americans. Poor and rural populations lack access, and the high expenditures are more a function of high-cost specialty care than of high-volume, quality care in general.

In the past decades, medical inflation has threatened to throw Argentine health care schemes into disarray because underlying weaknesses have been concealed under general inflation. A lot of progress needs to be achieved before the schemes can be brought under control.

Recently, the Argentine government has taken initiatives to improve quality, efficiency, and access. Programs now in place to redress the situation include the

National Quality Assurance Program (1992), Self-Management of Public Hospitals (1993), the Reconversion Program for *Obras Sociales* (1995), and the Obligatory Medical Plan (1995).

This chapter provides a background for understanding the Argentine health care system, describes system structure and organization, describes the new reform initiatives, and identifies future anticipated developments in the industry.

Background

Argentina has made a successful transition into a genuine democratic system, with two major parties vying for power: the *Justicialista* Party (reformed Peronists) and the Radical Party, which recently won the presidential elections; power was transferred from Carlos Menem to Fernando de la Rua in December 1999. The country is a federation of twenty-three provinces, with the capital, Buenos Aires, by far the largest in terms of population and concentration of decision making.

In the last fifteen years, Argentina's GDP has almost tripled, to around $350 billion, and health care spending has risen at a still faster rate. The stability plan that was introduced in 1989 to reduce hyperinflation has been highly successful. Three major processes underpin the plan: (1) the Convertibility Plan, regulated by a currency board to ensure parity of the peso with the dollar; (2) privatization of major state-held industries; and (3) deregulation, including the opening of Argentina's borders to free trade. Unparalleled stability has been achieved. On the downside, unemployment is high (14.5 percent in 1999), and the balance of trade is deteriorating.

Argentina's demography is markedly different from the demography in most of the rest of Latin America. Of the 36 million population, a mere 15 percent are younger than fifteen, whereas 13 percent are over sixty, with that number projected to rise to around 20 percent in the next couple of decades. With low birth rates, there is little overall population growth, so the burden for health care and pensions falls on a relatively few young people. And these young people are finding it difficult to obtain employment.

The country has a high level of education and thus a large middle class, but wealth distribution is becoming more skewed, to the detriment of the middle and lower classes. The urban population is a striking 89 percent of the total, with a concentration of health care services in the cities. The sheer size of Argentina's territory makes for gross asymmetries in income distribution, especially for provinces thousands of kilometers from the capital.

Per capita GDP has risen from $8,000 in 1995 to $9,200 in 1999, but recent reversals of fortunes suggest that this level will be hard to sustain, at least until

Brazil (Argentina's major trading partner) returns to its historic vigor. The challenge is to manage a return to a fairer level of equity in income distribution and employment opportunities.

Structure and Organization

Argentina has a three-tiered structure to its health care system: (1) social security, (2) the *prepagas*, and (3) the public sector. The largest tier, known as social security, serves those in the trade and professional unions through OSs. The highest tier in terms of spending caters to the white-collar wealthy through the *prepagas*, which are prepaid plans providing service. And poorer people are covered by the public sector. There is considerable overlap among these groups, as there is considerable cross-over. Members from all segments pay directly out of pocket.

Obras Sociales

Membership in an OS is mandatory, that is, members of trade or professional unions must belong to their organization's OS. All together, 11.5 million employees belonged to an OS in 1999. These groups are far too many in number (with 261 of them in mid-1999) and too small to create financial efficiencies and risk sharing. Close to 40 percent of OSs have fewer than 1,000 members. The top ten have the majority of the OS members, and there is increasing consolidation and competition among them.

Health care for pensioners (as well as for the poor) is funded from employer and active employee contributions, as well as through public debt; these funds are grouped as part of social security under PAMI, the national social services agency. PAMI covers some 4.5 million pensioners, and the regional OS (state employee fund) covers another 4.5 million. With 20.5 million OS members, then, health care funding has hitherto been managed on too small a scale.

Prepagas

Prepagas are private, prepaid plans that cater to the wealthy—some 2 million higher-level employees or voluntary independent subscribers. The largest *prepaga* is OSDE (*Obra Social para Direccion de Empresas*). These health plans provide service as in the traditional distinction between insurance and managed care but do not offer a far higher level of care and client choice than the other tiers of the Argentine health care system. Most are closed panels with freedom of choice within the panel, and the average premium paid each month by each *prepaga* beneficiary is an average of

$73, compared with the OS. A *prepaga* smaller than OSDE, Galeno, caters to mid-level subscribers. Galeno now belongs to venture capitalist Exxel, which is cutting costs dramatically and consolidating. Premiums vary from $40 per member per month (pmpm) with AMSA (which is skewed lower by covering some OSs) to over $100 pmpm for *Medicus* and *Qualitas*. Other *prepagas* premium rates vary from $40 pmpm for AMSA up to a high of $100 for *Medicus* and *Qualitas*.

All employees choosing to belong to a *prepaga* must still contribute to their OS, but moves are afoot to qualify *prepagas* for obligatory quotas and allow them the same tax-deductible quotas that OSs enjoy. When this happens, further competition will put the OS fight for membership quotas on a more level playing field.

Prepagas come in for criticisms similar to those of the OSs. There are too many *prepagas* (some 200 at present, although a mere nine cover more than half the total membership), and these are often criticized for medical underwriting practices such as excluding high-risk patients. The smaller *prepagas* are often single-hospital plans, something like the U.S. physician-hospital organizations. They are less regulated than the OS. *Prepagas* must contribute 15 percent of their income to solidarity funds (to provide coverage for low-income and high-risk employees), whereas OSs contribute 10 percent.

Both *prepagas* and OSs contract out a little more than 90 percent of their health care to private providers (doctors, hospitals, pharmaceuticals, and so on). *Prepagas* spend more on secondary- and tertiary-level care than OSs do, and this sector's medical inflation is much higher. Interestingly, medical inflation in the last seven years among this sector has been 25 percent, whereas for the public sector it has been 50 percent. Increased demand for services in the public sector probably accounts for the major difference.

Public Sector

The public sector is run by the Ministry of Health through a number of agencies: the pensioners' social service (INSSJ/PAMI), the regulatory agency ANMAT, and SSSalud, which supervises the OSs. Smaller agencies under the Health Ministry umbrella run preventive medicine (education, hygiene, and vaccination), as well as primary care clinics. In turn, each of these agencies is replicated at provincial and municipal levels.

Public sector funding comes from taxation (from federal, provincial, and municipal governments) and provides free coverage for any member of the population—in practice, for the poor. Public sector hospitals use 85 percent of these funds, although the hospitals are only part of the public sector health care responsibilities. The public sector operates 43 percent of the total number of clinics and hospitals in the country and 54 percent of all hospital beds but only 23 percent of total health care spending. More than 70 percent of the spending is in the provinces.

The public sector has been under severe strain, not only because of funding difficulties but also because of the increased demand on its services.

Providers

On the provider side, doctors—and above all, specialists—are in oversupply. Quality of service varies widely from center to center, and the race for higher patient volumes to compensate for a steady reduction in fee levels has led to overtreatment and excessive diagnostic procedures. At the same time, the fragmented providers are the weaker members at the bargaining table, with the real power in the hands of the payers. The OSs and *prepagas* represent between 60 and 70 percent of most providers' income.

Initiatives for Change

Major initiatives to redress the problems in health care funding and provision are discussed in the sections to follow.

National Quality Assurance Program, 1992

The National Quality Assurance Program focuses on accreditation, use of clinical protocols, and measurement of clinical outcomes and patient satisfaction.

Self-Management of Public Hospitals, 1993

In an effort to provide public hospitals with management expertise and to impose a level of accountability, public hospital services are now offered to the OSs and the *prepagas* in competition with private providers. The major faculties of medicine reside in some of these public hospitals, where they are able to offer a high degree of sophistication. So far, this program has met with limited success due, in part, to high levels of unemployment that have significantly increased the patient load in public sector hospitals.

Overhaul of the *Obras Sociales,* 1995

The overhaul program, known as PROS, is designed to introduce genuine competition among the OSs and thus improve quality and efficiency. The idea is to allow members of a given union to choose a different OS fund and thus oblige inefficient OSs to close or merge with others. The PROS legislation aims to reduce the number of OSs to around thirty or fifty.

Some OSs have truly overhauled themselves under PROS and are attracting new members by offering improved quality of service. In fact, the numbers have shrunk, from 350 OSs at the start of PROS to 261 in mid-1999. But the relationship between the OS managers and the Peronist Menem administration has slowed the transformation. The government also maintains a number of tax incentives, to the detriment of OS competitors.

The World Bank contributed $230 million, increasing PROS reconversion funding to $500 million since 1995. Reconversion funds are available to OSs that qualify, and it is hoped these soft loans will provide sufficient incentive to speed the much-needed transformation.

Obligatory Medical Plan, 1995

The Obligatory Medical Plan (PMO) defines the basic set of services that all health plans must provide. The law creates a comprehensive benefit package to include tertiary care. Reimbursement for drugs (40 percent for outpatients—more for certain chronic illnesses—and 100 percent for inpatients), and minimal copayments. Unlike other countries in Latin America with their basic medical coverage, Argentina has legislated virtually unlimited levels of care.

These reforms have led to increased costs over the past ten years, up from an annual per capita rate of $227 in 1986 to $710 in 1998 in 1996. In part, the aging population, the incidence of new diseases such as AIDS, and the use of new medical technologies can explain the increase in cost. But another factor plays a role. Notwithstanding the PMO, provider groups (hospitals, doctors, clinical laboratories, and so on) have to contract with a wide range of fundholders; each has its own demands. The perverse incentives are legion, based on fees for service, and such payments have given rise to duplication of services, further increasing costs.

A recent gradual introduction of capitation arrangements for organizations that offer integrated care should restore some order. It is important to keep in mind, however, that per capita rates are averages spent on health care for all Argentines. The total numbers conceal the inequities that exist between the poor and the rich, between the private sector and the public.

Mandatarias

Mandatarias are pharmacy benefit managers who handle reimbursement for medicines on behalf of the OSs. In 1998, as part of the drive for lower costs, PAMI capitated the entire pharmaceutical industry for a fixed annual sum, regardless of the variety and quantity of medicine provided by the manufacturers.

Work-Related Accident Coverage, 1996

Separate insurance for work-related injuries is now provided by private insurance companies and no longer falls under health care funding.

Investments and Opportunities

Given the enormous challenges and opportunities in Argentine health care, particularly in the private sector OSs and *prepagas,* new investors have entered the market. Venture capitalists, including Exxel, moved into the *prepaga* and indeed the provider side through its acquisition of Galeno, Vesalio, and TIM; likewise, Swiss Medical acquired CIM and *Salud y Diagnos Prepagas.* Recent arrivals from abroad include AMIL from Brazil, Aetna from the United States in a joint venture with AMSA, Principal with Qualitas, International Managed Care Advisors from the United States, with *Banco Provincia,* ADESLAS from Spain (buying *prepagas* and hospitals), and Intersalud from Chile (buying *prepagas*).

Under Argentine law, an OS cannot be sold but a *prepaga* can be. Furthermore, many opportunities exist for selling services to both: programs for home care, disease management, clinical protocols, and outcomes improvement; ambulatory and primary care clinics; and information technology and telemedicine are all needed. Within the giant tool chest of managed care, opportunities abound for processes to improve performance and client satisfaction.

Future Developments

We can expect to see a number of transformations, such as

- The Health Ministry becoming more of a policy-setting and supervisory body, with clear and enforceable game rules
- A shift toward demand-side subsidies
- More emphasis on primary care and less on specialization
- An improvement in the transparency, efficiency, and numbers of OSs and *prepagas*
- Tight controls and lower fees, the disappearance of fee-for-service plans in favor of prepaid plans, and more capitation
- A trade-off from quantity to quality under a managed-care philosophy

- A toning down of expectations of certain privileged income groups covered by health plans, but with a number of out-of-pocket alternatives persisting over time

A recent publication ("Una necesida," 1999) recognizes the vagaries of an unintegrated health care market and recommends creation of universal coverage for all Argentines. If introduced, this would break down the artificial barriers and could favor the flow of money to the most efficient providers by fostering individual choice of plan. If such a system were to become a reality, then a profound transformation of the health care scheme into a fully integrated system could occur.

Reference

"Una necesida, un derecho: Salud para todos" [A necessity, a right: Health for all]. *Acción por la República,* 1999.

CHAPTER NINETEEN

CHILE

Pat Vitacolonna, Franz Schenkel

Health care reform in Latin America has taken several forms, but nowhere on the continent has a model emerged that has been so widely discussed as the system adopted in Chile. Its funding mechanisms and its delivery system, quite progressive when they were designed twenty years ago, are now facing the new reality of a better-informed democratic society. This society has higher expectations and, in many cases, the financial wherewithal to support those expectations.

What is good about the Chilean system? What should be retained? What cracks in the system have been exposed, given the changing demographics of the population and Chile's position in the world economy?

We will give the reader a glimpse of the country's vital statistics and background, as well as an overview of Chile's current health care system and how its major players operate. We will also look at the regulatory climate and the opportunities that exist within the system. Finally, we will take an in-depth look at Salumax, a company founded to help insurance companies deliver a high-quality managed care product.

Background

Chile extends 2,600 miles along the southwestern edge of South America and averages about 110 miles in width. It is sealed off from its neighbors to the east by

237

the Andes Mountains, shares a northern border with Peru, and is separated from all countries to the west by the Pacific Ocean.

Eighty-three percent of the Chilean population of 15 million live in urban areas, and about 39 percent (5.8 million) live in the metropolitan region that includes the capital, Santiago. The country is experiencing a growth rate of 1.5 percent per year. Nearly 70 percent of the population is under forty years of age, and 38 percent are under twenty; just 7 percent are over sixty-five. By 2010, the population is expected to reach 17 million.

Chile has sustained a successful transition from military rule to a democratic government. Its fifteen years of open-market policies have paid off, and the country enjoys solid economic fundamentals. Both savings and investments have been at about 25 percent of GNP, though the savings ratio declined to about 22 percent during the recent Asian financial crisis, with its inevitable but temporary effect on the Chilean economy. (This is still the highest savings ratio in South America and among developed nations.)

The government has encouraged international trade and foreign investment with relatively lenient rules for repatriating profits and capital. The inflation rate has been low in the context of the region. A recent monthly report showed inflation to be at 0.2 percent per month, or 2.4 percent annualized. It is anticipated that the inflation rate in Chile will remain well below 5 percent for the near future.

Chile has a per capita GDP second only to Argentina in South America. Per capita GDP reached $5,700 for 1998. Although it is projected to decrease to about $5,000 in 1999, it is also expected to recover nicely in 2000. Similarly, the growth in GDP—as high as 8 percent in recent years—had declined to 3.4 percent in 1998 and was projected to be lower in 1999. A strong rebound is projected for 2000.

Health Care Structure

The Chilean health care system is a mix of public and private medical care. Public health insurance covers 52 percent of the population; private insurance, 27 percent; and institutional insurance programs (such as the armed forces or police health systems), 14 percent. The remaining population has no health care coverage but can access the public health care system as indigents.

Under Chilean law, employees must contribute 7 percent of wages and salaries, up to a ceiling income figure of approximately US$2,000 per month, to the state health care insurance plan (*Fondo Nacional de Salud,* or FONASA) or to a private insurance company (*Insitucion de Salud Previsional,* or ISAPRE). FONASA has generated a list of several thousand medical, surgical, and diagnostic procedures, which is used as the basis for establishing reimbursement rates for medical, hospital, and laboratory fees. The FONASA fee schedule regulates public sector reimbursement rates and serves as a nonbinding reference for private insurers. To secure the highest-quality physicians and hospitals, private insurance companies typically provide higher reimbursements than those established in the FONASA list.

Individuals with both private and public insurance plans can freely elect outpatient providers. Except in government hospitals, providers set fees and determine what reimbursement levels to accept without restrictions. This creates a pyramid of care, with private clinics and top-tier physicians at the peak. At the top, competence and technology are equal to that of North America and Europe. Physicians in this category, however, rarely accept the reimbursement rates set by the insurance companies. Patients pay the physician directly and recover reimbursable fees from the insurance company. At a second level, physicians provide services for a range of fees, accepting insurance company vouchers as payment. At the lowest level, physicians accept FONASA reimbursement levels.

Private Insurance Companies

As of December 1998, ten "closed" *(cerradas)* and seventeen "open" *(abiertas)* IS-APREs operated in the Chilean market. Employers run the closed ISAPREs, funding health care for their employees by adding their own voluntary contributions to the 7 percent payroll deductions. Only current and retired employees and their dependents may enroll in the closed ISAPRE—a limitation that makes this type of insurance company naturally inefficient in an industry that clearly benefits from critical mass. Today less than 4 percent of the privately insured population is enrolled in closed ISAPREs.

Open ISAPREs provide health insurance plans to the public. These companies account for 96 percent of the population covered by the private sector, with the three leading companies alone holding a market share of nearly 60 percent.

Over the past several years, low rates of membership growth and declining profit margins have driven a wave of consolidations in the industry; fewer than ten viable ISAPREs are expected to remain in the market, with no more than three dominant firms holding a market share of 65 percent or more.

The Chilean ISAPRE system, with funding tied to wages, has created a cumbersome product portfolio for the various insurance companies. The contract holder's salary determines how much premium the individual contributes to the ISAPRE, so the insurer must offer a broad range of benefits packages to cover the complete spectrum of income groups. Each company markets at least several dozen benefit packages and may easily have hundreds of packages active in its portfolio at any given time.

The most common variables of the ISAPRE health plan are (1) coverage levels as a percent of ambulatory and hospital care fees and (2) maximum allowable fee schedules. Essentially an indemnity product, the ISAPRE plan thus determines to which provider the member will have access. The maximum allowable fee caps the ISAPRE's reimbursement. Hence, a lower-income member is unlikely to use the services of a provider whose fees exceed the maximum allowable fee schedule for that member's health plan. The resulting copayments—that is, the difference between the provider's fee and the insurance plan reimbursement level—would be prohibitive for that member.

In order to control the provider fee schedule, several of the largest ISAPREs operate their own medical facilities, matching the insurance plan's coverage level with their own benefits packages. The advantage of these plans is a predictable copayment for the member. Most ISAPREs have replicated these proprietary PPOs in that they contract with independent providers. The participating provider in the PPO accepts the ISAPRE voucher as full payment for services. This ensures the member, who purchases the voucher from the ISAPRE, a transparent and predictable copayment.

The ISAPRE's benefits packages are required by law to include all of the services listed by FONASA, but the level of coverage required for each service is not specified. Notable gaps in the ISAPRE health plans are mental health care, dental services, and outpatient pharmaceuticals.

ISAPRE contract holders can purchase supplemental coverage either by increasing the amount of premium above the 7 percent wage contribution or by purchasing products offered by life insurance companies. These insurers offer a type of gap insurance that covers all or part of the difference between a provider's fees and the ISAPRE reimbursement rates and that also covers services not included under the ISAPRE, such as dental care and outpatient pharmaceuticals. Gap insurance products are typically available only to groups and cannot be purchased by individuals. An estimated 16 percent of the population covered by ISAPREs are enrolled in one of the gap insurance products offered by life insurance companies.

Managed Health Care

Managed care systems such as those operated by HMOs in the United States are new in the Chilean market but have relatively little enrollment to date. Noteworthy is the fact that these managed care plans have been embraced most successfully not by the large ISAPREs, with their proprietary provider infrastructures, but rather by medium-sized ISAPREs that have not integrated vertically. These medium-sized ISAPREs have contracted with IPA-type organizations or have created alliances with provider groups (such as the joint venture between ISAPRE Vida Tres and the medical group Integra Medica).

As a whole, the ISAPRE industry appears to lack sophistication in cost management and quality control on the provider end. Statistical measures of system efficiency tend to be rudimentary, focusing on isolated claims data such as sick days granted by preferred providers. Insurance companies are well aware of the need to improve efficiency and control costs in order to prepare for future market-share battles and restore profitability. Without exception, leading ISAPREs are exploring and in some cases attempting to implement increasingly closed provider systems, in which patients must first contact a primary care physician.

A number of factors will drive changes in the way medical care is offered and insured in Chile and in the manner in which it will be delivered.

Status of Services

Although economic growth in Chile has slowed somewhat in the past two years, it is rebounding and is expected to regain its high-single-digit rate over the next decade. Together with economic growth, improving basic health indicators (for example, decreased infant mortality, increased life expectancy, and reduced number of deaths from infectious diseases) will dramatically increase the demand for health care services in the years to come. The following dynamics are particularly relevant:

- The decreased death rate, increased life expectancy, and reduced number of deaths related to acute diseases such as infections result in a higher proportion of chronic adult diseases in the population. Treating these diseases increases the consumption of health care resources.
- Education and information improves the recognition and self-reporting of medical problems. In developing markets, this phenomenon means that consumption of health care services per unit far exceeds population growth. Paralleling this increased demand, the quality of the service provided gains in importance.
- Developing nations have demonstrated a high-income elasticity of demand for health care. Per capita expenditure for health care in Chile today is very low compared to Europe and the United States. Quickly rising personal income levels in the coming decade will likely result in even greater growth in the demand for health care.
- The health insurance system of Chile, a model for other Latin American countries, has significantly increased access to health care services.

Insurance Market Consolidation

From the mid-1980s until recently, enrollment in private insurance companies grew, on average, at a rate of 15 percent per annum. Growth rates have now come to a standstill, however. As enrollment rates drop, competition for market share has grown among insurance firms. Some are meeting this challenge by vertically integrating; others are resigned to being acquired. Seven to ten dominant organizations are likely to survive in the long term, each competing for enrollees based on the cost and quality of insurance plans.

Insurance for Retired Persons

Compared with developed nations, the population of Chile is relatively young; 65 percent of Chile's inhabitants are thirty-five years of age or younger. Since 1995, the age groups of forty to forty-nine and fifty to fifty-nine have grown 17 percent. The age group of sixty-five and older will grow by 12 percent. Overall population growth during this same period has been less than 8 percent. Hence, age groups that consume a relatively high proportion of care are experiencing strong growth. This trend is expected to accelerate in the years between 2000 and 2005.

With a life expectancy of seventy-two years, Chile is approaching developed-nation norms in survival. To date, however, no plan exists to provide insurance to retired persons. Private insurers raise premiums sharply at the time of an insured individual's retirement, making postemployment health insurance unaffordable for most Chileans.

Whatever the solution to this problem, it appears certain that the elderly population will, over the coming years, fall under a formal insurance scheme. A health system designed for the young will have to be modified to meet the needs of this elderly patient population. This age group is certain to have a high impact on the demand for and consumption of health care.

The Future of Health Care in Chile

The Chilean health insurance system is recognized as a leader for implementing private health care concepts in a continent traditionally dominated by public health care schemes. Nevertheless, local politicians from the center-left parties are concerned about an increasing separation between the standards and resources in private and public health care. Private insurers have attracted the top third of the population in terms of income. The 7 percent salary contributions thus diverted from the public to the private health funds represent a disproportionate loss of revenues for the public sector.

Insurance System Reforms

Although the importance of the private health sector is not likely to be diminished, some level of health reform may be implemented in Chile within the next two to three years. A proposal for the creation of a basic benefits package that all insurance companies would have to offer is now under consideration. The aim is to prevent private insurance companies from enrolling lower-income individuals in plans that may in fact contain less coverage than the public insurance provider would offer. Also under consideration is a proposal to impose a general employer-employee tax to support the public insurance fund.

Opportunities

The environment created by the Chilean health care system generates a number of opportunities. New services will be required to accomplish the following:

- Reduce the incidence of high-cost chronic disease
- Increase the efficiency of health care service providers
- Introduce services and products to meet the health needs of Chile's growing elderly population
- Reduce workers' health care costs in order to stay competitive in the international economic market place in which Chile has chosen to participate

These opportunities may be rewarded by exploiting the benefits of the following:

Preventive Medicine. Although Chile's national health bill stands at a comparatively reasonable 7 to 8 percent of GNP, demand will predictably increase the absolute amount of health care expenditures as well as the percentage of GNP consumed. Employers, insurance companies, and the state will be motivated to increase investment in the prevention of disease, particularly of high-cost, chronic diseases for which preventive measures have been shown to be cost-effective.

Disease Management. Both public and private insurance systems could benefit from applying integrated, standardized approaches to the clinical management of conditions such as asthma, cardiovascular disease, and diabetes, to name a few. Cost-control measures will make optimizing resource allocation mandatory.

Disease management may be the best vehicle to accomplish this. Many of the disease management techniques developed in the United States could be applied in Chile. Case management techniques would also find fertile ground in both public and private sectors.

Information System Services and Associated Products. Technology must be aimed at improving operating efficiency of health care providers, particularly as related to disease and case management. The use of database technology early on may lead to a system in which clinical outcomes are evaluated in ways still not possible in larger health care systems, as in the United States, where the population is much more mobile and difficult to track.

Elderly Care Services. In Chile's relatively young society, it may be possible to initiate programs for the elderly and learn from the experience while avoiding the extraordinary expenses usually associated with long-term care and home care services.

Services to Improve the Efficiency of Physicians. Group practice, as well as more sophisticated models of office management widely used in the United States, must be implemented.

Pharmacy Benefits Management. Several private insurance companies sell pharmaceutical products coverage. These plans call for 60 to 80 percent reimbursement of any prescribed pharmaceutical. The insurance companies employ no formulary, no databases, and no management system with which to administer the product. The plans are relatively rare because of their high cost to the beneficiaries. A well-managed plan employing all available techniques would surely increase enrollment at a reasonable cost. In fact, in 1998 the first pharmacy benefits management company in Chile (Pharma Benefits) launched its services. To date, Pharma Benefits has introduced pharmacy coverage to nine ISAPREs.

Founding of Salumax

The structure of the Chilean health care system, its emerging problems, the stagnation of growth in the ISAPREs, the changing demographics of the Chilean population, and the realities facing Chile as a player in the international economy made it clear to some that a form of managed care was needed. In 1996 a group of U.S. investors and sixty Chilean physicians provided the seed capital to create Chile's first IPA network-based HMO, with operations in the metropolitan region of Santiago and the port city of Valparaiso/Vina del Mar, Chile's second largest population center.

The objective of Salumax and its related companies is to implement and operate managed care programs in Chile and other South American markets. The company applies accepted principles to create and administer managed care health plans tailored to meet local needs. Provider groups, physician participation, information technology, and professional management are combined to develop and commercialize health plans that offer access to quality health care services and comprehensive coverage.

The health plans are positioned to compete with private sector indemnity products, as well as with government-sponsored health plans, by offering markedly improved coverage at similar costs. This advantage is possible with the application of managed care tools: emphasis on primary care, patient education and preventive medicine, risk sharing with providers, case management, utilization review, clinical guidelines, and quality control.

Salumax has created a series of assets unique to the region. Its staff of physicians, nurses, information systems specialists, administrators, and customer service and commercial personnel is the single largest team in Chile that is focused exclusively on developing and administering managed care operations. A proprietary, integrated, managed care information system based on client-server and Oracle database technology supports operations. The system, developed by the company with help from U.S. consultants, operates with a Spanish language interface.

To date, Salumax has introduced managed care by completing the following steps:

• It has recruited, credentialed, and contracted with an IPA network and established the information and management systems necessary to administer network operations.

• It has created managed care plans based on IPA network services and commercialized them as private-label products. This process required actuarial and underwriting skills. The utilization data required and its translation into costs on a PMPM basis were not readily available in a useable format. Nevertheless, with the help of a U.S. consulting firm and the company's local managers, the first health plan was launched in 1997 by the Chilean ISAPRE Vida Tres, and additional plans were added in subsequent years. In 1998 and 1999, several new private-label products were launched with other Chilean health insurance companies.

• The company is currently applying its managed care expertise and technology to carve out services in the areas of pharmaceutical benefits, mental health, oncology, transplantation, and dental care.

Salumax and Pharma Benefits currently cover more than 70,000 members through various private-label and ASO (administrative services only) plans.

Continuing with the current non-ISAPRE status gives the company greater credibility in Chile and allows the company to provide consulting and development services outside of Chile, providing new sources of revenue. This strategy also allows continued growth of the pharmacy benefits company in and out of Chile. In short, international opportunities are more realistic with this new model and its accompanying financing requirements.

CHAPTER TWENTY

MEXICO

Neelam Sekhri

The Mexican Constitution explicitly recognizes the right of all persons to health protection. In principle, the country has achieved near-universal coverage of its population under various public and private schemes. The Ministry of Health (MOH) and the Social Security System operate integrated financing and delivery systems for specific populations and act as both purchasers and providers of care.

Although most Mexicans have access to some basic health care services, these services are often limited in accessibility, quality, or scope. As a result, despite the well-developed public system, many Mexicans choose to pay out of pocket to private providers for health care. Forty-four percent of health expenditures occur through private sector providers. Government providers for the uninsured account for 13 percent of health expenditures and social security providers for the remaining 43 percent (National Economic Research Associates, 1998; World Bank, 1995).

According to Mexico's 1994 National Health Survey, 23 percent of those enrolled in social security agencies and 46 percent of those with no social security benefits reported a private provider as their usual source of ambulatory care, indicating dissatisfaction with public alternatives for health services (Sistema Nacional de Salud, 1994).

This chapter is adapted from Neelam Sekhri, Octavio Gómez-Dantés, and Tracy MacDonald, *Cross-Border Health Insurance: An Overview* (Oakland: California HealthCare Foundation, 1999). Copyright 1999, California HealthCare Foundation.

Out-of-pocket spending constitutes 43 percent of outlays on health. The largest public purchaser is the social security system (43 percent), which is largely financed through individual and employer payroll taxes. Private insurance only represents 2 percent of health purchases.

Components of the Health Care System

As shown in Figure 20.1, the health system in Mexico is made up of three major components. Two of these are public (or publicly mandated) and one is private.

The largest of the public components, in terms of expenditures, is the social security system, which finances and provides services for workers and their families in the formal sector of the economy, both private and public. Formal sector workers constitute about 52 percent of the Mexican population (Fundación Mexicana para la Salud, 1996). Coverage is purchased through the Instituto Mexicano de Seguro Social (IMSS) for private sector workers and through separate organizations for federal and state civil servants (the Instituto de Seguridad y Servicios Sociales de los Trabajadores del Estado, or ISSSTE), the armed forces, and employees of the national oil company (PEMEX).

The second component includes governmental organizations providing services for the uninsured population (MOH, IMSS-Solidaridad, and so on), which cover approximately 43 percent of the total population, mainly the rural and urban poor (National Economic Research Associates, 1998; World Bank, 1995). The most important institution involved in the provision of services for this population is the MOH, which is responsible for meeting the health care needs of almost half the population. However, MOH spending represents only about 12 percent of national expenditures.

The third component, the private sector, is made up of a diverse collection of health care providers working in hospitals, pharmacies, HMOs, ambulatory clinics, and physicians' private offices. The private sector also includes practitioners of folk medicine. Financially, this sector is about the same size as the social security system, accounting for approximately 44 percent of all expenditures, financed largely through direct out-of-pocket, fee-for-service payments.

Financing and Flow of Funds

Mexico has a population of approximately 92 million persons, making it the third-largest country in the Western Hemisphere. Although 75 percent of its inhabitants live in urban areas, approximately 12 percent dwell in 140,000 scattered and very small rural communities. According to the World Bank classification, Mexico is an "upper middle-income country," with a GNP per capita in 1995 of US$3,320—the eighth highest in Latin America and the Caribbean (World Bank, 1997).

Mexico devotes about US$20 billion per year or 5.3 percent of its GDP to health care services (World Bank, 1997). This translates to per capita annual health spending of US$223.

Over the past ten years, the Mexican government has made steady progress in increasing health expenditures, in real terms, although this trend was reversed during the 1994–95 recession. Mexico's spending on health is low relative to industrialized countries but is similar to most other middle-income nations in Latin America.

Public Sector Financing

Public institutions in Mexico are financed through three basic mechanisms:

1. The agencies for the uninsured population are almost completely financed with resources from the federal budget.
2. IMSS, the agency for workers in the private sector, draws its resources from worker and employer contributions and a federal subsidy. Until 1997, approximately 25 percent of this agency's revenues came from worker contributions, 70 percent from employer contributions, and the rest from the federal government (Banco Interamericano de Desarrallo, 1997).
3. Social security benefits for civil servants, the armed forces, and other government-related groups are financed through employer-employee contributions and a federal subsidy.

The relative contributions of various funders are shown in Figure 20.2.

The largest public funder is the federal government (20 percent of expenditures), which finances health care services through the following mechanisms:

- Direct provision of health care services to the poor and uninsured
- Contributions to social security benefits for civil servants
- A subsidy to IMSS for private workers

State spending on health care in Mexico is relatively minor, accounting for less than 5 percent of overall expenditures. Most of this goes toward the states' share of operating MOH public health clinics based on agreements with the federal government.

FIGURE 20.1. THE MEXICAN HEALTH CARE SYSTEM.

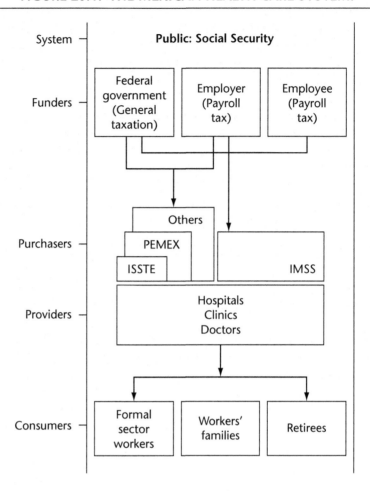

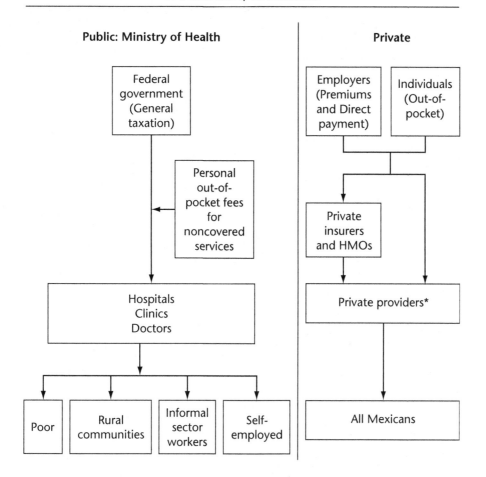

Public: Ministry of Health

Private

*Many of these providers are also employed by the social security system and by the Ministry of Health.

FIGURE 20.2. PUBLIC HEALTH CARE EXPENDITURE BY INSTITUTION.

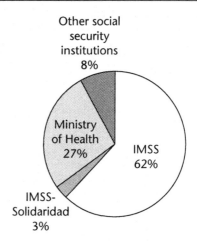

Private Sector Financing

A payroll tax is levied on employers and employees in the formal economy (for example, industrial workers, service sector employees, and bureaucrats) to help fund social security benefits, including health care, for a large segment of the working population and their families. In the future, a greater proportion of the burden for this program will be shifted to the federal government through social security reforms.

A large percentage (43 percent) of health care expenditures in Mexico are made by individual consumers (Frenk and Gonzalez-Block, 1997). Most of this spending represents out-of-pocket payments to private providers. This burden appears to have a disproportionate impact on the poor, with the poorest households spending 5.8 percent of their incomes on direct payments for medical care, compared with only 2.8 percent spent by the wealthiest ones (Frenk, 1997).

The private health insurance industry in Mexico is currently very small, accounting for only 2 percent of all expenditures. Health insurance is much more common in the north of Mexico and in urban rather than rural areas. Overall, private health insurance coverage is about 3 percent in urban areas and 0.7 percent in rural areas (Knaul, Parker, and Ramírez, 1997). Observers see tremendous opportunity in this relatively undeveloped market, with potential growth of up to ten times its current status. Because of concerns with the social security system, some employers offer additional or duplicate coverage to employees or absorb the costs of workers purchasing care in the private sector. Nearly 70 percent of those having private health insurance also have coverage under one of the social security agencies (Frenk and Gonzalez-Block, 1997).

In response to a growing demand for private health coverage, several managed care organizations (MCOs) have appeared in Mexico over the past five years. The largest of these—Meximed and Premedica—have benefited from foreign investment, primarily from the United States, Spain, and Chile.

Public Purchasers and Providers

In contrast to the separation of purchasing and delivery functions in the United States, public agencies in Mexico both finance care for their populations and provide that care directly in their own independent "vertically integrated delivery systems." Each of these systems has its own network of hospitals, physicians, and clinics that theoretically cover the entire continuum of care, from prevention to tertiary care services. Hospitals are owned by each system, and doctors are salaried employees. Many publicly employed physicians also operate their own private practices, catering to those who can afford to pay out of pocket for medical care.

Social Security

Several social security agencies finance and provide health care services for specific groups of Mexicans working in the formal economy, most of whom live in urban areas. These are discussed in the sections to follow.

Instituto Mexicano de Seguro Social (IMSS). Of the nationally financed health care systems, IMSS is by far the largest. It provides health coverage for approximately 40 percent of the Mexican population (about 36 million persons), including workers in the formal sector, their families, and retirees.

Although IMSS does not finance care for self-employed persons or workers in the informal sector (for example, small businesses or agricultural workers), it does offer a voluntary "buy-in" program. Until recently however, few Mexicans took advantage of this program due to high premiums (US$38 per month) and cumbersome enrollment paperwork, as well as a preference for private sector care.

Social security reforms are attempting to increase IMSS coverage by introducing a substantial public subsidy toward the cost of purchasing coverage and simplifying the enrollment process (Fundación para la Salud, 1995).

Primary care in IMSS is provided through over 1,400 family care units; secondary and tertiary care are provided in the system's 215 general and 41 specialty hospitals. IMSS also operates 10 medical complexes, where as many as 30 hospitals are grouped together (National Economic Research Associates, 1998; World Bank, 1995).

In managing such a large health care system, IMSS faces multiple service delivery problems, many of which are being addressed by current reforms. Consequently, many employers and employees neglect to pay their full contributions to IMSS through under-reporting salaries. About one-third of eligible beneficiaries pay out of pocket to receive their care in the private sector. This is further encouraged by the fact that many physicians who work in IMSS use the system as a referral mechanism for their private practices, where they earn direct fees for service (National Economic Research Associates, 1998).

Instituto de Seguridad y Servicios Sociales de los Trabajadores del Estado (ISSSTE). ISSSTE covers employees of the federal government, several government-owned *parastatals,* and municipal and state governments. Approximately 10 percent of the population, or 8.8 million persons, receive services through ISSSTE. ISSSTE is not as well funded as IMSS, with spending of US$58 per member per year (National Economic Research Associates, 1998).

Other Agencies. Other social security agencies include those for the armed forces (SEDENA for the army and air force and SDM for the navy) and Petroleos Mexicanos (PEMEX), which provides health services to employees of the national oil corporation. Together these schemes cover about 2 percent of the population.

Ministry of Health (MOH)

The MOH is at the heart of the Mexican public health system. In Mexico it is known as the Secretaria de Salud (SSA) and serves multiple roles, including setting national health policy and regulating the health care system. The MOH also provides direct medical services to approximately 27.5 million poor Mexicans through an extensive network of facilities ranging from small, rural primary care clinics to highly specialized tertiary hospitals (Poder Ejecutivo Federal, 1995).

Funding for the MOH comes from general federal tax revenue, with a small contribution from state governments. In 1996 MOH spending was approximately

US$19 per covered person and US$51 per user (National Economic Research Associates, 1998), highlighting how few of those who are eligible for the system actually use it.

The MOH has accomplished a great deal in recent years. It has provided access to care for millions of the rural poor, dramatically increased immunization levels for children, and created salary incentives for physicians to serve in rural areas. Patients, however, have limited choices of providers, and they complain about the quality of services, availability of drugs, and long waiting times.

On average, only half of hospital beds in MOH-run hospitals are occupied due to low demand and poor management. Doctors working in these hospitals and clinics often see fewer than one patient per hour, further aggravating the system's chronic problems of quality, accessibility, and low productivity (Fundación Mexicana para la Salud, 1995). Like IMSS, the MOH has a highly centralized structure that contributes to inefficient operation and allocation of resources.

Recognizing the inefficiencies in its system, in 1983 the MOH began to devolve responsibility for health care services to the states. All thirty-two states now receive funding from the MOH and in turn operate their own health care clinics and other facilities for the poor.

IMSS-Solidaridad

The Special Basic Health Program for the Uninsured, or IMSS-Solidaridad, provides health coverage and services to 11 million Mexicans living in poor rural communities. Funding for IMSS-Solidaridad comes almost exclusively from the federal government. Annual expenditures per covered person are only US$21. The program operates 3,450 clinics and 67 hospitals in more than 1,000 localities (National Economic Research Associates, 1998; World Bank, 1995).

Private Providers

The private sector, which includes physician practices, outpatient clinics, and hospital facilities, receives nearly half of health spending in Mexico. This sector, which is more heavily concentrated in the ambulatory care market, is growing rapidly with minimal regulation from any formal body. Most private providers charge patients or purchasers on a fee-for-service basis.

Approximately one-third of working physicians are employed in the private sector, with many working simultaneously in IMSS or MOH. These physicians are highly "atomized," that is, operating independently and often contracting with multiple hospitals and clinics (Fundación Mexicana para la Salud, 1995).

Thirty-six percent of Mexican hospitals are private, but only 20 percent of hospital beds are private. Private hospitals, many of which are maternity clinics, average only twelve beds per facility. Private hospitals may be for-profit, nonprofit, or religiously affiliated. A small charitable sector provides services to the poor through the Red Cross and other organizations (Fundación Mexicana para la Salud, 1995).

Many Mexicans, especially those living in rural parts of the country, continue to rely on indigenous folk healers to treat their medical problems. Unfortunately, few estimates are available on the numbers of these practitioners, the proportion of Mexicans who visit them, or payments for their services.

Health Status

Like most middle-income countries, Mexico is undergoing an economic and demographic transition that affects all sectors of society and will have a significant impact on health care delivery.

Mexico's population is growing, but the growth rate has decreased considerably in the last two decades. Life expectancy is increasing, and the elderly population is rapidly growing in relative and absolute size (Banco Interamericano de Desarrallo, 1997). Mexico will witness important changes in its age structure in the decades ahead. The proportion of people under fifteen is expected to decrease from 39 percent in 1990 to 30 percent in 2030. In contrast, the number of adults over sixty will triple to 11 million during this same time period (Fundación Mexicana para la Salud, 1995). The population under age five still accounts for one-third of the disease burden, with losses mostly due to premature death from communicable diseases (Frenk and Gonzalez-Block, 1997).

Over the past fifty years, the Mexican health care system has made significant headway toward solving many of the problems associated with poverty and development. Sixty years ago, one out of every two deaths occurred before the age of five; today, only one out of seven deaths occurs in this age group (Frenk and Gonzalez-Block, 1997).

Like many countries, Mexico now faces a protracted epidemiological transition. Common infections and other pretransitional ailments, though decreasing, have not been fully controlled, while noncommunicable diseases and injuries already represent the main causes of death and disability. The country is also confronting emerging and reemerging problems (for example, the HIV-AIDS epidemic and the health effects of environmental pollution), all of which compete for the scarce resources of the health care system.

As a result, the Mexican health care system must address diseases associated with underdevelopment, such as common infections, malnutrition, and maternal and perinatal deaths, as well as reemerging problems such as cholera, malaria, dengue fever, and tuberculosis (Frenk, Gonzalez-Block, Lozano, 1997). At the same time, health problems associated with industrialization and urbanization, including cardiovascular disease, chronic conditions, mental illness, substance abuse, and violence, are rapidly emerging as important public health threats. In 1991, the three major causes of death were cardiovascular diseases, accidents, and cancer (Fundación Mexicana para la Salud, 1995).

Health Care Regulation

The Mexican government, through the MOH, has the responsibility of regulating the health care system. There is minimal enforcement, however, of MOH rules and regulations. The private sector in particular operates with very little outside monitoring. Responsibility for licensing health professionals falls on institutions of higher education rather than on the MOH. Licensure of general practitioners—a legal requirement for practicing medicine—requires only a professional examination administered by the school of medicine of origin, which is eventually endorsed by the Ministry of Public Education. In 1994, the National Center for the Evaluation of Higher Education was created. It developed the National Examination of Professional Quality for several professions, including medicine, which is already being used by several universities as a graduation requisite and by others as a graduation option (Luna, Barrera, and Mandujano, 1998).

Certification of specialists is conducted by specialty boards that are coordinated by the National Academy of Medicine. A physician's lack of certification in a specialty, however, poses no legal restriction for practicing in that or any other specialized field of medicine.

Observers and participants in the Mexican health care system have noted the need to improve the quality of training for health care professionals and to improve the balance of nurses to physicians and generalists to specialists. Currently no agency attempts to formally or informally shape the medical workforce.

Certification of health care facilities in Mexico has been limited to registration. In 1993, the Mexican Commission of Hospital Certification was created. It is a nongovernmental, nonprofit organization that is promoting voluntary certification using standards for three different complexity levels for health care facilities: low, medium, and high.

In terms of the regulation of other key inputs, few policies exist to regulate medical technology, most of which is imported from other countries. The Mexican government regulates neither the safety nor the efficacy of medical devices or medical equipment, resulting in the indiscriminate adoption of technologies that may or may not be safe, useful, or cost-effective (Freeman, Gómez-Dantés, and Frenk, 1995).

Although a structure is in place to regulate the use and distribution of pharmaceuticals, intrasectoral systems for purchasing and distributing medicines are regarded as highly inefficient and the cause of periodic shortages.

Challenges

Mexico has made considerable progress in reducing mortality, expanding coverage, providing financial protection through the social security system, training capable health care workers, and conducting scientific research. The health care system, however, still faces several challenges.

• *Shortages of infrastructure and support personnel.* Compared to the United States and to other Latin American countries, Mexico has fewer hospital beds (.8 beds per 1,000 population) (World Bank, 1997). Although the absolute number of beds may be appropriate given the average length of stay and admission rates, the distribution of these beds is highly uneven, with most facilities concentrated in urban areas. This can result in acute shortages in southern states with a high proportion of the indigenous population.

The supply of nursing staff in Mexico is relatively scarce and, as is true of hospitals and physicians, nurses are more prevalent in cities.

• *Lack of access to basic health care services and inequity.* A consequence of the shortages described is that many Mexicans have limited access to health care services. According to official figures, 10 percent of the population in 1995 had no regular access to basic health care services (Fundación Mexicana para la Salud, 1995). If economic and organizational barriers are considered, at least 20 percent of the Mexican population has no regular access to basic health services (Frenk, Lozano, and González-Block, 1998).

• *Inefficiency and duplication.* Because each public sector system operates its own independent delivery system, there is significant duplication of resources, particularly in urban areas. Excess capacity is especially problematic given the scarcity in nurses. Parallel and fragmented systems create waste where planning and coordination could help to stretch these resources.

At the same time, the distribution of physicians in Mexico is unequal. More than 15 percent of qualified doctors are either unemployed or underemployed; many physicians, particularly those in the public sector, exhibit low levels of productivity (Frenk and Gonzalez-Block, 1997).

Inefficiencies are also manifest in the centralized organization of the major public programs. Centralized "top-down" management and inflexible line-item budgeting tends to inhibit local innovation; this prevents the creative use of strategies to improve health status and perpetuates outdated approaches.

There is also little incentive or accountability for performance or efficiency. Mechanisms for referring patients and for purchasing and distributing medicines and supplies are widely regarded as ineffective.

• *Quality of care and service.* Each of the public sector systems operates like a monopoly, providing little consumer choice and few incentives for responsiveness or quality of care. Many public sector hospitals are deteriorating in terms of infrastructure, personnel, essential drugs, and supplies. Neither public nor private facilities are subject to any process of accreditation that verifies their capacity to provide an acceptable standard of care; consequently, the quality of hospital services varies widely.

Plans and Proposals for Reform

A reform process to address the challenges began in the early 1980s. Political and economic difficulties in the late 1980s and early 1990s, however, hindered its progress. Renewed efforts are now under way. Past administrations have attempted to improve the quality, efficiency, and equity of the system through the implementation of health sector reform, which includes changes in the social security agencies and the Ministry of Health.

Social Security Reforms

The recently approved changes in the social security system may lead to a gradual separation between financing and delivery of services and a shift to a more pluralistic delivery system that enhances consumer choice. The goals of these reforms are to stimulate competition, improve equity, enhance patient satisfaction, reduce employer financial burdens, and raise the efficiency of service delivery.

Most important, the reforms will facilitate the following:

• *Expanded health coverage.* Members of the informal economy (for example, self-employed persons, small business owners) will be encouraged to participate in IMSS through a new plan financed with workers' contributions and a subsidy from the federal government. In the first four months of its implementation, this measure allowed the incorporation of 20,000 new families to the IMSS. An additional incorporation of 300,000 families is expected in the next three years (Institute Mexicano del Seguro Social, 1998).

- *Shift in financial burden.* A new financial scheme will be introduced for IMSS that will increase the government's subsidy of this agency from 5 percent of its annual budget to approximately 39 percent. Employer and employee contributions will be reduced from 70 and 25 percent to 52 and 9 percent, respectively (Institute Mexicano del Seguro Social, 1998).
- *Strengthening managerial and financial systems.* IMSS is preparing to improve the efficiency and productivity of its network of providers through several measures. Financing and provision are being separated, and decentralization will be achieved through the creation of local medical zones that will serve the health needs of defined geographical populations of approximately 200,000 (Institute Mexicano del Suguro Social, 1998). In addition, IMSS hospitals will move gradually toward greater financial and managerial autonomy. In support of this, hospital financing will move from fixed historical budgeting to reimbursement based on DRG (Institute Mexicano del Seguro Social, 1998).

Ministry of Health Reforms

The reforms of the MOH include the following (Poder Ejecutivo Federal, 1995):

- The decentralization of health services for the uninsured population, which was initiated in 1987, has been restarted with the allocation of federal resources to the states based on a formula that includes mortality and poverty indicators.
- The delivery of a package of twelve interventions to Mexicans who have limited access to basic health services will be developed.

Private Sector Reforms

The government is encouraging the private sector to develop new models of health care fund management and provision of care. Legislation outlining the rules for health plan insurance, risk allocation, and managed care organizations have been approved by the senate.

Opportunities for Investment

Mexico offers one of the best potential markets for new investment in health care within Latin America. Although it is not the largest market, the government is focused on reorienting its health care system and exploring new models for health care delivery. The market is opening to fresh investment in health care to increase access to the country's large population (Doulton, 1998).

Managed care models still have potential in Mexico, although, as Paul Doulton points out, the opinion of one Mexican leader is that "HMOs have long passed their sell-date, so don't foist them off on us" (Doulton, 1998). Doulton goes on to argue, however, that managed care may offer a "bulging tool chest of well proven processes, such as outcomes improvement, metrics geared toward client satisfaction and many others that new and existing investors in Mexico can use to enormous advantage in building a differentiated health care business."

Trade liberalization through the North American Free Trade Agreement (NAFTA) has significantly increased the interest of U.S. firms in the Mexican health care sector. Several U.S. firms that have established and are managing health care facilities in Mexico have decided to extend their operations to all twenty Mexican cities with populations greater than 500,000. In these cities, about 20 percent of the population can afford to purchase private health care services (Gómez-Dantés and Frenk, 1995; Bryant, 1994; Carlino, 1994).

Eighty percent of the respondents to a Mexican Health Foundation survey agreed that NAFTA had favorably changed the investment horizon for conducting business in the Mexican health care sector (Gómez-Dantés and Frenk, 1995). Ninety percent of these respondents also felt that there was potential for significant market share in Mexico for their service or product. Survey respondents identified hospitals, clinics, and HMOs as the most profitable sectors of the Mexican health care market (Gómez-Dantés and Frenk, 1995).

Conclusion

As a strong middle-income country with a government committed to enhancing its health care system, Mexico offers good investment potential for insurers and providers. However, the country has a powerful trade union structure and is rooted in the philosophy that access to health care is the right of every citizen. Recent attempts to privatize the power industry have met with strong union protests, and attempts to introduce market forces into health care have even stronger opponents. Political pressure to protect the rights of the poor and of workers will remain a critical issue; strong controls on the market are likely to be introduced, along with liberalizing legislation. All of this, however, should not deter those who are interested in a long-term investment horizon and are committed to building Mexico's capacity to provide affordable, quality health care services for its population.

References

Banco Interamericano de Desarrallo. *Progresso económico y social en América Latina: Informe 1997: América Latina tras una década reformes.* Washington, D.C.: Banco Interamericano de Desarrallo, 1997.

Bryant, J. "Mexico Ready to Ride the NAFTA Wave." *Clinica,* 1994, *620,* 10–11.

Carlino, M. "Outpatient Care: U.S. Companies Respond to Mexican Demand for Quality Health Care." *El Financiero* (international ed.), 1994, pp. 10–11.

Doulton, P. "Latin America: Building Business in Pharmaceuticals and Healthcare." *Financial Times Reports,* 1998.

Freeman, P., Gómez-Dantés, O., and Frenk, J. *Health Systems in an Era of Globalization: Challenges and Opportunities for North America.* Washington, D.C.: Institute of Medicine, 1995.

Frenk, J. (ed.). *Observatorio de la Salud: Necesidades, serviccios, politicas.* Mexico City: Fundación Mexicana para la Salud, 1997.

Frenk, J., and González-Block, M. A. "Health Reform in Mexico." *Eurohealth,* 1997, *3,* 38–39.

Frenk, J., González-Block, M. A., and Lozano, R. "The Latin Progression." *Odyssey,* 1997, *3,* 14–21.

Frenk, J., Lozano, R., and González-Block, M. A. "Seis tesis equivocadas sobre las politicas de salud en el combate a la pobrecia." *Este País,* 1998, *84,* 28–36.

Fundación Mexicana para la Salud. *Health and the Economy: Proposals for Progress in the Mexican Health Care System.* Mexico City: Fundación Mexicana para la Salud, 1995.

Fundación Mexicana para la Salud. *Health and the Economy: Proposals for Progress in the Mexican Health Care System.* (2nd ed.) Mexico City: Fundación Mexicana para la Salud, 1996.

Gómez-Dantés, O., and Frenk, J. "NAFTA and Health Services: Initial Data." In P. Freeman, O. Gómez-Dantés, and J. Frenk (eds.), *Health Systems in an Era of Globalization: Challenges and Opportunities for North America.* Washington, D.C.: Institute of Medicine, 1995.

Institute Mexicano del Seguro Social. *55 años: Hacia el siglo XXI, hechos y perspectivas.* Mexico City: Instituto Mexicano del Seguro Social, 1998.

Knaul, F., Parker, S., and Ramírez, R. "El prepago por servicios médicos privados en México: Determinantes socio-económicos y cambios a través del tiempo." In J. Frenk (ed.), *Observatorio de la salud: Necesidades, servicios, politicas.* Mexico City: Fundación Mexicana para la Salud, 1997.

Luna, A., Barrera, O., and Mandujano, L. "Capacidad universitaria en duda." *Universitarios,* 1998, 12–18.

National Economic Research Associates. *The Health Care System in Mexico.* London: Pharmaceutical Partners for Better Healthcare, 1998.

Poder Ejecutivo Federal. *Programa de Reforma del Sector Salud,* 1995–2000. Mexico City: Poder Ejecutivo Federal, 1995.

Sistema Nacional de Salud. *Boletin de información estadistica, recursos y servicios,* no.14. Mexico City: Sistema Nacional de Salud, 1994.

World Bank. *Staff Appraisal Report, Mexico: Second Basic Health Care Project.* Washington, D.C.: World Bank, 1995.

World Bank. *Sector Strategy Paper: Health, Nutrition and Population.* Washington, D.C.: World Bank, 1997.

CHAPTER TWENTY-ONE

CULTURE CLASH

A Case Study of Mexico

Keith F. Batchelder, Laurence Dene McGriff

Valuable lessons can be learned by assessing an international business that failed—a start-up HMO that at one time was positioned to become a major managed care company in Mexico. Millions were spent on the project, and some of the richest, smartest, and most successful people in the world were involved. It started in 1994 with a flourish and faded away to nothing four years later, with the trial and imprisonment of the mastermind who conceived and developed the project. Ultimately, this is a lesson in the clash of cultures and plans gone awry.

The U.S. Board of Directors

The business began when a group from Harvard University, from both the medical school and public health school, formed a company to develop international health care businesses in Latin America. The board of directors of the company was very high-profile and included a prominent Harvard physician with public health credentials and international contacts, a full professor and former department chairman, an MIT professor who is one of the better-known experts in finance and IPOs, a deputy attorney general of the United Nations, and a prominent businessman. The leader, Yamil Kouri, was a well-trained Cuban American physician who was a master communicator in English and Spanish—a man who was able to sell his vision and gain access to some of the wealthiest men in the world.

The Corporation

The Cambridge, Massachusetts-based corporation was developing a variety of businesses in different countries in Latin America. It had successful radiology businesses in the Dominican Republic and had expanded in Mexico from its radiology practice in the third-largest hospital in Mexico City by purchasing a network of radiology centers. The corporation was actively developing business in Puerto Rico and other countries. The goal was to bring high-quality health care and technology transfer to Latin America by technology, medical organization, practice, and health care financing—specifically, managed care.

The Mexican Corporation

The Mexican Corporation, known both as Harvard Health Care de Mexico (HCC) and Harvard Salud Integral, was the entity formed to run the HMO. It consisted of representatives from the U.S. corporation and "local" Mexican partners: a very wealthy Mexican banker, a Mexican businessman who owned a variety of firms and industries, and prominent local physicians. The project consumed a lot of financial resources prior to beginning operations and was always looking for new business partners. Discussions occurred with wealthy individuals and large insurance companies, and eventually secured additional funding from one of the wealthiest families in Mexico and Latin America.

The Vision

The project was driven by the vision of one man—the Cuban American physician. The business plan was broad and at one time was projected to cost in excess of $100 million. This resonated with both the investors and physicians who were recruited to build the organization. The plan included the purchase of two managed care networks that were already in operation in Mexico, a PPO, and a staff model HMO. The plan included the construction of multispecialty and primary care clinics around Mexico City and other major cities. The details of the "reversion" in the Mexican health care system required enrollment at the employer level, not the individual level. Wholesale contracts could be negotiated for (theoretically) millions of covered lives at once. Not included in this investment was the acquisition of or partnership with a tertiary hospital such as ABC Hospital in Mexico City. The plan would focus attention on the proprietary network where there would be greater control of costs. It was anticipated that lower-income people from the social security reversion would enroll in the "closed" Harvard network. The idea was that the wealthy (fee-for-service patients) would enroll due to the availability of state-of-the-art, multispecialty centers where the finest doctors in Mexico would practice.

The Provider Network

The HMO had a unique method of building the provider network. The idea was to approach the finest, most prestigious physicians in the country and obtain their support by allowing them to manage the medical side. This was a unique strategy and was incredibly persuasive; commitments were secured from the leaders in the academic and hospital community. These physicians were going to be given space in a new, deluxe, state-of-the-art, six-story center where they could continue with their private practice (mostly for the elite, private fee-for-service). In addition, they would be responsible for bringing in young physicians. This was very important for Mexico, where credentialing did not follow any objective criteria. To maintain quality health care, the personal endorsement of an elite physician was needed in order to hire a new physician who would be delivering services. In this sense, the HMO understood the Latin mentality very well, that is, the importance of getting the medical elite on the side of the project rather than opposing it in order to get the cooperation of the young physicians. Kouri also understood the importance of having all medical affairs managed by physicians answering to physicians. The elite physicians would function almost like department chairs of a large medical center, handling most of the problems (quality and cost) with physicians in their department or specialty. Construction began on an expensive, luxurious, state-of-the-art clinic in one of the most elite districts of Mexico City.

It will never be known whether this approach would have worked. The physician leaders would have had to move their existing practice to the new facility and taken on the tremendous job of recruiting and overseeing doctors, not just in Mexico City but across the country. In exchange, they were offered stock options, salaries, free space, and staffing. There was much speculation over how it would have worked, as other "external" events led to the derailment of Harvard Health Care de Mexico.

Because Mexico is the closest Latin country to the United States, both physicians and patients were very familiar with managed care, including all of the horror stories and bad press that HMOs were getting in the United States. It was not an easy sell to the average physician. The doctors were skeptical, but again, they were promised so much. Promises of future profit sharing were made to investors, physician leaders, staff, and providers. Although the HMO had good intentions, the reality was that premiums were low for many participants. The optimism of Latin America allowed this scheme to move forward, with all the parties believing that if only some expectations were met, it would be a great enterprise.

Model Questioned

This HMO was a "mixed model," involving components of an IPA and staff model health plan. In order to build confidence in the health plan, the management team recruited independent outside experts to conduct an analysis. One group hired to review the plan was United HealthCare. When United HealthCare began its work, the HMO and the delivery system were intermingled, and it was impossible to determine whether either would be profitable. When at the insistence of the UHC consultants the two were separated, the staff model was still paramount. Despite recommendations that a staff model was an expensive and risky strategy, it was still promoted as the center point of the plan. The consultants pointed out that even Harvard Community Health Plan (HHC's model) had failed and Kaiser in California was struggling. The HMO leadership decided to retain the original business approach, despite seasoned international advice to alter some core strategies.

Consultants explained that the difficulty with a "closed model" is that the elite want freedom of choice and do not want to be forced into a clinic setting, no matter how well appointed. HHC countered that patients would go to the elite multispecialty clinics because the doctors were the "best" in Mexico. Arguments suggesting that unless "their" doctor was in the network patients would stay away were ignored. At this point, it became clear that HHC's leadership did not appreciate how intensely the elite patient wants freedom of choice. The plan was to develop multispecialty clinics strategically in the capital and major cities of the country.

HHC was idealistic, naïve, and based on American models of twenty years ago. Enrollment included a proposed multiphasic screening for nearly everyone, with treadmill testing, extensive laboratories, and more. After a careful analysis of the costs, the consultants told them it would take 40 percent of their premium just for "prevention." A problem often observed in Latin America is the belief that appropriate care means that every person, of no matter what age, should have a complete physical every year. Although noble, this idea was based on what HMOs in the United States did thirty years ago and is highly impractical.

HHC proposed building several large, multispecialty centers in Mexico City in the higher socioeconomic areas. Many consultants, including those from UHC, tried to explain that the elite, no matter how good and modern these centers were, would not go there unless their physician was there. The same centers would be too expensive and elegant for the "middle class," which could be directed to more practical centers, and the HHC could never recover their construction and operational costs. In Latin America, the lower classes will accept the trade-off of being limited to a network in exchange for more comprehensive coverage. The problem is the huge difference between what the elite can pay (U.S. rates, essentially) and what those with middle incomes—less than $20 a month—can pay.

The real volume for any HMO in Mexico is in the population that comes from the social security "opt-out" (new legislation allowing a *reversión de quota*). The elite class will not mix with the working class; they live in different neighborhoods and use different providers. Harvard Health Care remained steadfast in their failure to integrate the different socioeconomic classes of people they were serving. Yes, the elite would expect to go to ABC hospital, but the average person would not. If they had that expectation, the health plan could not afford the high cost of care in these expensive facilities.

Again, there is a huge difference between an elite hospital such as ABC, which charges almost U.S. rates, and an average hospital that charges around $100 a day. The problem with many health plans abroad is that the providers running the health plan want to provide high levels of care with limited budgets. They want to use the best specialists and the best hospitals, pay the doctors very well so they will give better or "preferred" care to their patients, provide the most comprehensive preventive services, and so on, with little insight into the impact all that would have on their budget.

Medical Management and Systems

Harvard Health never had the opportunity to put medical management into effect beyond the networks they purchased. These networks represented the opposite of what they were developing—providers who were willing to see patients at a low negotiated fee and willing to accept the restrictions the medical director put on them in terms of authorizations and length of stay. One would suspect that they would have had much more difficulty getting their "elite" physicians to accept the same limitations.

The United HealthCare advisers tried to convince the plan to buy adequate information systems. The claims processing, clinical information, and business management systems were originally expected to run from Microsoft Access Databases. After demonstrating the failure of the existing systems to manage costs and risks, and explaining the problems of scaling to millions of lives, a novel mix of

U.S. and Mexican systems was selected. Problems associated with localization (for example, Spanish as opposed to English, the peso as opposed to the dollar) and multisystem integration were defined and work was begun. A contract was signed with ERISCO to purchase their client-server claims processing system. Demonstration production systems were implemented, but fully licensed versions waited for funding that was never put into place. Money was allocated for infrastructure but was not spent. MIS installation waited for patient enrollment.

Again, a weakness in Latin America is the lack of use of diagnosis and treatment codes, criteria, protocols, and so on. The typical way to control costs is to preauthorize treatment and then have an auditor-physician follow each inpatient. This can be done because these doctors do not earn much money, although the process is labor-intensive, involving regular physician visits to the hospital. It can also cause a lot of strife with the admitting physician, just the way it does in the United States. This form of medical management only focuses on the high-cost items, not the high-volume items such as primary care and specialist outpatient visits, laboratory, X-rays, and drugs. As patient care volume increases, standards-based, automated systems are necessary to capture and interpret utilization data. A major point of the UHC review of HHC was that the only way to get their "arms around" utilization and referrals and be able to educate their providers was with a system that would give them comparative data.

Conflict

HHC leadership had sold the idea to the Mexican staff, investors, and leaders that the model was the best approach—building clinics, buying hospitals, and so on. However, it was repeatedly pointed out that the model would not work due to the high cost of bricks, mortar, equipment, and salaries. Further, the staff model side, including the cost of all of the facilities, salaries, and so forth, were still intermingled in the minds and accounting books with the HMO. Another concern of the consultants was the need for the HMO and staff model to be separated, not only to avoid conflicting incentives but to be able to manage each business and know how it is performing as a stand-alone entity. HHC's response was to create separation in terms of budget pro formas but not staffing. The same people were in charge of the delivery and insurance side of the business, so HHC understood the importance of separating the business in practice, but only for the investors.

One of the biggest areas of conflict with the Mexicans was over the way care was delivered. Once the clinics and centers were separated from the rest of the business, it became obvious from the spreadsheet models that HHC was going to lose a lot of money. So they finally compromised. Consultants suggested proven workflow models using at least three exam rooms per doctor so people could be moved through rapidly. HHC countered, saying that was not the way they practiced in Mexico—only one exam room, off to the side of the doctor's spacious office, was needed; no compromise was ever in the offing. Consultants proposed that a physician should see a patient every ten minutes. HHC argued for thirty minutes and compromised at twenty, probably the maximum for one exam room per physician. U.S. data were presented supporting the concept that it was not necessary to have a laboratory and an X-ray department in each primary care center because there was not enough volume to justify it. At least a nurse could be assigned to do the job rather than hire a full-time laboratory technician as well as a full-time X-ray technician. HHC disagreed and got their way. It was very difficult for elite physicians who wanted to build a quality system for their privileged friends to understand that this model would not work as a business that must deal with many average people with very little money.

Conflict arose continually over the shortage of money during the "establishment" of the HMO. Harvard Health had hired some talented and experienced staff from within Mexico (and these businessmen, doctors, actuaries, and so on were expensive). The staff would expand from a core group of ten or so up to fifty or sixty and then retract again when money ran short. The company was liquidated twice in order to get rid of old investors and make room for new ones. This also allowed them to get out of debts, either by not paying them or settling for cents on the dollar. This restructuring affected both of the authors, as they worked with HHC.

Plan Unravels

The start-up phase continued for nearly four years. Money to finish the construction of the showplace clinic in the Santa Fe region of Mexico City came in spurts. Staffing fluctuated. Meanwhile, the visionary promoter made presentations to one investment group after another. But any company who did due diligence discovered that Dr. Kouri was under investigation by a federal grand jury for offenses that were unrelated to HHC. This was enough to scare off most institutional investors from the United States, but not Mexican investors. We estimate that over the four-year start-up period, about $20 million went into the project.

Once Kouri received a formal U.S. federal indictment, the HMO began to unravel quickly because no one else could hold the project together once he was gone. There was certainly a cloud over the entire undertaking. HHC tried to hold it together for a few months, but without Dr. Kouri's leadership and vision, the project crumbled.

Conclusion

Thus ends what was conceived to be the dominant managed care company in Mexico. At one time Grupo Nacional Provencial (GNP), the largest insurance company in Mexico with 800,000 lives covered by health insurance, as well as other companies, was in heavy negotiations and considered contracting with Harvard Health. ABC Hospital considered a joint venture. Other hospitals were to be purchased by Harvard Health. Some of the most prestigious physicians in the country were courted by the plan and almost persuaded to join in the scheme. It was a unique mix of U.S. and Mexican formulas and would have been an interesting experiment if carried out, especially when it came to the concept of organizing the providers from the top down. It also shows the power of a Latin personality, in the right milieu, who is able to impose his vision on others and sell a very ambitious project to people who pour millions into a plan and then move on to attract more investors once that money is exhausted. Even though Americans with international experience were brought in, HHC seemed to accept advice only on trivial matters or where it was blatantly obvious that the HHC model was unworkable. The Mexican entrepreneurs focused too much on building a staff model while seeking to deliver care in the traditional, inefficient Mexican way.

PART FOUR

PACIFIC BASIN

The Pacific Basin is a region of diverse nations, ranging from the islands of New Zealand and the Philippines to Malaysia to the continent-country of Australia. In this section, contributors analyze the widely varied health care systems of these four countries.

With only about 3 percent of its GDP going toward health services, Malaysia has considerably lower health care expenditures than other developing countries, yet its system is recognized as being the most comprehensive among developing countries. In fact, the level of health enjoyed by its population is almost comparable to that of some developed countries. In Chapter Twenty-Two, Tan Sri Dato' Dr. Abu Bakar Suleiman and Rohaizat bin Yon describe Malaysia's system, which is focused on health promotion and preventive health care programs. The contributors also look at factors likely to influence future development, including Vision 2020—the nation's goal of becoming a developed country by the year 2020.

The Philippines shares many qualities with other developing countries in health care: it has limited sources for funding, and large segments of the population cannot afford access to care. In Chapter Twenty-Three, Benito R. Reverente Jr. discusses the development of HMOs in that country as a viable, sustainable, and cost-effective alternative for the delivery and financing of health care. He notes the differences between HMOs in the Philippines (now numbering thirty-five companies) and in the United States. Finally, he makes a case that what the

Philippines has started may be the wave of the future for health care financing in other developing countries.

Australia is in a unique position in its health care policy environment. It has both a large public sector and, in terms of percentage of population covered, one of the largest private sectors outside the United States. In Chapter Twenty-Four, Russell J. Schneider details the current movement in Australia of private health insurers from their traditional role as passive payers to a position of being active purchasers. Finally, Schneider discusses potential opportunities for growth in the system: managed care, information technologies, effective quality measurement, and management of an aging population.

New Zealand, a member of the Commonwealth of Nations, has modeled its health care system after that of the United Kingdom. State reforms in the 1980s, however, tightened accountability for expenditures of public funds and refocused priorities to reduce disparities in health status between Maori (indigenous New Zealanders) and non-Maori. Chapter Twenty-Five authors Mary-Anne Boyd and Nicolette Sheridan give an overview of New Zealand's heath care system and assess possible reforms for the near future.

CHAPTER TWENTY-TWO

MALAYSIA

Tan Sri Dato' Dr. Abu Bakar Suleiman, Rohaizat bin Yon

Malaysia occupies a central position within Southeast Asia and includes two land masses separated by the South China Sea. Peninsular Malaysia, comprising eleven states, forms the southern tip of the Asian mainland. The states of Sabah and Sarawak lie on Borneo Island along the northern border of Indonesia.

This chapter describes the Malaysian health care system, its systems of delivery and financing, health sector achievements, and the planning and policy framework of the Ministry of Health. The development of the Malaysian health care system reflects the nation's economic well-being and the availability of resources.

Background

The population of Malaysia is multiethnic, with the Malays, Chinese, and Indians forming the major community groups. The population was estimated at 22 million in 1997 and is projected to increase to 32 million by the year 2020. Malaysia's population is relatively young, with 34.5 percent in the zero-to-fourteen age group,

---

Unless otherwise indicated, the statistics cited in this chapter were provided by Malaysia's Ministry of Finance and Ministry of Health and by the World Bank.

61.7 percent between fifteen and sixty-four years of age, and the remaining 3.8 percent in the age group sixty-five and older. Annual population growth rate is 2.3 percent, based on 1997 figures. The poverty rate was 5.3 percent for urban households and 18.6 percent for rural households. Per capita income is US$4,320, with economic growth at 7.8 percent. Inflation and unemployment remain very low.

Health Care

The World Bank estimates that Malaysia's per capita health expenditures in 1990 were about US$67. Malaysia spent about 3 percent of GDP on health services, considerably less than the health expenditures of other developing countries. These low expenditures are attributed to the emphasis on creating a rural health infrastructure and implementing health promotion and preventive health care programs. The budget of the Ministry of Health (MOH) has increased in real terms, but the allocation remains more or less constant, at about 5 percent of the national budget and 2.5 percent of GNP.

Provision

Three levels of government exist in Malaysia: federal, state, and local; public and private health services coexist. In 1995 the country had 8,432 health facilities of different types. The MOH owns 40.5 percent of these facilities, whereas the private sector and non-MOH government ownership make up 59.5 percent.

Rural health services are provided through rural health units designed to cover a population of two to four thousand. People in rural areas have access to comprehensive health services ranging from outpatient curative care to preventive and health promotion services. These relatively inexpensive services are delivered free of charge to the rural population by a mix of personnel, ranging from multipurpose community nurses in rural clinics to trained "health team" members in health centers.

In urban areas, a significant percentage of the population seek care at private clinics and hospitals. Services provided at these facilities are paid for on a fee-for-service basis either by the patients themselves or by a third-party employer. Larger employers provide privately funded medical reimbursement schemes for their workers and family members. The benefits vary greatly, and no comprehensive study of these reimbursement schemes exists.

Primary care in urban areas is delivered through maternal and child health clinics and through general health clinics. To increase the efficiency of service delivery, the concept of a one-stop urban health clinic, similar to the ones in the rural areas, was introduced in the years between 1991 and 1995. These urban health clinics with comprehensive services support a policy separating general outpatient departments from hospitals, thereby permitting hospitals to concentrate on secondary and tertiary care. Although services provided at rural health clinics are free of charge, a nominal user fee is levied at urban health clinics and hospital facilities.

Financing

The majority of health and health-related facilities in Malaysia belong to the public sector and are funded through general taxation from public revenues. In fact, the government provides 76 percent of the funding for health services, with the MOH providing most of that. User fees collected in government hospitals contribute only about 5 percent of the total MOH expenditure.

Other government agencies complement and supplement the role of the Ministry of Health to safeguard the health of the people. The Ministry of Education is responsible for the operation of university hospitals as teaching hospitals. The Ministry of Human Resources inspects factories to enforce regulations designed to protect the safety and health of the workers. Estate hospitals also come under the jurisdiction of the Ministry of Human Resources. The Ministry of Defense provides health services for its own personnel and for the local population around its military cantonments. The Ministry of Home Affairs is involved with ensuring the health of the aborigines through its hospital and jungle medical posts.

The Social Security Organization (SOCSO) has implemented a scheme to provide certain benefits to workers for occupational injury and diseases. The scheme covers only those earning less than about US$800 per month in the private sector, however. The Employee Provident Fund (EPF) allows members to withdraw some of their savings for medical expenses.

Malaysia does not have a national health insurance scheme at this time; nor are private health insurance and managed care organizations (MCOs) in Malaysia currently well developed. Individuals may purchase personal insurance, but out-of-pocket expenditure for private sector care is the norm.

The Ministry of Health

In 1997, the MOH operated a total of 111 hospitals and 7 medical institutions throughout the country. MOH hospitals operate 24,773 acute care beds for secondary and tertiary care, and medical institutions provide 6,692 chronic care beds. The ratio of acute care beds to population is 1.2 to 1,000, compared to a target ratio of 2 to 1,000.

The MOH has adopted a national referral system of ascending technological complexity of hospitals to augment the basic care provided in clinics. Patients who require treatment in a hospital may be referred to the appropriate level (basic or specialist hospital care) based on need. A key objective is to provide equitable service; as a result, basic specialist services are decentralized peripherally to hospitals in the districts.

Private Health Providers

Four decades ago, private health care in Malaysia consisted of a limited number of small private clinics and individually operated family practice or general practice (GP) and specialist clinics, or small private hospitals with only a few beds.

In the last decade, the private sector has begun complementing the government's efforts in health care. In 1980 there were fifty private hospitals with 1,171 beds; by the end of 1997 this number had increased to 197 hospitals with 8,963 beds. Private beds, concentrated in state capitals and urban locations, now represent about 29 percent of the total number of acute care hospital beds in the country. In addition, more than 3,000 private GP clinics in Malaysia provide a range of primary health care services.

The unprecedented growth of Malaysia's private sector in recent years has wide-ranging implications for the public sector and overall health care costs. In conjunction with higher income levels, the expectation of and demand for quality health care have increased, resulting in higher costs for facilities and treatment. The private sector has taken advantage of this demand and is providing the necessary services to meet it. The private sector is able to attract more doctors—especially specialists—from the public sector, causing perennially acute staff shortages in the public sector.

Alternative Medicine

Traditional healers continue to play a significant role within the health care system. The government accepts the practice of these traditional forms of therapy along with orthodox health care. Traditional systems of therapy, including homeopathy, naturopathy, ayurveda, sidha, unani, and ethnic traditional medicine (Malays, Chinese, Indians, and aborigines), are widely practiced and accepted both by rural and urban populations. This is evident from the presence of almost a thousand Chinese *sinseh* shops all over the country and, for the Malays, from the continued existence of traditional healers *(bomoh or dukun),* traditional circumcision attendants *(tok mudim),* and traditional birth attendants *(mak bidan).*

Organizations

Nongovernmental organizations (NGOs) are also important players in the provision of health care services. NGOs are usually associations and societies. They make up the voluntary or informal sector and are often nonprofit organizations.

Health Sector Achievements

Malaysia has greatly improved the health status of its population, dramatically reducing mortality indicators and increasing life expectancy. It compares favorably to other countries in the region. The life expectancy at birth of males and females has increased to 69.5 years and 74.5 years, respectively, while the infant mortality rate has declined from 13 per 1,000 live births in 1990 to 9.5 per 1,000 in 1995. Basic immunization coverage of infants has also improved, from 86 percent to 100 percent (Sarji, 1995).

Morbidity and mortality data indicate that disease patterns are changing. Noncommunicable diseases, which occur most often in urban areas, have supplanted communicable diseases as the leading causes of death. Diseases of the heart, accidents, and cancers are among the most common reasons for admissions to the hospital, whereas diseases of the heart, prenatal complications, accidents, cerebrovascular disease, and cancers are the most common causes of medically certified deaths.

Basic health care through facilities is currently available to and accessible for more than 95 percent of the Peninsular Malaysia population and about 70 percent of the population in Sabah and Sarawak. These coverage estimates would be higher if outreach services such as traveling dispensaries and riverine services, the flying doctor service, mobile health teams, and dental clinics were taken into account.

The MOH has adopted a pragmatic approach to health planning, incorporating a strategy of setting priorities. This strategy has made optimal use of the limited resources available for health. Improvements in the health status of the population are evidence of the success of this approach.

Quality

Quality of care has been an important concern of the MOH. The Quality Assurance Program (QAP) was introduced in 1985 and started with a focus on patient care services. It is gradually being expanded to all services, including public health, pharmaceutical, dental, health engineering, and pathology services. Today, QAP incorporates the principles of TQM to ensure a comprehensive approach to the issue of quality of care.

The government has consistently emphasized quality, most recently with the decision to implement the International Organization for Standardization of 9000 (ISO 9000) in the civil service. ISO 9000 is being implemented in the Health Engineering Division, Planning and Development Division of the Ministry of Health, and some MOH hospitals. A progressively wider application is planned for in the MOH. Some private hospitals have also achieved ISO 9000 certification.

Information Technology

The MOH is building an information technology system for hospitals. To create a truly "paperless hospital," a fully computerized system will be introduced for electronic medical records, telemedicine, and teleconferencing. Application of telemedicine and teleconferencing will be extended in phases to all hospitals to support the government's efforts to develop the Malaysian Multimedia Super Corridor (MSC). The MSC has seven "flagship applications": an electronic government, a smart school, telemedicine, research and development clusters, a national multipurpose card, borderless marketing centers, and worldwide manufacturing webs.

The increasing demand for quality care, continued innovation, and the introduction and acceptance of advanced technology will enable the health sector to become a profitable market for various types of new technologies and products. To guide this development, the MOH has established the Health Technology Assessment Unit, which will work toward ensuring appropriate and cost-effective technology suitable for the country's health care system.

Privatization and Quasi-Market Policies

The Privatization Policy, launched in 1983, initiated the transfer to the private sector of activities traditionally vested with the government. It signaled the government's intention to reduce its presence in the economy, reduce the level and scope of public spending, and allow market forces to govern economic activities. Privatization forms one component of the government's strategy of strengthening the role of the private sector as the engine of economic growth and development.

In line with the government's commitment to encouraging the privatization of government activities, as an initial step the government has privatized nonmedical hospital services at state specialist hospitals and some smaller hospitals in the country. The distribution of drugs and the management and maintenance of Central

Medical Stores have been privatized, as have hospital support services such as cleaning, laundry, waste disposal, and maintenance of engineering and biomedical services. This quasi-market approach is widely known as *corporatization.*

The National Development Policy

The National Development Policy (NDP) stresses the need for balanced development and emphasizes growth with equity that will enable all Malaysians to participate in mainstream economic progress. This is to ensure political stability and national unity. The NDP also references equity, the overcoming of inequalities, human resource development, science and technology development, and protection of the environment.

Health initiatives under the NDP give priority to human resource development and take into account the role of the private sector as the engine of economic growth. The public sector is expected to play a supportive and regulatory role, to maintain quality and standards, and to promote avenues for socioeconomic expansion. The emphasis will be on training and developing a skilled workforce to achieve the targets of the accelerated industrialization program and promote standards of excellence in science and technology.

The Seventh Malaysia Plan (7MP)

During the Seventh Malaysia Plan period (1996–2000), health sector development will continue with the objective of improving the health status of the population. Primary health care continues to focus on equality in health care and equity in health for all groups. A greater emphasis will be placed on health promotion and preventive services in order to balance future expenditures on curative and rehabilitative health care. The mass media and community-based health programs will promote the maintenance of a healthy lifestyle.

Telemedicine is key to transforming Malaysia's health care system and realizing its vision for health. In the future, the health care system will focus on people and services, with technology playing a key enabling role. This will require reshaping a system currently focused largely on illness, facilities, and health care providers into one focused on wellness, people, and the capacity to deliver services directly to where they are needed, including in people's homes.

The technologies involved in telemedicine will enable a more person-focused, integrated, and productive health care system. Through the seamless and almost universal availability of information virtual services, telemedicine will dramatically change the way consumers and health care professionals interact with the health care system of the future. Individuals will access health care services and manage their personal health in an empowered and knowledge-rich environment. As new technologies and services are introduced to directly support front-line personnel, telemedicine will also reshape the working environment of health care professionals.

As telecommunication networks and multimedia technologies develop, health-related transactions will increasingly be provided virtually, maximizing the benefit of new technologies in providing fast, cost-effective services directly to users, regardless of time or place. The dynamic information environment is also expected to create a completely new range of health care and health-related products and services delivered directly to users through multimedia networks.

Vision 2020

Malaysia's progress for the future is now guided by the strategic challenges of Vision 2020, launched in 1991. The ultimate aim is that "by the year 2020, Malaysia can be a united nation, with a confident Malaysian society, infused by strong moral and ethical values, living in a society that is democratic, liberal and tolerant, caring, economically just and equitable, progressive and prosperous, and in full possession of an economy that is competitive, dynamic, robust and resilient" (Sarji, 1995).

To achieve the health component of Vision 2020, policies need to be developed to give priority to and emphasize the creation of health in its broadest sense. As a result, the MOH has formulated its Vision for Health, stating that "Malaysia is to be a nation of healthy individuals, families and communities through a health system that is equitable, affordable, efficient, technologically appropriate, environmentally adaptable and consumer-friendly with emphasis on quality, innovation, health promotion and respect for human dignity, and which promotes individual responsibility and community participation towards an enhanced quality of life" (Sarji, 1995).

Conclusion

The Malaysian health care system, recognized as being the most comprehensive among developing countries, has progressively improved population health status and quality of life since the country attained independence. Both external and internal forces—Vision 2020, Malaysia's development policies, the Multimedia Super Corridor objective, and others—are influencing reforms to the Malaysian health care system. With comparatively low health expenditure, the country has achieved a far better level of health for its population than some other developing countries and a level almost comparable to that of some developed countries.

Reference

Sarji, A.H.A. *Malaysia's Vision 2020*. Kuala Lumpur: Pelanduk Publications, 1995.

CHAPTER TWENTY-THREE

THE PHILIPPINES

Benito R. Reverente Jr.

The Philippines is a developing country in a region that has experienced rapid economic growth in the past fifteen years. The Asian economic crisis of the last two years has caused negative GNP growth in most countries of the region; however, the Philippines has successfully weathered the crisis far better than other countries in the region.

Demographic, Economic, and Health Indicators

The country's population of 74 million people is distributed among 7,100 islands in the eastern part of Southeast Asia. The people are mainly of Malay stock, are predominantly Catholic, and have the highest literacy rate in the region. The Philippines is the largest English-speaking nation in Asia and has a GNP per capita of US$907. Forty-six percent of the population lives in urban areas. Other economic indicators are shown in Table 23.1. Health-related statistics are shown in Table 23.2.

Table 23.2 shows that the Philippines spends 2.5 percent of GNP for health, which is relatively low compared to other developing countries. The population growth rate has been reduced considerably from a high of over 3 percent in the 1980s to its present level of 2.3 percent. The Department of Health is continuously pursuing a vigorous maternal and child health program to reduce popula-

TABLE 23.1. DEMOGRAPHICS AND ECONOMIC INDICATORS IN THE REPUBLIC OF THE PHILIPPINES.

Population	73.9 million
Urban population	46.0%
Population growth	2.3%
Literacy rate	94.0%
GNP per capita	US$907
GDP per capita (purchasing power parity)	US$3,475
GDP growth	1.2%
Inflation	5.7%

Source: Asiaweek, June 30, 1999.

TABLE 23.2. HEALTH-RELATED STATISTICS FOR THE PHILIPPINES.

Life expectancy	68 years
Infant mortality rate	40 per 1,000 live births
Share of GNP spent for health	2.5%
Shareof national budget spent for health	2.4%
Percentage of households with potable water	76%
Percentage of households with sanitary toilet	67%
Hospital bed–to–population ratio	1:835
Physician-to-population ratio	1:1,016
Primary care health unit–to–population ratio	1:4,200

Source: Department of Health, Manila.

tion growth below 2.0 percent and infant mortality rate (currently at 35 per 1,000 live births) to fewer than 30 per 1,000 live births. Life expectancy has increased to seventy years from sixty-seven years three years ago. In contrast to many developing countries, four of the five leading causes of death are no longer infectious and communicable diseases. Cardiovascular diseases and cancer now top the list.

The Philippine Health Care System

Health care delivery in the Philippines is a mix of government (public) programs and private sector initiatives. The affluent and middle classes (anyone who can afford to pay) normally access private sector providers. The majority (medically indigent) receive their health care from government institutions. One of the objectives of past and present health care reforms has been to reduce the medically indigent population significantly so that meager government resources can be spent on the "truly indigent." One of the initiatives to achieve this intended shift is to generate and draw resources from the private and employed sector through risk-sharing mechanisms such as medical insurance and managed care. Other reform initiatives by the government are to shift from branded to generic drugs, from socialized to free-enterprise financing, and from out-of-pocket payments to a risk-sharing, managed care delivery system. Table 23.3 shows these government initiatives.

Health Care Delivery

Health care is delivered through public and private sector providers. The public health care system follows the political and geographical boundaries of the country.

The first level of care is at the *barangay* (village) health station or rural health unit, which is usually staffed by a midwife or nurse and occasionally by a rural health physician. Only primary health care is rendered in these units, along with the dispensing of basic drugs. The next level is at the municipal or town level, where a municipal health center run by a municipal health officer (usually a physician) is the primary provider. In some towns there may be a small primary care hospital of ten- to fifteen-bed capacity that handles simple cases needing one- to three-day confinements. Cases that are more serious are referred to the provincial, city, or regional hospitals where secondary and limited tertiary care can be given. The more complicated and catastrophic cases are sent to the regional or national referral hospitals located in the major urban centers such as Manila and Cebu City. The government also runs a few specialty centers of excellence such as the Philippine Heart Center, the National Kidney Institute, and the National Children's Center. All physicians of these government facilities are on salaries.

Private sector facilities consist of individual clinics of private practitioners and hospitals that are mostly owned by physicians or religious organizations. These

TABLE 23.3. HEALTH CARE REFORM INITIATIVES IN THE GOVERNMENT SECTOR.

From	To
Public sector	Private sector
Hospital care	Primary care
Branded drugs	Generics
Regulation	Liberalization
Socialized	Free enterprise
User fees	Risk sharing
National health insurance hospital indemnity	Managed care

hospitals range in size from primary hospitals of ten- to fifteen-bed capacity to tertiary hospitals with one hundred to five hundred beds. A few medical centers, located in major cities, offer the latest modalities of treatment and diagnosis that include invasive cardiovascular procedures, organ transplantation, and steriotaxic neurosurgery. There are also freestanding outpatient facilities like polyclinics, renal dialysis centers, and diagnostic laboratories.

Service quality is perceived to be much better at private sector providers, except in the specialty and referral hospitals run by the government. That is why individuals and their families who are not covered by some form of health financing normally try to raise funds from various sources to secure health services from private providers for the more serious cases.

Health Professionals

Physicians are licensed after passing a board examination at the end of an eight-year premedical and medical course, followed by a one-year internship. The certification of specialists follows the American model of residency training: a residency is served in an approved institution, and a specialty board examination that is given by the particular specialty medical society must be passed. A large number of specialists had training and fellowships abroad, mostly in the United States. Nurses and other paramedical professionals (midwives, medical technologists, X-ray technologists, nutritionists, and pharmacists) are required to pass board examinations before licensure.

There is consensus that the quality of care and the professional skills of these health professionals, especially the specialists, are comparable to what can be found in most advanced and industrialized countries in the world. These skills, in addition to a facility in the English language, are the main reasons why thousands of these health professionals have easily found jobs in the United States, Europe, and the Middle East.

Health Care Financing

Financing for health services comes from both public and private funds. Table 23.4 shows the mix of funding sources for health services. The largest source is still user fees or out-of-pocket expenses from the private sector, amounting to 49.7 percent of total expenditures. The share of insurance is a meager 11.8 percent, from both social (7.2 percent) and private (4.6 percent) insurance. Government expenditure for health constitutes 45.7 percent of funding and is a mere 3 percent of its budget. One of the objectives of health sector reform undertaken by the Department of Health is to increase insurance funding to 34 percent in three to

TABLE 23.4. PHILIPPINES HEALTH EXPENDITURES BY SOURCE OF FUNDS.

Government sources	40.5 (45.7%)
National and local expenditures	34.1 (38.5%)
Social insurance	6.4 (7.2%)
Private sources	48.0 (54.3%)
Out of pocket (personal and corporate)	44.0 (49.7%)
Private insurance (indemnity and HMOs)	4.0 (4.6%)
Total	88.5 (100%)

Source: National Statistical Coordination Board, Republic of the Philippines.

five years. The projected increase will be generated from both the public sector through the National Health Insurance Program (NHIP) and the private sector through managed care initiatives.

Government Financing

The Philippines spends only 2 percent of the GDP for health—far less than most of its neighbors in Southeast Asia and other developing countries in the world. Although the government has been increasing the health budget for the last three years, the percentage of the budget devoted to health services has remained relatively constant. With the Asian economic crisis of late 1998 and 1999 causing significant currency devaluations, health care costs have escalated two to three times more than general inflation, due to the heavy reliance on imported health care supplies and equipment. Budget shortfalls resulted, causing shortages of drugs in government hospitals; the replacement and repair of hospital equipment was also deferred.

The government budget is spent mostly on personal health care (curative) services (50 percent) and administration (20 percent). Expenditures for public health accounted for (30 percent) of the budget. Part of the health reform agenda is for the Department of Health to reduce expenses for curative services and increase allocation for public health services.

National Health Insurance Program (NHIP)

The Philippine Health Insurance Corporation (PHIC) is the other major source of health funds. PHIC is the implementing agency of the NHIP, which aims to achieve universal coverage in ten to fifteen years. PHIC took over the previous

Medicare program—a compulsory program that covered all private sector and government employees as well as their families. Self-employed persons can enroll voluntarily. Employers and employees contribute equally to health care premiums, with each paying 1.25 percent of monthly salary; the maximum cap is 3,000 pesos. Benefits have recently been doubled and are now at approximately 50 to 70 percent support level of the average hospitalization costs in a ward bed. Any excess is a copay, or it can be covered by a supplemental insurance such as an HMO plan. Coverage is limited to inpatient services and outpatient surgery, paid on a traditional fee-for-service basis, like indemnity health insurance. PHIC is mandated to extend coverage to the entire population and has started pilot projects to cover the indigent population from funds generated by local government units (LGUs) and a portion from national government subsidies (the third source of public sector funds).

The law and the implementing rules governing the NHIP mandate a number of managed care features especially directed toward quality assurance, cost containment, and fraud prevention. Some of the features of the law allow the PHIC to contract with HMOs. The NHIP is therefore shifting from a pure indemnity insurance to a managed care system, with features such as capitation, DRGs, case payments, a gatekeeper-triage system, practice guidelines, and utilization and peer reviews. To enhance and support these initiatives, a sophisticated information system will be installed in two to three years.

Other significant shifts in health care policies to be implemented are reference pricing for drugs, use of the essential drug list, and the adoption of a relative value system (RVS) as the basis of payment of professional fees. Administration of the NHIP will be decentralized to the LGUs through regional, city, and provincial health boards.

Private Sector Financing

Financing from the private sector comes mainly from three sources: (1) out-of-pocket payments, (2) employee benefits, and (3) private insurance.

Out-of-Pocket Payments

Out-of-pocket payments by individuals and corporations in the form of user fees constitute the largest source (64 percent) of health care expenses for curative or personal care services due to the perceived better quality of such services in the private sector. With the low support level for hospitalization expenses of the NHIP at present, even the middle-class, employed sector is forced to dip into savings to purchase health services from private providers. Persons covered by insurance and employer benefits are burdened by out-of-pocket payments due to limitations of their health benefits. This segment of private sector financing is the primary market for medical insurance and managed care companies.

Employee Benefits

The Labor Code of the Philippines mandates certain levels of health benefits for all employees from employers. Coverage by the NHIP is compulsory, as previously mentioned. In addition, companies are required to have on-site outpatient clinics to render primary care consultation and emergency care. All employers are also required to provide workers compensation insurance for workplace and work-related injuries and illnesses through the government-run Employees Compensation Commission (ECC).

Except for these benefits, employers are not required to provide additional coverage. However, most large employers and a growing number of small- and medium-scale enterprises are giving additional health benefits to employees and their dependents through various financing mechanisms, which can range from self-insured to managed care plans.

Large enterprises usually run self-insured plans, and most of them have comprehensive coverage. A few large companies have contracted the management of their self-insured plans to an ASO (administrative services only) at a managed care company. The great majority purchase traditional indemnity health insurance or HMO plans for their employees. There has been an increasing shift from self-insured and indemnity insurance plans toward managed care or HMO plans. This trend is mainly management-driven, due to the growing practice of outsourcing noncore businesses and activities to third-party entities. In addition, corporations perceive HMO plans as being of better value because of its more comprehensive benefit package.

Health care coverage by employers is also increasing due to pressure from labor unions. A recent survey showed that health benefits were running a strong second to wage benefits in the list of demands from unions during collective bargaining negotiations.

Indemnity Insurance

Before the advent of HMOs, indemnity insurance was the only available health insurance in the country. Its market, however, has been limited to an enrollment of fewer than a million lives. The few insurance companies that offer it have not marketed it aggressively. They, in fact, offer it in most cases as a rider to group life and accident insurance. Insurance companies have incurred heavy losses from their indemnity insurance plans. As a result, they formed or invested in managed care or HMO companies and gradually shifted their health care portfolios to the latter.

Managed Care Companies (HMOs)

The first HMO in the Philippines was established in 1978, but the attempt failed. In the early 1980s, five HMOs were formed. Since then, the industry has grown to thirty-five operating companies. With a few exceptions, all the HMOs are for-profit companies. Table 23.5 shows the present status of the HMO industry in the Philippines. Even though HMO enrollment has grown steadily over the last ten years, enrollment in indemnity insurance has remained stagnant, below a million. Profitability is low, with only five of the top ten HMOs showing profits. What drives the market is the potential of 25 million enrollees, as estimated by the industry association.

The HMO industry developed entirely through private sector initiatives. No laws gave incentives to its formation nor were there any regulations to govern the industry. In 1990, the industry association initiated moves to introduce an HMO regulatory bill in Congress. Due to difficulties encountered in enacting a law, an alternative mechanism through an administrative order of the president was implemented. Such an order mandates the Department of Health to regulate HMOs in conjunction with the Securities and Exchange Commission. Stakeholders in the health care sector, however, have clamored for stricter controls following the financial failure of two small HMOs. The industry association has

TABLE 23.5. STATUS OF HMOs IN THE PHILIPPINES.

Number of HMOs	35
HMO members of industry association (AHMOPI)	19
Estimated enrollment	2.6 million
Percentage of enrollees with AHMOPI members	90%
Percentage of enrollees from corporate accounts	95%
Estimated revenues	3.0 billion pesos
Return on revenue, top ten HMOs (1997)	2.3%
Return on equity, top ten HMOs (1997)	10%
Enrollment growth	15%–20%
Estimated market	25 million

Note: Only five of the top ten HMOs were profitable.

Source: Association of HMOs in the Philippines Inc.

supported these moves and has conducted a dialogue with the Insurance Commission, which is charged with formulating new regulations and eventually acting as the regulatory body.

The industry association was formed in 1987 and incorporated as the Association of HMOs in the Philippines Inc. (AHMOPI). It is composed of nineteen of the largest HMOs in the country and accounts for 90 percent of total enrollment and revenues of the industry. The Department of Health has given AHMOPI the task of being the primary arbitration body to resolve complaints of HMO members, providers, and the public. The association has also introduced a code of ethics for the industry and is in the process of developing standards and benchmarks. It serves as the industry spokesperson in matters of legislation, taxation, regulation, and public relations.

Differences Between U.S. and Philippine HMOs

HMOs in the Philippines were patterned after U.S. HMOs. There are, however, many differences between them. HMOs in the United States were formed as an answer to escalating health care costs, and the primary concern was cost containment. In the Philippines, the driving force for the formation of HMOs was the need for financial access to quality health services in the private sector through a risk-pooling mechanism among the enrolled members. The risk pooling took place in the private sector because public health facilities can be accessed free for most services. As a result, managed care features and tools that control costs, such as capitation, DRG, per diems, utilization review and, to some extent, gatekeeping, were not vigorously pursued initially. The much lower cost of hospital services in the Philippines did not warrant the use of some of these cost-containment features of HMOs at the start. Providers were also reluctant to accept risk-sharing schemes.

Other conditions led to the establishment of managed care in the Philippines. Corporations needed a cost-effective system that would ensure the delivery of quality care. The government was unable to fill the need due to lack of resources and, to some extent, the political will to implement meaningful reforms. In addition, escalating health care costs due to new and expensive technology, as well as dependence on imported drugs and equipment, fueled this need for an efficient and cost-effective system. Finally, it was the entrepreneurial spirit of the pioneers in the managed care industry that brought about the establishment of HMOs in the country.

Premiums were pegged at levels that were affordable to the target market—the middle class and corporate groups. Affordable premium levels were not sufficient to cover comprehensive benefits as in the United States. Philippine HMOs had to carve out some of the more expensive benefits such as outpatient drugs, maternity, and mental health. They also had to put maximum caps on the more serious and catastrophic diseases. Some HMOs have offered optional riders to cover those carved-out benefits and, through re-insurance, have increased the maximums.

Payment of providers is mainly through negotiated, discounted fee-for-service arrangements. Specialists are paid using a relative unit value system (RUV). Outpatient services are mainly through salaried or retained primary care physicians. There are no nurse practitioners in the country; utilization review nurses or their equivalent are merely data gatherers and liaison personnel. Provider relations and case management issues are handled by medical managers who are all physicians, resulting in better rapport between HMOs and the medical profession. The other reality in the Philippines is that HMOs do not have much negotiating influence with hospitals. Most major cities in the Philippines are underbedded, and occupancy rates of tertiary hospitals are high.

Other Funding Sources

There are other, minor sources of funds for health care. Charitable, religious, civic and nongovernmental organizations (NGOs) occasionally conduct charity clinics and medical missions to rural and slum areas. International funding agencies have supported a number of health projects in the country. Most of the funds, however, are spent on family planning and maternal and child health, as well as on health financing projects.

The Emerging Role of HMOs

The Philippines was the first developing country that was able to successfully introduce managed care into its health care system through private sector initiatives alone. Managed care is now firmly entrenched in the country, and its thirty-five operating HMOs offer an alternative system for delivery and financing of health care.

Developing countries have limited resources to fund health care and spend a lower percentage of their GNP for health. The Philippines is no different. Large segments of the population with limited incomes have no financial access to health care, so there is a need to generate additional resources for health and spend them in a cost-effective manner. Managed care, with its cost-containment and risk-sharing features, may be the answer to such a need. In the Philippines, teachers, factory workers, laborers, and farmers, as well as middle-income people who are enrolled in HMOs, are now able to access private providers without dipping into their savings. They no longer must compete with the truly indigent for health services in government institutions. The limited resources of government can therefore be allocated to the poor and to public health.

Presently, HMOs cover approximately 2.6 million people and generate 3 billion pesos in revenue (see Table 23.5). Enrollment and revenue growth have averaged 15 to 20 percent yearly for the past three years. Ninety-five percent of HMO members come from corporate clients, with premiums mostly paid by employers as part of employee benefits. Most of these group accounts come from small- and medium-sized companies. In the past five years, there has been a continuing shift from indemnity insurance and self-insured plans to HMOs. It is worth noting that all the HMO benefits are supplementary to NHIP benefits due to the inadequate coverage of the latter.

The decision of the PHIC to include HMOs as possible providers, managers, or contractors of the NHIP, as well as its inclusion of managed care features in the implementing guidelines of the law, signify the growing importance of HMOs in the country. PHIC is also pilot testing new policies that will shift its operation from a pure indemnity insurance to a managed care plan using risk-sharing payment schemes to providers and cost-containment measures such as utilization review, utilization management, peer review, and preauthorization for hospital access.

The entry into the Philippine managed care market by multinationals such as Aetna, Cigna, AIG, United Health Care, and CMG, as well as the three largest life insurance companies in the country, is proof of the emerging role of HMOs and managed care in the country. There has also been interest shown by some health care companies from Singapore and Europe for possible joint ventures in the health care business.

On a negative note, there have been an increasing number of newspaper articles and opinions by columnists critical of HMOs. This development parallels the experience in the United States. The industry association (AHMOPI) has taken urgent measures to reverse this trend through a public relations campaign.

Conclusion

The successful implementation of managed care in the Philippines has shown that it can be a viable, sustainable, and cost-effective alternative of delivery and financing of health care in developing countries. It generates new resources for health from the private sector. Besides managing cost and quality, it organizes and rationalizes the provision of health care. Its foremost model, the HMO, is a variant of the U.S. model, modified to adapt to local conditions of the country. It is now the fastest-growing segment of the health care market in the Philippines.

Neighboring countries in Southeast Asia have started to show interest in managed care. Several multinational companies have started joint ventures in managed care companies in Singapore, Malaysia, Hong Kong, and Indonesia. What the Philippines started may be the wave of the future for health care financing in developing countries.

CHAPTER TWENTY-FOUR

AUSTRALIA

Russell J. Schneider

Australia's health care system is in an exciting state of evolution, as private health insurers move from their traditional role as passive payers for care to active purchasers. Although some private sector payers had flirted with active purchasing arrangements earlier, the change in the system only received formal government blessing in 1995 and is still very much embryonic.

Australia is in a unique position in its health care policy environment: it has both a large public sector and, in terms of percentage of population covered, one of the largest private sectors outside the United States. Privately owned hospitals, operated by religious or charitable institutions, doctors, or large corporations, provide about 23,000 beds—or 30 percent of total beds; private bed days (either in private or public hospitals) that are funded by health insurance total 6 million, or about 30 percent of overall hospital occupancies. Private health insurance contributes more than $4.4 billion in benefits each year, most ($3 billion) on hospital-related services, with the remainder going to "ancillary" health services (which are not covered by Medicare) such as dental care, physiotherapy, optometry, natural therapies, and so on.

Unlike most other countries, health insurance is rarely employer-purchased. The contract is between the individual and the health insurance fund, which facilitates employment mobility. With the inclusion of community rating, many older persons can retain insurance after retirement; about one person over sixty-five has private health insurance. This, of course, puts upward pressure on rates.

Health Spending Complexities

Health spending as a percentage of GDP is in mid-range—about 8 percent, compared with 4 percent in the United Kingdom and 14 percent in the United States. Health outcomes, as measured by mortality rates, longevity, and other factors, are very close to the best of world standards. However, health care policy remains a matter of significant political debate. Conflicts between levels of government are an almost permanent feature of the policy landscape. The private health sector, particularly the health financing industry, is at enormous sovereign risk, even though it is currently the beneficiary of a favorably disposed government that is both philosophically and pragmatically committed to encouraging the expansion of the private sector.

This position is further complicated by the iconic status of Medicare, which provides all Australians, regardless of means, with virtually unlimited cheap or even free (at point of service) access to both primary health care and to leading teaching hospitals. Private health insurance is limited to in-hospital episodes in "private" (that is, nongovernment) institutions, and legislation forbids health insurers from interfering in clinical judgments.

Such an apparently complex service system is, in fact, much simpler than it first appears. It is replete with opportunity as well as challenges, although there are many threats to it and an almost inevitable conflict with sections of the medical profession who see the evolution now under way as representing a serious threat to their traditional freedoms. This conflict is likely to become more in the next few years as governments, insurers, and providers experiment with new forms of funding and of providing care in a nation in which "managed care" has become a pejorative.

Understanding the Past

To understand the direction in which Australia's health care system is going, we need to take a brief look at the past. Traditionally, the government or charitable or religious institutions provided hospital care in Australia. Although basic funding was available from government, it seemed in everyone's interests to encourage private financing. Today's health insurance funds (effectively the only source of private third-party payment for health care) grew from two main sources: (1) the friendly societies and trade unions, who established health insurance arms to provide their members with affordable access to health services, and (2) providers, who established health insurance bodies both to guarantee their bills would be paid and to protect doctors from the dreaded "lodge" (or friendly society-capitated system). Indeed, so great was the antipathy of the medical profession to the attempts by the fraternal bodies to place them on a semi-salaried basis that "Lodge Patients Treated Last" became a commonplace sign in many GP surgeries. Managed care died in Australia before it was born in many other places.

By their very nature, the established insurance organizations, whether by providers or benevolent bodies, had a strong mutualist culture. This coincided with government philosophy in the late 1940s and 1950s, when much of the constitutional framework for today's health financing arrangements was established. As a result private health insurance is very much a part of the national policy, and private hospitals are an important part of the overall hospital system. As noted, most elderly persons retain private insurance. Although they represent only about 14 percent of the overall privately insured population, they account for more than 46 percent of claims. For government the challenge has been maintaining an appropriate balance of utilization and funding between the public and private sectors.

The historical separation of power between the Commonwealth or central government and state territorial governments is an important component of Australian health financing. This separation effectively limits the roles of federal and state governments. For example, the federal government can pay for hospital services, but state governments (or the private sector) provide them; the federal government can pay for medical services but cannot control the fees charged; state governments have the power to control medical fees but choose not to exercise them.

At the end of World War II the then-Labor government, put forward proposals that would allow it to directly fund medical and hospital services. Aware of similar moves in the United Kingdom, the Australian Opposition refused to support the enabling referendum unless the resulting constitutional amendment provided a firm guarantee that any such funding would not allow "civil conscription." Labor, anxious to commence its social program, agreed and the referendum was carried. The civil conscription ban, however, prevented any federal government from controlling doctors' prices or practices; its power was limited to the payment of benefits. It did, however, have an unlimited power over insurance, which it has used ever since as an oblique weapon to influence medical charging and practice patterns.

Under a Liberal (comparable to a U.K. Conservative or U.S. Republican) government in the 1950s, a shift occurred from Labor's collectivism to more emphasis on self-help, resulting in the introduction of the Earle Page Scheme, which in many ways remains today. Under this scheme, the Commonwealth government was prepared to provide health welfare benefits to those (other than the mendicant) who made some contribution of their own. Given the existence of mutual cooperatives (the health funds), the government had a built-in delivery mechanism. The insurers, once independent servants of either providers or patients, became agents of government in delivering a social welfare program.

This scheme remained intact until the early 1970s, when discontent with the gaps between medical benefits and doctors' charges encouraged the Labor Party to renew its commitment to semisocialized medicine. By 1983 this dissatisfaction had grown to the point where a newly elected Labor government was able to claim a mandate for the introduction of the lynchpin of its program, Medicare. Despite some changes, Medicare has not only survived until today but has become fundamentally accepted by both major political groupings and the Australian community. Indeed, any politician who attempts to make dramatic changes to Medicare (or promises to do so) risks losing his or her seat.

Medicare

Medicare is really two programs: one providing outpatient medical benefits and the second providing in-hospital benefits. Third-party funding of outpatient services (both GP and specialist) is, in effect, a Medicare monopoly administered by the Health Insurance Commission (HIC). It is an offense to offer to pay an insurance benefit for a medical service that is eligible for funding under the Medicare Benefits Schedule (MBS)—a fee list determined by the government. Under Medicare, all Australians are entitled to care in public hospitals (that is, those owned by state governments), provided they accept treatment by doctors paid by the hospital (either full-time employees or doctors working on a contract basis that allows rights of private practice). This treatment is free to the patient and is funded by a combination of state and federal taxes, the sharing of which is a source of constant friction. Because demand outstrips supply, patients may opt for "private" status, which allows them to choose their own doctor (who can provide treatment either during his private-patient access times at the public hospital or in a private facility). Medicare does not reimburse hospital costs for such a patient, although a proportion (75 percent) of the MBS is reimbursable.

Private Insurance

The role of private health insurance is, therefore, to act as third-party payer for the hospital component and a proportion of the medical fee. (This is currently limited to 25 percent of the MBS unless the health fund has an agreement with the doctor on fee capping, in which case the insurer can cover all medical costs or even provide for a limited and predetermined patient copay. This requirement for an "agreement" between insurer and doctor has led to three-party (doctor, health insurer, and government) conflict over provider claims that "managed care" is about to be introduced.

Private health insurance membership has dropped from 70 percent of the population prior to the introduction of Medicare in 1983 (the remainder were in most cases covered by social welfare programs) to 31 percent in 1999. The government was alarmed by the financial consequences of an ongoing slide—not merely to government but to the private hospital sector, which provides about 30 percent of total beds, and to the general sustainability of private medical practice. Therefore, the government introduced a succession of incentive measures, including a 30 percent rebate on private health insurance premiums and a 1 percent tax surcharge on higher-income earners who chose to be uninsured.

Health insurance is itself highly regulated by the Commonwealth government, which restricts payment of benefits to organizations registered (and therefore approved) by it. These organizations must "community rate" members (Australia has probably the purest community rating system in the world) and require government approval for premium changes and are subject to very strict solvency requirements. It is an offense for an unregistered organization to undertake liability for the reimbursement of hospital or medical services.

This complex regulatory mechanism sends confusing signals about what is and may be required of insurers; the confusion is compounded by the lack of a bipartisan agreement on health care financing beyond the fundamental principles of Medicare. The net effect is to lock health insurance activity inside the hospital gate, denying health fund managers opportunities to seriously negotiate better care arrangements with doctors and totally unable to negotiate alternate care provision outside the hospital setting. A recent attempt by the government to allow registered health insurers to pay medical benefits for outpatient procedures or treatments (for example, psychiatric consultations) was rejected in the Upper House (Senate), leading to a curious coalition of the medical lobby (claiming it would lead to the introduction of managed care) and the Labor Party (claiming it would be the end of Medicare).

Cost Containment

Because of these restrictions, cost-containment activities have been relatively limited and aimed at negotiating prices with hospitals. The reluctance of most private hospitals to be seen as influencing the clinical (or fee-setting) activities of the doctors who use them (most hospitals see their client base as being the medical profession, not the patient) has limited progress in this area.

However, one significant organization—now owned by AXA—has embarked on a preferred provider system, and other health funds have or will soon follow suit. Under these arrangements, patients are encouraged to use the participating providers on the basis that their costs will either be fully covered or their own co-payment known in advance. The industry has watched this experiment with interest, and a number of other insurers have now either announced similar plans or are looking seriously at emulating this move.

A total of forty-four registered health funds now operate in the Australian marketplace. All are registered to act nationally; most still operate in either state or regional markets or, in some cases, specific employment segments. For example, teachers, banks, and police each have their own health funds and are termed "closed" health funds, whereas those accepting members from any walk of life are known as "open" organizations. The need for specialist human resources, data analysis, and IT systems has led to smaller health funds establishing purchasing alliances, in which a group of health funds agrees to use a common agent to negotiate contracts with providers. As a result there are only nine separate "buying" agencies, and in most states only two to four significant ones. More aggressive buying on the part of the health funds has slowed the rate of growth of benefit expenditures but has not halted it. In 1999, premium growth was under 10 percent—the lowest in several years.

Nevertheless, the private hospital industry has reacted strongly against benefit constraints. This is, in part, a reaction to the fact that previous years had seen ongoing increases in hospital income from health funds brought about both by benefit inflation and a dramatic upsurge in the use of private hospitals. Recently the private hospitals lobbied aggressively for a Code of Conduct. An earlier push for "any willing provider" legislation has been dropped, however. Hospitals now officially accept the concept of selective contracting—at least publicly.

Of the forty-four health funds the largest—the Commonwealth government—in fact owns Medibank Private. Established in 1975 as the Health Insurance Commission, Medibank Private was operated conjointly with Medicare from 1983 to 1998, which facilitated its maintenance of a large (25 percent) market share. Now separated from Medicare, Medibank Private operates as a stand-alone health fund in competition with nongovernment entities. Despite its large market share, however, Medibank Private's membership is largely concentrated in Victoria (44 percent of the market).

Hospitals

Hospitals range from small cottage-type facilities to large corporations. The largest, Hospital Care of Australia (HCOA), is a subsidiary of the large transport group Mayne Nickless and now represents a significant component of the group's balance sheet. Health Care of Australia operates forty-six hospitals (4,950 beds), representing 21 percent of the private acute and psychiatric hospital market.

Health Care Politics

The politics of health care continues to be a source of conflict. The major political parties support Medicare, but the universal access (for those prepared to wait for elective surgery) system puts considerable pressure on resources, particularly at the state level. State governments operate public hospitals, whereas the Commonwealth provides funds and influences delivery at the state level. State leaders have for many years demanded a review of Medicare, which the Commonwealth has consistently rejected. At the national level, the debate is about the extent to which the Liberal Party (now in power) plans to shrink Medicare and promote the private sector, while the Labor Party (creators of Medicare and now out of power) is accused of wanting to nationalize services and destroy private health care.

Disturbed by the decline in private health insurance numbers, the federal government has introduced a number of incentive and assistance measures. These include a 1 percent income tax surcharge on incomes above $50,000 (single) or $100,000 (family); average weekly earnings are about $35,000 for a single male. These measures are aimed at ensuring that higher-income earners use private health insurance rather than the "free" Medicare (which their taxes largely pay for). The government also provides a 30 percent rebate on health insurance premiums, which can be taken as a premium reduction or claimed via tax. This will cost the government an expected $1.5 billion a year, depending on collections. Initial reaction to the rebate has been an upturn in private health insurance numbers for the first time in many years.

However, a major impediment to higher collections is the existence of unpredictable "gaps" or copayments above the government's Medicare benefits schedule. Given the option of using their private health insurance and being faced with unexpected bills or exercising their entitlement to be a Medicare patient and receive "free" treatment, many Australians exercise the latter option—and often drop their insurance as well.

In 1995 the Labor government introduced legislation allowing health funds to pay above the schedule, provided they had a fee-capping agreement with the doctor. The Australian Medical Association (AMA) bitterly opposed this provision, claiming it would force doctors to sign "U.S.-style managed care contracts." As a result of a vigorous AMA campaign, few doctors agreed to contracting, even though the incoming Liberal government supported "no gap" deals and further expanded the legislation to allow "no gap" coverage if doctors entered into agreements with the hospital or hospitals in which they received visiting privileges, still with little progress.

Political concern about copayments reached a point at which the 30 percent rebate legislation was amended by the powerful Senate, with a demand that health insurers only be able to deliver the rebate as a premium reduction if they had "no gap" or "known gap" policies in place by June 2000. Although this motivated health insurers to offer full-coverage policies, it remains to be seen whether the medical profession will accept the arrangements. It is likely that the government will be forced to take further action, although constitutional difficulties will make this hard to achieve.

Response of "Organized Medicine"

Organized medicine in Australia (something of an oxymoron) has always resisted reform or any threat to its independence. One particular difficulty is the way it is structured—still very much on an individual practice basis. There are few group practices; usually *group* means two or three specialists in the same specialty sharing rooms. Anesthetists are moving to larger practices, however, and radiology and pathology services are being offered by both individual practitioners and large corporate groups. There is an oversupply of general practitioners and a shortage of specialists, especially in some key specialties. The colleges control specialist supplies with an iron fist, thus ensuring that strict limits on numbers are perpetuated.

Although public hospitals increasingly impose constraints—both budgetary and nonbudgetary—on physician behavior, many private hospitals seem less willing to do so (although some of the larger chains are now looking to more performance measurement). This is largely because a tradition exists in which the doctors provide the hospital with patient flows. The threat by surgeons to take their business elsewhere inhibits private hospital operators from imposing rigid quality requirements on the surgeons to whom they grant visiting privileges, which seem to be regarded more as rights. This situation is of particular significance in that it reduces the capacity of the private sector to distinguish itself favorably from the public sector.

At this stage hospitals that seem to be aggressively ensuring quality of care cannot proclaim their initiatives without risking the loss of medical manpower. Until this situation changes, many believe that the private health care sector will find it difficult to substantially expand the privately insured patient base.

An even greater threat to private health care comes from the development of "coordinated care" trials that are being enthusiastically promoted by state and federal administrations. These trials are aimed at overcoming difficulties created by the lack of coordination of health and welfare programs offered by different tiers of government. The trials provide a pooling of funds available under these programs to maximize patient well-being, particularly for those who have chronic illnesses or are at high risk—diabetics, the elderly, asthmatics, heart disease sufferers, and so on. The care coordinator, normally a GP or a GP's delegate, can access various services to ensure that the patient receives the most appropriate care. Although still in the trial stage, anecdotal evidence suggests that these trials will prove significantly beneficial.

A publicly run program that emphasizes health promotion and illness prevention obviously expands the attractiveness of Medicare relative to private health insurance and health care, especially if private health insurance is restricted to retrospective payment for hospital treatment. As a result, the government is being urged to allow similar trials in the private sector. Health insurers are anxious to be allowed to provide an all-embracing, quality-based comprehensive health care product. Any such move, of course, risks clashing with the die-hard supporters of Medicare, who would resist any change in the status quo.

Opportunities

Although "U.S.-style managed care" is a threatening concept to most providers and many consumers in Australia, opportunities nevertheless abound for those willing to share expertise with appropriate Australian partners.

Australian insurers and software houses are relatively well advanced in IT systems, but hospitals are far less IT-literate. Although there are forty-four insurers, there are only eight buying agencies; these are moving toward episodic payment systems but are at different developmental stages. Hospitals complain that the demands of the insurers (even though there only eight real buyers) create unnecessarily complex reporting and billing systems and that much has to be handled manually. Insurers and hospitals are currently exploring the possibility of downloading insurer business rules to hospital billing systems to facilitate information and payment exchanges.

In many hospitals the purchase of information systems is seen as an added cost rather than a rational business investment. Those who can convince smaller hospital operators of the benefits of improved information should open up opportunities.

Advocacy of the benefits of better-managed care systems also represents an opportunity within the Australian environment, where the population has been conditioned by provider propaganda to see managed care as threatening. Without this education any attempt to launch innovative products is unlikely to succeed.

Talent scouting is also totally open in Australia, with health funds and others interested in developing coordinated care or managed care arrangements unable to find the willing providers who can make such systems work. Prospective funders need much more information on incentives, payment systems and, most important, ways of convincing GPs of the benefits of new delivery arrangements to their own incomes and lifestyle.

Effective quality measurement is still embryonic in Australia. Although all parties are committed to improving quality, hospitals, especially in the private sector, are reluctant to look at appropriate benchmarking arrangements. The development of a nonthreatening quality measurement system for the private health care sector is an issue of major importance.

Finally, as in most Western countries, Australia's population is aging. Because of the high cost of care for the elderly, most insurers have seen this as a potentially risky business. However, more older people will be enrolled with health insurance firms whose survival will depend very much on managing the costs of their care. Organizations with expertise in holding down the cost of care for older people while enhancing outcomes should find plenty of opportunities "down under" over the next decade.

CHAPTER TWENTY-FIVE

NEW ZEALAND

Mary-Anne Boyd, Nicolette Sheridan

New Zealand, sometimes called Aotearoa (Land of the Long White Cloud), is an independent island country in the South Pacific Ocean and a member of the Commonwealth of Nations. Governmental, legislative, and health care systems have evolved from United Kingdom models. New Zealand comprises large north and south islands and numerous smaller islands, covering a total of 104,450 square miles. The population of 3.7 million is spread across urban and rural communities. Tokelau in the Pacific Ocean is a territory governed by New Zealand, and the Cook Islands and Niue are self-governing territories in free association with New Zealand.

In 1840, the Treaty of Waitangi was signed between chiefs of the indigenous Maori race and the British Crown. The treaty provided for a transfer of sovereignty, a confirmation of existing property rights, and citizenship rights to Maori.

State sector reforms in the 1980s reactivated the formal recognition of the treaty and its integration into health services. Consistent with principles of the Alma Alta Declaration (1978), health reforms have tightened accountability for the expenditure of public funds and refocused health priorities to reduce unacceptable disparities in health status between Maori and non-Maori.

History

Health care spending remains at around 7 percent of GDP. Government-owned organizations purchase services as part of a tax-funded system of universal coverage that accounts for about 77 percent of all health expenditures. A complementary private system is supported by insurance premiums and direct payments, and charitable and voluntary organizations provide important services.

A social security scheme launched in 1939 provided New Zealanders with free medicines, free hospital care, and a universal subsidy for primary care physician visits for over twenty years. Initially, many doctors did not charge a copayment. By the 1960s, public hospital waiting lists were long, and medical insurance schemes grew to help people pay for private hospital admissions, particularly for nonacute surgery. The basic framework of the health system that was set up in 1939 remains (Bassett, Sinclair, and Stenson, [1985] 1997).

Primary care physicians have continued to function as independent, fee-for-service practitioners receiving some government subsidies. In 1983, fourteen area health boards, with elected and later partially appointed boards, brought together many of the publicly funded services and devolved much of the decision making. Boards had a duty to convene service development groups, and providers and communities were encouraged to integrate services regionally.

The late 1980s and 1990s saw a move to the general management of publicly funded health services and an expansion of privately owned services as technology proliferated and waiting lists lengthened. Then in 1993, state reforms separated trading activities from regulatory and nontrading functions in the publicly funded health sector.

Reforms and Recent Changes

With the separation of purchase and ownership, as well as provision responsibilities, contestability and business disciplines took a higher profile, and commercial secrecy became accepted in the public sector. Service contracts were intended to keep day-to-day service delivery at arm's length from government ministers. A compromise policy framework retained state ownership of forty-four hospitals, including all major, acute care hospitals. Efficiency gains were expected to result from competition and limited funding and from more explicit rationing criteria.

Reforms increased competition in areas such as pharmaceutical supply, elective surgery, continuing care and rest homes, urgent twenty-four-hour primary care, laboratory services, radiology and maternity services, primary care services for Maori, and (for Pasifika people) rehabilitation and work-related injury insurance.

Overall, the reforms of the 1990s failed because of poor implementation, market failure due to lack of scale, poor sector information for purchasers and providers, and the government's deficit funding of acute care hospitals. Communities were not engaged in the design and development of dynamic health centers to replace hospitals suited to former decades. There was insufficient investment in educational and change management support to enhance immature clinician-manager relationships and resolve confused accountabilities.

The very high focus on financial and commercial performance of government-owned organizations was balanced just ahead of the new millennium by the government encouraging providers and communities to cooperate and collaborate for more efficient and effective services. A new center-left government is merging central agency roles and is promoting local collaborative and accountable cultures, as well as community involvement in decision making through district health boards. Broad objectives include reducing inequalities.

Structure

The government is the predominant funder of health services and sets supply side limits, with resources nominally allocated on a per capita basis adjusted for age, sex, ethnicity, and relative mortality. Actual funding is influenced by geography, population density, and politics. The Ministry of Health is the government's principal policy adviser, as well as its agent in managing relationships with funders and purchasers and in regulating health and disability sectors. The central government agency responsible for purchasing known as the Health Funding Authority (HFA) is programmed for disestablishment during 2000. In 1998 and 1999, spending was NZ$6.2 million, including disability support services. The HFA is not permitted to own service facilities, deliver services, or provide gap insurance. There is an obligation to consult; principles for purchase include equity, effectiveness, efficiency, safety, and acceptability. Core benefits are not clearly defined—a factor that has limited the development of competing purchasers.

Health Expenditures

Some 70 percent of HFA contracts are for personal health services, and half of these are purchased from state-owned providers. The contracts cover specialist trauma services, most technology-dependent and intensive inpatient services, ambulatory consultations, mental health services, and treatment for alcohol abuse, as well as secondary care, home-health services. The insurance industry's reimbursements are also substantially directed to secondary care, with 18 percent to specialist practitioners and 51 percent to hospitals in 1997 (Aetna, 1999).

Anderson (1998) found that 59 percent of New Zealand's total spending was on hospitals, whereas most countries spent between 42 and 46 percent on hospitals. However, health status statistics do not show New Zealand's population to be better off, comparatively. Although total expenditures, as well as the definitions of the term *hospital* vary, studies such as this stimulate debate and creative thinking.

Population Health Gain

It is no longer assumed that delivering personal health services will result in population health (Marmor and Mashaw, 1994), and New Zealand is among the countries rethinking the demands, issues, and incentives that drive health service priorities. Currently, these include decreasing smoking, improving nutrition, and preventing infectious disease. Also included are improved functional outcomes from adequate elective surgery, integrated services for people with long-term disorders, and Maori health.

Emphasis is being placed on population health policies to improve health for all New Zealanders, especially those with poorer health. A paradigm change of this order brings, in everyday practice, tension between the medical ethics of the individual and the social ethics of population health (Lamm, 1994). Participating communities, self-management, and effective primary care are the bases of such a model.

Better and more integrated information is enabling citizens to gain a clearer overview of expenditures and results. Consumer consultant roles are expanding, and the voices of informed communities and service users are expected to strengthen as a key element in shaping the future.

Primary Medical Care

Citizens are encouraged to choose a primary care physician, or general practitioner, many of whom are now in independent practitioner associations (IPAs). State subsidies and contracts include primary care services for children under six years, immunization programs, primary care for people with low incomes and high need, and some community nursing services.

In 1999 there were thirty-two IPAs in New Zealand, involving, along with other primary care organizations, some 2,000 primary care physicians. The IPAs covered between 10,500 and 500,000 people, with a mean of 130,000 citizens covered and 87 medical practitioners (Houston, Coster, and Wolffe, 1999). Smaller IPAs are tending to amalgamate.

Almost all IPAs manage a budget for laboratory and pharmaceutical expenditures. In some cases, savings in the initial years were up to 23 percent of total previous expenditures, and this was shared equally between the IPA and the HFA. IPA savings have been used in a number of ways to benefit patients (consumers) (Coster and Gribben, 1999).

Primary Health Care Teams

To support community knowledge and self-determination, dietitians, physiotherapists, occupational therapists, counselors, traditional healers, and community workers may increasingly be included in multidisciplinary primary care teams, and there are opportunities for the more appropriate utilization of nurses. Government subsidies of NZ$30 million a year for nurses who work directly with primary care physicians are expected to better align incentives for collaborative and effective teamwork.

Primary care capitation (see Scott, 1998), based on health needs, age, gender, ethnicity, socioeconomic status, and chronic disease, has been proposed but barely implemented. Copayments and fees-for-service would continue for some of the population. Regulatory and risk-management strategies for adverse selection have been proposed (see Keating, 1998; Bowie, 1999). The existing fee-for-service system has poor incentives that promote cost shifting between primary and secondary care, and the new millennium is a good time for change.

Specialist Referrals

Primary care physicians have a key role in relation to specialist services. They are gatekeepers, or sources of referral, as well as partners in the management of care with and for individuals. Specialists in publicly funded services increasingly are expected to balance reactive treatment for individuals with a proactive approach to the health of populations. Citizens are in geographical catchment areas for publicly funded specialist services. Since the mid-1990s, an ambitious multiyear project has aimed at the nationally consistent use of priority criteria for publicly funded, nonacute procedures such as cataract surgery and coronary artery bypass grafts. The criteria are intended to provide a framework for clearer definition of publicly funded services and client certainty of care plans. Most specialists in the private and insurance market are referred patients from primary care physicians, although clients self-refer for some dermatological, ophthalmic, and cosmetic procedures.

Specialist practitioners in the private sector (for example, those in surgery, diagnosis, dental care, and mental health) are moving toward larger groupings to support infrastructure and modern facilities. Publicly owned companies hold the majority of public health contracts.

State-owned hospital and health service companies are subject to oversight by a monitoring and advisory unit, and they function as discrete companies rather than as a chain under common ownership. Facilities development requires commercial loans or partners, or special government loan vehicles or equity input. NZ$920 million was invested in the five years prior to 2000, and the government plans spending of a further NZ$1 billion between 2000 and 2003. Major hospital redevelopment is planned in the capital, Wellington, in Auckland, as well as facilities throughout the country.

Insurance

Over one-third of New Zealand's population is covered by private health insurance, which has a history of meeting the cost of services outside the taxpayer-funded health system. Although reforms promised a more explicit system, the government has failed to define core benefits and clinical thresholds so people can judge the need to insure. Insurance coverage usually means greater choice of provider, reduced waits, convenient booking times, and enhanced hotel services. Numbers have fallen in recent years, while the proportion of health spending attributable to private health care has been growing. Key players in the market appear to be moving from passive claims paying to more active service management; they are offering wellness incentives for policyholders and vending management services, and are building relationships with health service providers. The health insurance industry in New Zealand has a code of practice and currently operates under a relatively liberal regulatory regime. In addition to complying with normal commercial law and disclosure requirements, insurers are subject to the Fair Trading Act 1986, the Consumer Guarantees Act 1993, and the Insurance Companies Deposits Act 1953 (Davies, 1999).

The Accident Insurance Act of 1998 created a new accident insurance and rehabilitation environment in which private insurers compete for the accident insurance business of employers and self-employed people. Continuation of this policy is in doubt with a center-left government. The Accident Compensation Corporation (ACC) for personal injury automatically covers every New Zealander while they are not working. The legislation limits legal actions against registered health professionals, so New Zealand has not experienced the level of defensive medicine and legal activity seen in some other countries. Nonetheless, there is an increasing focus on quality, and practitioners are strengthening self-regulatory procedures.

Investment

New Zealand's economy is diversifying from an agricultural base. Import controls and export subsidies have markedly declined in number; state-owned activities such as telecommunications have been privatized, and industries such as electricity and banking have been deregulated. Tourism, knowledge-based industries, horticulture, fisheries, and manufacturing are among the bases of the economy. Education and health are significant sectors.

Across the range of health service providers, noncore business activities such as the maintenance of facilities, infrastructure, and hotel services are often outsourced. The competitive market spans birthing facilities, rest homes, continuing care, retail and courier pharmacy services, most primary and specialist dental surgery, much elective surgery, podiatry, audiology, optometry, and a range of services outside the scope of conventional Western medicine. Private sector investment is evident in the design, construction, purchase, and lease of health care properties. Hospitals and clinics, diagnostic centers, rehabilitation, geriatric, and continuing care facilities are examples. Health property is currently regarded as an attractive long-term investment because of the sources of service funding and increasing demands associated with an aging population.

New technologies and skills are both marketed into and exported from New Zealand. As a small country with a culture of innovation, New Zealand exports considerable consulting expertise and is also successful in international markets with certain software products such as clinical and management software for dental services.

Management and Information Technology

Leadership and management expertise are in relatively short supply, so international job-search and contracted management services will probably be used. Executive and clinician leadership education is competitive and sourced nationally and internationally. Maori primary care providers and primary care services for Pacific peoples have set new standards and more appropriate choices and services.

Effective information and management systems are essential if providers are to adhere to strict privacy legislation and yet exchange critical patient information that is basic to integrated and effective services. The creation and maintenance of electronic health and medical records are best undertaken within primary care settings (Schloeffel, 1998). Ironically, the health reforms appear to have weakened the potential for a nationally coherent system of unique identifiers for use across all services with electronic tracking of cumulative outcomes and costs. For many years, hospitals have used "national health index" numbers, giving the Ministry of Health an ability to analyze and synthesize nationally secondary and tertiary services data.

This system started and has so far stayed in the secondary sector. It has formed a record of transactions rather than a dynamic accurate profile of the current living population. It is therefore a massive exercise to link the concept with the practicalities of primary care enrollment in an environment with privacy and consumer concerns. At the end of the 1990s, the New Zealand government invested NZ$4 million on trials of health information systems to support integrated providers. The Australian version of the ICDC10 is used, and Reed codes are used in many primary care settings.

There is a lack of integrated patient management systems. All major providers are engaged in refining or developing effective information systems. Those imported from offshore typically are created for other uses; adaptation is lengthy and problematic. Those developed locally often are challenged to provide enough timely expertise to maintain momentum. This is a significant area for continuing development in the immediate future.

New Zealanders value opportunities for mutual exchanges of expertise and learning; benchmarking is of particular interest. Although the sharing of ideas and partnerships across geographical boundaries and cultures can add to knowledge and profitability, New Zealanders have a do-it-yourself culture and reservations about ventures perceived as threatening the welfare state or depleting New Zealand ownership.

Future Reforms (2001–2005)

The government has set a target of 2005 for New Zealanders to conduct dealings with all government agencies on-line, and all government services will be available through a single portal. This will also affect consultation, which is built into processes at national and local levels. Intermediate purchasing through "care plans," "integrated care organizations," or Maori organizations will continue to be considered in the early 2000s; there is the potential to develop integrated systems locally. These could build on existing child health and other initiatives that involve mainstream infant services, local Maori providers, and IPA and public hospital specialists and services. Better-informed citizens, both as individuals and through special interest organizations, will drive changes toward improved customer service.

Summary

Since the mid-1980s, New Zealand has seen radical change, with purchaser-provider separation, improvement in primary-secondary integration, and more explicit rationing and access criteria. Positive results have been limited due to the lack of workforce and change management planning, confused accountabilities, and immaturities within the system.

At the beginning of the new millennium, private financing accounts for 23 percent of expenditures on health and on much service. Publicly funded universal services are always under pressure; there is a healthy focus on reducing hospital admissions and stays (New Zealand Health Technology Clearinghouse, 1998) without the addition of a utilization management layer. A shift from fee-for-service payments to a new emphasis on provider cooperation, value-based informed decisions, and a population perspective could balance primary and secondary care interventions and strengthen prevention and self-management. Maori health priorities require focus on asthma, diabetes, smoking cessation, injury prevention, hearing, immunization, mental health, and oral health.

Stronger leadership, particularly in areas such as health information systems, could ensure national standards, appropriate methods, and commonality among clinical computing systems, electronic records, and clinical messaging.

Payers and citizens want results, and combinations of publicly and privately owned organizations will together provide services of the future.

As with ventures in all countries, the attitudes and competencies of people are critical to success. Off-shore organizations are likely to be successful only if they have the patience and skills to partner with locals to ensure that value is added and implementation is relevant to New Zealand and its peoples.

References

Aetna. *Trends in Private Health Insurance Reimbursements*, Sept. 1999. [http://www.aetna.co.nz/misc/privatefund.html]

"Alma-Ata Declaration." International Conference on Primary Health Care, Alma-Ata, USSR, September 1978.

Anderson, G. F. *Multinational Comparisons of Healthcare, Expenditures, Coverage, and Outcomes.* New York: Commonwealth Fund, 1998.

Bassett, J., Sinclair, K., and Stenson, M. *The Story of New Zealand.* Auckland: Reed, 1997. (Originally published 1985.)

Bowie, R. "The Role of Health Insurance in New Zealand: A Brief History and Future of Health Insurance. *Healthcare Review—Online,* Apr. 1999.

Coster, G., and Gribben, B. "Primary Care Models for Delivering Population-Based Health Outcomes." Discussion paper on primary health care, National Health Committee, National Advisory Committee on Health and Disability, Aug. 1999.

Davies, P. "The Role of Health Insurance in New Zealand: Health Insurance in New Zealand." *Healthcare Review—Online,* Apr. 1999.

Houston, N., Coster, G., and Wolffe, L. "Quality Improvement Within Primary Care Groups: Lessons from New Zealand." Unpublished manuscript, 1999.

Keating, G. "Integrated Care: The Role of Policy and Government: A View from the Ministry of Health." *Healthcare Review—Online,* June 1998.

Lamm, R. D. "The Ethics of Excess." *Hastings Centre Report,* 1994, *24*(6), 14.

Marmor, T. R., and Mashaw, J. "Strategy for Survival: Change and Stability in the Management of Health-Care Institutions." *Health Management Quarterly,* 1994, *16*(4), 5.

Schloeffel, P. "Integrated Care: Information Management: Information Management and Information Technology (IM/IT) for Integrated Care. *Healthcare Review—Online,* Oct. 1998.

Scott, G. *The Next Five Years in General Practice.* Wellington: Health Funding Authority, 1998.

PART FIVE

ASIA

The health care of the citizens of China has improved significantly over the past half century, with life expectancy increasing from about thirty years at the end of World War II to sixty-nine years by 1990. But today, while the government continues to provide most health care services, individuals are being forced to absorb an increasingly large proportion of the expense. In Chapter Twenty-Six, Richard G. Schulze looks at what led to China's improved health care, how things are changing now, and what this means for potential investors.

In Hong Kong, the government commissioned Professor William Hsiao and associates of Harvard University in 1998 to assess both the public and private sectors of the present health care system. Hong Kong native Yanek S. Y. Chiu, in Chapter Twenty-Seven, examines the history of health care and Hsiao's findings; he also reviews possible future reforms. Chiu argues that the current secretary of health and welfare, E. K. Yeoh, has the extensive training, vision, and energy to move ahead with reforms.

India's health care system is pluralistic, which is unusual in that nearly 80 percent of it is financed by the private sector. Whereas the rich can afford high-priced private health care, the middle class and the poor often cannot find affordable care of reasonable quality at all. In Chapter Twenty-Eight, Neelam Sekhri analyzes the various types of public and private health care providers and payers in India and looks at potential for future investment there.

Japan's rapidly aging population is on the verge of forcing reconsideration of the largely fee-for-service health care system the Japanese have liked for many years. In Chapter Twenty-Nine, Aki Yoshikawa describes the organization and financing of the country's universal health system and recommended reforms; he also offers an in-depth review of the *kenpo*—the managed health insurance associations for employers.

CHAPTER TWENTY-SIX

CHINA

Richard G. Schulze

At the end of World War II, China's population was among the least healthy in the world and had one of the world's worst life expectancies: only about thirty years. By 1990 this had increased to sixty-nine years. During the same period, infant mortality had dropped from 265 deaths per 1,000 to 41. Today, though most health care services are provided through public hospitals and medical facilities, the payment mechanisms that permitted such an improvement in the health of the population have been eliminated. Now the individual pays for his or her own health care services.

How did the country get to this point? What are the implications for the quality of health and health care in the future? What are the implications for those seeking to invest in providers, medical equipment and supplies manufacturing (or to export to China), or pharmaceutical production? This chapter will provide the background to the current situation of the Chinese health care system, the factors that influence the direction in which the industry is moving, and implications for investors and others interested in this fascinating market.

Unless otherwise indicated, the facts and figures in this chapter are drawn from *China Human Development Report: Human Development and Poverty Alleviation, 1997* (New York: United Nations, 1997) and from *China 2020: Issues and Options for China* (Washington, D.C.: World Bank, 1997). Additional information was obtained in personal communication with various government officials.

Historical Developments

Because of the dismal state of public health care at the time of the Communist revolution, the new government made improved health care a major focus, along with adequate food, education, and so on. This was accomplished through development of a rural cooperative medical system and by requiring state-owned enterprises (SOEs) to have their own health care delivery structure (physicians, clinics, hospitals). At the same time, the government undertook a substantial redistribution of health care resources toward the countryside—to "barefoot doctors" and a proliferation of local clinics. The benefit of the rural cooperative medical system was to encourage preventive care, which reduced the use of medical facilities and hospitals at county levels. This reduced the overall cost of care.

In urban areas, there was a growth of smaller hospitals and clinics to serve the more common medical problems of the population. More financing for tertiary and quaternary care hospitals of more than 500 beds became available. The latter started as an effort to treat more acute illnesses and diseases, as well as to be able to say that China had a quality of medical care of world-class standards available to its people.

China has made major inroads against infectious diseases and malnutrition. However, it is now facing a "second health revolution," resulting from the growth of noncommunicable and chronic diseases—diseases of developed rather than developing countries. These partly stem from environmental problems, such as pollution, and from lifestyle issues, such as smoking. Nevertheless, large parts of the countryside continue to be burdened with malnutrition, high infant and maternal mortality rates, and victimization by infectious and endemic diseases.

Devolution of power and an increased focus on self-funding has resulted in an overlap, and therefore duplication, of facilities between those of the Ministry of Health, state-owned enterprises, traditional Chinese medicine (TCM), and public works facilities. This has led to an increased focus on hospitals and less attention to public health services such as immunizations and tuberculosis treatment (which are paid for out of pocket), and on testing food and water in urban areas. Hence, a relatively small number of infectious diseases, most of which are inexpensive to prevent and treat, currently cause most deaths of children.

Development of Payment Mechanisms

The dramatic success in improving health conditions between 1950 and 1982 resulted from two factors. First, the government provided comprehensive insurance coverage for urban residents, required SOEs to provide health care services and to cover all their costs, and developed a rural cooperative medical system that reached close to 90 percent of the rural population. And second, the financing of health care was combined with the delivery mechanism so that costs could be contained. As a result, in 1981 health care costs were just over 3 percent of the GNP.

By 1978 the "Great Leap Forward" and the "Cultural Revolution" had not been successful. On the contrary, about 250 million rural people, or about 31 percent of the rural population, lacked adequate food and clothing. As a result, the government started to move from a centrally planned economy toward a more competitive market system, which led to the devolution of power from Beijing to the provincial governments. In rural areas this led to the weakening of the financial base of the cooperative medical system (funding went from 20 percent of national health spending in 1978 to 2 percent in 1993).

The share of health spending from the government budget (excluding amounts spent for government employee care) declined from 32 percent in 1986 to 14 percent in 1993. Out-of-pocket payments rose from 20 percent of the health care sector's revenue in 1978 to 42 percent in 1993. As a result, while government health care spending almost tripled between 1978 and 1993, private spending increased ten-fold. In other words, the government was very successful in causing people to pay an increasing share of the sector's revenue out of their own pockets rather than having government pay.

It should also be pointed out that although the percentage of the government budget spent on health care significantly declined between 1986 and 1993, only about 4 percent of the latter was under the direct control of the central government. Spending by the provinces, prefectures, counties, and township accounted for the rest, resulting in increasing inconsistencies in policies across China.

As the percentage of the health care sector's revenue from out-of-pocket expenditures significantly increased, the cost of routine, basic, outpatient health services appeared low enough that most non-poor Chinese households could pay for them out of current income or savings. However, a 1992–1993 survey found that of those who had been referred to a hospital for care, 40.6 percent did not seek hospitalization on grounds of excessive cost and inability to pay.

In trying to better control the quality and costs of health care services, the Chinese government conducted an experiment beginning in December 1994, in two towns on the Yangtzi River, Jiujiang and Zhenjiang (nicknamed the "Two Jiangs" experiment), that provided promising results for a new insurance scheme. Essentially, it split the funding of health services from their provision. Specifically, the experiment

- Collected insurance payments from enterprises and public agencies and split them between individual and group accounts. The individual accounts were also combined with large copayment amounts.
- Introduced an essential drug list of 1,100 Western and 500 traditional Chinese medicines that it was willing to reimburse.
- Combined the government and the state-enterprise insurance systems into a single insurance center.
- Bundled fees per outpatient and inpatient admission, setting the rates prospectively.

The result was that

- Coverage gaps were eliminated.
- Rates of overprescription and use of expensive diagnostic tests were cut significantly.
- Aggregate hospital expenditure annual growth rates declined by 23 to 28 percentage points from the average annual rate of 33 percent in 1991–1994.
- Quantity of service utilization declined 9 percent, and bed occupancy declined 2 percent.
- Inpatient and outpatient visits fell for enrollees.

The success of the demonstration project attracted the attention and visits of more than 600 officials from provinces and municipalities, and the project will be extended to fifty more cities and prefectures.

Current Financing and Delivery System

Whereas many countries are moving toward a curative health care system that is financed publicly but provided privately, China is moving in the opposite direction. Contrary to the situation for the nonpoor who cannot afford acute care treatment, the growing middle class, particularly in urban areas, values high-quality, private, urgent and acute care and is prepared to pay for it.

As pointed out earlier, private spending to pay for care has skyrocketed, whereas the portion of health care costs paid for by the government has significantly declined. Although the government operates almost all of the hospitals, it is not paying for the majority of care.

Other than the health care budget, the government spends about 8.8 percent of total health spending on government employees and retirees, disabled veterans, and university students, or about 2 percent of the population.

The government is concerned about inadequate insurance coverage and the lack of good-quality medical care for the rural population and for those put out of work through the privatization of SOEs. The government will be pushing for improved health care insurance programs such as the Two Jiangs experiment.

Hospitals

China today provides almost all health care services through public hospitals and medical facilities. There are over 200,000 health establishments providing health services to the population of 1.2 billion. Although most hospitals are part of the Ministry of Health, of provincial or county health care systems, or of SOEs, private practitioners operate an estimated 161,000 clinics in urban areas.

The country has about 3 million hospital beds, or 2.4 per 1,000 people—a ratio nearly as high as in Latin America and the Caribbean. Of these, about 700,000 beds are operated by SOEs. In 1994 the bed occupancy rate was 69 percent.

The almost 70,000 hospitals that are owned and managed by the government are categorized in three levels: Level 3, with more than 500 beds, of which there about 700 in China. About 4,000 hospitals are Level 2, with 100 to 500 beds. About 65,000 are Level 1 hospitals, with fewer than 100 beds—almost exclusively rural or in cities with a population under 1 million.

Level 3 hospitals (tertiary care) are considered the strongest, and generally most financially sound, although some are expected to go bankrupt (to the extent that bankruptcy is possible in China). With the government's push for increased reliance on out-of-pocket fees for paying health care costs, Level 1 and Level 2 hospitals will be much more at risk.

In rural areas, the collapse of the cooperative medical system, including insurance programs, has weakened referral patterns between health organizations, resulting in the underutilization of facilities. At the same time, in urban areas there is an overcrowding in some tertiary care hospitals, with an average stay of fifteen days for patients, which is excessively long by international standards.

Prices for health services are set under guidelines established by the Price Commission, often at levels well below costs, especially those with large labor input. In Shanghai actual costs for some routine procedures are two to four times the allowed fees of patients paying out-of-pocket, and two to three times for insured patients. This leads to under-the-table payments to physicians and a strong incentive to rely on generating fees from pharmaceutical sales and diagnostic testing using expensive equipment, the pricing of which is not regulated in the same fashion by the Price Commission. All this results in the misallocation of spending, medically inappropriate services, and upward pressure on health care spending, without improving health. This is not only an urban problem; it is also rural, although rural hospitals primarily overuse pharmaceuticals because they do not have access to expensive equipment.

Fee-for-service reimbursement is another factor leading to drug overprescription and to the overprovision of services. Costs can be better contained by the use of DRGs, which is payment-by-disease instead of payment per service rendered, or payment on a capitated basis, that is, on a given amount per covered person on a per month basis.

Because of the revenues generated by high-technology equipment, hospitals organize investor groups or borrow from banks to buy diagnostic testing equipment or lease it from international equipment suppliers. Diagnostic testing centers are often structured as specialty clinics. Today a hospital's reputation is said to depend on its possessing the latest and most expensive equipment.

At the end of 1993, China had 1,300 CT scanners, 200 MRIs, and 1,200 color Dopplers. Beijing, with 80 to 100 CT scanners, reportedly has the highest concentration of any city in the world. Many specialists believe these are not the most cost-effective investments for a country at China's stage of development, or even for more wealthy countries.

Because they are so reliant on public funding to meet operational costs, large public hospitals have started to add private wings for foreigners or wealthy Chinese. By paying fees of 300 to 400 yuan per day as opposed to 40 yuan (about US$37 to US$50 versus US$5), one gets a private room, treatment by department head physicians, better nurses, an unlimited pharmaceutical formulary, and priority in testing. These wings are reportedly full, with longer waiting lines than for the other wings of the same tertiary care hospitals.

Despite generally excess capacity in hospitals, one of the largest tertiary care hospitals in a major city in the south is seeking to increase its beds by two-thirds. Although construction has already started, it is seeking funding from the private sector because government funding has run out. This reflects poor planning at the hospital level and poor oversight by the regional Department of Public Health.

Medical inflation has become a serious problem in recent years. The medical inflation rate of 11 percent per annum between 1986 and 1993 exceeded the GDP per capita growth of 7.7 percent per annum Although this is similar to what happened in the West, when combined with a focus on fee-for-service reimbursement, it will lead to unsustainable cost escalation. To attempt to control these escalating hospital costs, in July 1994 Shanghai established a limit for medical cost inflation in hospitals, increased fees for visits and surgeries to better reflect costs, and cut CT and MRI test prices by 12 to 15 percent. The program was effective in cutting medical inflation from 53 percent the previous year to 24 percent. This experience suggests that coordinated pressure on medical inflation can be successful.

Private Providers

Of the 5.3 million health professionals in China, about 1.9 million are physicians (about 1.6 per 1,000 population) and 1 million are nurses. Government institutions under the Ministry of Health employ more than half of the workers. These numbers do not include about 1.4 million village doctors, many of who have only rudimentary training.

The private sector is mostly made up of physicians providing care from small offices or clinics, and of specialty services. Private practitioners operate an estimated 161,000 clinics in urban areas.

Some hospitals are also establishing their own private clinics in collaboration with foreign partners. One such example is a joint venture clinic of U.S. investors and a Shanghai hospital that focuses on providing primary, secondary, and some tertiary care for expatriates and overseas Chinese. The majority of its staff of physicians and dentists come from an American university.

State-Owned Enterprises

China's state-owned enterprises operate 700,000 hospital beds and employ 1.4 million health workers. In 1993, SOE health facilities provided 18 percent of outpatient care and 13 percent of inpatient treatment. Some of the large SOE-owned hospitals and clinics serve third parties on a fee-for-service basis. As an example, the Taiyuan Machinery Works in Shanxi Province operates a 300-bed hospital that receives one-quarter of its revenue from patients not affiliated with the enterprise. It plans to expand the hospital to 500 beds.

The government is now requiring all SOEs to divest themselves of their hospitals, as they are outside of their principal line of business. Currently, only Chinese nationals can bid to buy such facilities; foreigners may not.

At the same time, the ability of SOE employees to now use other hospitals for care and still be reimbursed will lead hospital management of SOE-owned hospitals to be more competitive and will improve their efficiency and quality of care. Some believe privatization of SOE hospitals will permit management to be less fettered by government regulation, thus more efficient. Others believe such hospitals will be sold to regional governments, thereby exacerbating management problems.

Health Plans and Health Insurance

Although most of the population can afford the costs of primary care treatment, paying for visits to hospitals or for higher-acuity treatment is generally beyond their ability. Usage is dropping, with a resulting impact on public health issues and on the demand for insurance. The government has two major concerns for China's health sector: (1) declining health insurance coverage and (2) inadequate access to health services for the poor.

In its attempt to avoid the rapidly escalating costs of providing health care services, China, over the past twenty or so years, has had significant success in cost-shifting from the government to the individual. Most of this shift has been in the form of out-of-pocket payments by individuals, not through a risk-pooled system.

Only 10 percent of the rural population (as opposed to 85 percent in 1975) and 50 percent of those in urban areas (as opposed to almost 100 percent) have health care insurance, principally from government insurance systems. The two largest systems cover only 15 percent of the population, yet account for 66 percent of public spending on health care and about 36 percent of all health spending. As a result, about 700 million rural Chinese, must now pay out-of-pocket for virtually all health services.

Although the situation is serious, there are some mitigating sources of financing. For example, the Medical Insurance Bureau provides extensive plans for students and the very young. The former costs about 100 yuan per year (US$12) and covers 50 percent of all medical costs, whereas the latter is quite inexpensive and covers all care, including immunizations, for the first few years of life. Employers generally pay the premiums for these policies.

The government has recently developed a new insurance scheme that includes medical savings accounts (MSAs) and is aimed at more affluent urban residents. As the government is concerned that the urban residents to whom such a program is targeted can be politically vocal, it is motivated to ensure that any such scheme is attractive and will work. The MSA scheme will require a 2 percent salary contribution by an employee and 6 percent by the employer. Self-employed individuals will pay the full 8 percent. These funds will go into an MSA, from which medical expenses will be deducted. Expenses greater than what is in the MSA will be paid out-of-pocket, be covered by a general fund, or a combination of the two, depending on the person's income level.

The largest life insurance company in China, which is publicly held, predicts a tremendous demand for health insurance for three reasons: (1) the growing urban middle class, (2) the limiting of government insurance to use in public hospitals and for basic services, and (3) the aging of the population. A private insurance market could foster the development of private clinics for physicals and urgent care services, and could eventually improve the overall quality of services available in public facilities. However, the government is reluctant to open the health insurance sector to foreign companies; insurers that wish to enter the market need to take a long-term view.

At the same time, the ability of insurance companies or programs to control health care spending costs is limited, as government hospitals oppose payment reforms that might reduce their revenues or force their closure or downsizing. Some agreement will be needed if very many foreign insurance companies are to enter the Chinese health care insurance business.

Opportunities for Investment

Currently, the government does not permit foreign investors to take majority ownership control of general hospitals—a position not expected to change for the next five years. One reason is that the Department of Public Health claims it cannot control the quality of care in government hospitals, so it would have even less influence over foreign-owned hospitals. However, it sees no problem with foreign management of hospitals.

Companies that are completely Chinese-owned are permitted to buy hospitals from the government or from SOEs. If the department continues its view on foreign-managed hospitals, this might provide investors an opportunity to come into China, initially in a management role, with some informal agreement for a future joint venture.

Majority foreign ownership is permitted of specialty hospitals or clinics. Such structures often are used as vehicles for making specialty equipment available to hospitals or providing a superior quality of care for private-pay patients.

Specialty Services

Opportunities for private investment are varied, particularly for specialized services. One example is renal dialysis. Only about 10 percent of those with end stage renal disease receive dialysis treatment, as dialysis centers are generally located only in larger cities. Cost is also a factor; it is about US$260 to US$300 per treatment. If the cost dropped significantly, families could afford to pay for treatment out of pocket and would consider this an obligation. Dialysis equipment in many hospitals is in need of upgrading, so joint ventures with operators or manufacturers may be welcomed.

Another segment for potential investment may be in diagnostic laboratories. Some public hospitals are interested in outsourcing these services to joint ventures with foreign operators on a profit-sharing basis. One foreign hospital operator, for example, has established a diagnostic lab in a provincial capital and expects to do the same in a hospital in another provincial capital. As diagnostic labs in many developing countries are among the most profitable segments of the health care industry, more investment can be anticipated. Quality control will be a critical issue in the future, so relationships with reference labs of world-class standards will be necessary.

Eye care may provide investment opportunities. One-quarter of the population in China has myopia; in Shanghai, it may be as high as one-half. Sixty million people in China have cataracts; if not treated properly, one-tenth of them will go blind.

Long-Term Care

As in most countries, the aging of the population will increase health spending in China. People age sixty-five and older currently make up 6 percent of China's population; that is expected to grow to 11 percent by 2020. To control costs, the government will have to introduce effective health promotion and disease-prevention programs to improve the health outlook for China's elderly people.

Long-term care facilities are almost nonexistent in China, as families have traditionally kept elderly members at home. However, these family values have eroded with the increased pressure for all family members to work, the rapid aging of the population, and the one-child-per-couple policy.

The government is becoming aware of the demographic issues affecting the need for serving the elderly but has yet to formulate a solution. Although few know what the government will do, it would appear that there will be an increasing demand for quality assisted living and skilled nursing facilities, as well as for more home health care.

Medical Equipment

There is a significant demand for the purchase of imported medical equipment, ostensibly to improve the quality of diagnosis and treatment. However, hospitals are not permitted to price basic services to be profitable, so they rely on generating fees from diagnostic testing with expensive equipment (required to be paid for in cash, as for most other services); therefore, the demand for expensive imported technology remains high. This leads to misallocation of spending, medically inappropriate services, and upward pressure on health care spending. This is not only an urban problem but also rural, although rural hospitals overuse pharmaceuticals. They do not have access to expensive equipment. It also gives cause for concern that the government's current approach on pricing of services and medical equipment imports may change over the next few years. This could affect the future demand but should not hurt the credit quality of existing borrowers.

This tremendous demand is only partly mitigated by local production. Foreign manufacturers see great potential in China, and most hospitals find that expensive medical equipment has about a three-year payback. However, few manufacturers appear ready to openly extend credit to buyers or even to provide financing of five to seven years against import letters of credit (LCs) from the few Chinese banks permitted to issue them. Most decline to accept import LCs with expiration dates in excess of six months from shipment.

The process is complicated by the fact that hospitals operate in local currency and have no foreign currency earnings; hence they are not permitted to import goods themselves. Instead, they must go to an authorized medical equipment distributor, of which there are about 2,000 throughout the country; all are government-owned. Reportedly, a number are losing money, but the government has not closed any down.

Pharmaceuticals

The pharmaceutical industry in China is a highly dynamic and diverse market; for a foreign manufacturer there are many challenges. For example, there are large discrepancies between regions, populace, wealth, and accessibility to health care, not to mention the varying disease profiles associated with the respective locale and economic conditions. All this creates fifty separate markets rather than a single, cohesive market. Further, distribution is limited to regionally focused domestic players, omitting national distribution capabilities, and channels are very localized; 85 percent of all drug products are channeled through hospital pharmacies. Moreover, competitive products differ in China. In addition to Western medicines (WM), there is a substantial selection of traditional Chinese medicines, or herbal-based medicaments.

Hospitals are motivated to overprescribe pharmaceuticals to compensate for below-cost fee levels for physician visits, which are regulated by the government. As the price structure for drugs allows markups of 15 percent at both the wholesale and retail levels, there is added incentive to overprescribe drugs, especially expensive drugs, to supplement their income. This has led to spending on pharmaceuticals being remarkably high—52 percent of all health care spending in 1993, as opposed to about 14 percent in OECD countries and 15 to 40 percent in most other developing countries. Even so, per-capita expenditures on drugs are only about $5 a year in China.

Pricing for pharmaceuticals is about double the manufacturer or importer sales price, as opposed to about 15 to 20 percent above the sales price for manufacturers in the United States. This is because there are almost 10,000 distributors, with the resulting lack of efficiencies in distribution.

Eighty-five percent of pharmaceutical sales in China occur in hospital inpatient or outpatient settings. The remainder are sold through retail outlets, mainly pharmacies that are normally "mom and pop" operations. This percentage is growing in the South however, and some distributors now own pharmacies. New regulations covering over-the-counter (OTC) drugs were published in July 1999, which has led to an explosive expansion of pharmacies. This will undoubtedly put pressure on hospital revenues that are generated from pharmaceutical sales.

As the Chinese government attempts to convert from a centrally planned economy to a free-market-based system, all the while balancing social stability, domestic companies are consolidating into fifty large domestic conglomerates, and legislative changes are being implemented to control escalating health care costs. In addition, TCM products are being developed as "new drugs," supported by Western structured clinical trials, to increase quality profiles in China and to allow domestic companies access to Western markets. These changes are forcing companies to introduce technologically advanced products while placing them under increasing pricing and real substitution pressures.

Despite these challenges however, China remains a good market for investment in pharmaceuticals. The Chinese government aims to develop its market into the second-largest pharmaceutical market in the world. It intends to improve the general condition of manufacturers by substantially improving quality requirements and weeding out defunct SOEs. This will provide a platform for three types of companies: (1) fifty large, domestic conglomerates; (2) foreign joint ventures or wholly owned companies (multinational or medium-sized) that have a strong product foundation or are entering the market with new technology; and (3) to a lesser extent, the TCM manufacturers focusing on product innovation and expansion into Western markets.

These players should additionally benefit from the substantial increase in health care spending that results from (1) the new measures that allow expansion and development of new distribution channels (retail pharmacies and supermarkets) and (2) new product markets such as OTC and herbal products. These changes, coupled with traditional market drivers such as increasing wealth, aging, increasing life expectancy rates, and shifting disease profiles, underpin the projected 13 to 15 percent per annum growth rate predicted for the US$5 billion pharmaceutical market.

Strategies for survivors will focus on tapping into the new market segments, expanding geographically, and strengthening key relationships, as China relies on such relationships to promote business opportunities.

Besides the China market, the pharmaceutical industry in Hong Kong is growing. The Hong Kong pharmaceutical market is currently only one-quarter of the size of Chinese market. However, Hong Kong has more strategic importance to the Chinese market, as it is the portal for many pharmaceutical companies. Large multinational corporations use Hong Kong as a re-export base (less so since 1997) and a main administrative hub for both China and the South East Asian countries (Leland, 1999).

The 10,000 pharmaceutical distributors in China are all state-owned. Foreign ownership is not permitted, although some close relationships with foreign companies are developing. Many of the existing distributors are losing money due to poor management, but it will be some time before the local Ministries of Health will force a consolidation of distributors, if they ever do.

Manufacturing is fragmented; although the top twenty companies produce 60 percent of production, there are about 2,000 manufacturers. R&D expenditures of 1 percent of turnover compare poorly with an average 12 percent in the United States, 13 percent in Europe, and 10 percent in Japan. Government pressure on pharmaceutical prices to reduce the portion of revenue of hospitals generated from pharmaceutical sales, as well as pressure on the quality of production, will lead to the merger or closure of a number of pharmaceutical manufacturing facilities. Because few are in compliance with international manufacturing regulations, they are not likely to be of interest to buyers. Some, however, may have permits worth purchasing.

China is helping pharmaceutical companies improve the quality of their clinical trial research. If a foreign company were to do its clinical trials in China, that would reduce the time needed for registration of a pharmaceutical in China, which is normally about two years from when it is approved for use in the United States or in Europe. As good clinical practices expertise is still lacking in China, research should be done parallel to trials in the West. However, China is rapidly improving its practices.

The Chinese pharmaceutical market has the potential to develop into one of the top markets in the world. Hence, it has expected to become a playground for multinational companies and a potential platform for the powerhouses within China to develop. Usually Hong Kong is the first step for foreign companies into China and the first step for Chinese companies out of China (Leland, 1999). Rabobank is already in discussion with some potential investors in local manufacturing operations.

As a method of controlling pharmaceutical costs, the concept of a pharmacy benefit plan with a set formulary is not understood in China but could potentially cut such costs almost in half. This is something that insurance companies should be discussing with the medical insurance bureaus in some of the larger cities; insurance companies could help them develop an approach to the issue and to the software needed to formulate a rational plan.

Patent law is tricky. For China to get into the WTO it must show compliance with international patent law. Although China has said it will comply with all patents issued in 1996 and later, those are on products not yet being marketed. Hence, companies will be in the difficult position of determining whether they want to register patents originating before 1996, with the risk of their being copied.

Role of Traditional Chinese Medicine

It has been estimated that about half of the Chinese population use traditional Chinese medicine rather than Western medicine techniques. As the cost of providing TCM is significantly below that of providing WM and technology, the government vastly prefers to emphasize the former. However, the increasingly educated young people in China vastly prefer WM, thus driving up the cost of health care services. It is this rapid cost escalation that the government wants to avoid so is pushing the consumer to pay an increasing portion of health care costs.

Interestingly enough, the Hong Kong government has indicated that it wants to establish a center for analysis of TCM, determine what properties in those medicines can be extracted and put into Western medications, and then produce the latter. The Chinese government seems much less enthusiastic about such an idea, however. They have targeted ten TCM products to run through clinical research to determine their efficacy, which would be required to permit registration in the Western countries.

Summary

China is a market with tremendous potential for health care providers and for equipment and pharmaceutical manufacturers seeking to export to or invest in China. However, many issues need attention; these include the disproportionate spending on pharmaceuticals and diagnostic testing (which will likely receive government attention in the next five years) and the foreign ownership of providers (which likely will not change significantly in the near future). These issues should be addressed before becoming actively involved in the market. A long-term approach to the market is needed in order to eventually become successful.

Reference

Leland, S. *China and Hong Kong: The Pharmaceutical Industry.* Amsterdam: Rabobank International, 1999.

CHAPTER TWENTY-SEVEN

HONG KONG

Yanek S. Y. Chiu

Changes in the Hong Kong Specialized Administrative Region (SAR) health delivery system are taking place, and the pace of reform has quickened under the new secretary of health and welfare. who took office in September 1999. As is true with most Southeast Asian countries, political and economic vagaries can be irrational and unpredictable. Hong Kong is no exception. The only difference is that Hong Kong has enjoyed a very long period of sustained economic boom. It has been the last major area to be affected by the recent economic downturn that started with Thailand and Indonesia in 1997; it is partially protected by its large cash reserve. Conversely, its economic recovery may also be the last to materialize.

The debate on the health care reform process in both the public and private sectors, as well as within the government, has taken center stage over the past few months. Experts have voiced their opinions almost daily, both in the Chinese and English daily newspapers and on television (English and Chinese channels). The stimulus for all this discussion has been the government's decision to commission Professor William Hsiao and his associates from Harvard University to assess the current system and to propose alternative options for improvement, as appropriate.

The *Hsiao Report*, which has been available to the public since April 1999, is comprehensive and well researched. Health statistics are not usually readily available in Hong Kong, particularly in the private sector, but the Hospital Authority (HA) has maintained a good bookkeeping record, as mandated by the government, and has provided plenty of data from the public hospitals for this important study (Hospital Authority, 1999).

The think tank of the current Hong Kong government is staffed by highly educated and experienced experts, with assistance from international consultants. There is a high level of sophistication in the formulation of ideas for reforms for the future, as evidenced by reports of many public debates over the past few months. Several options are available, and these are presently being debated within the inner circle. The stakes are high.

Inevitably, some self-serving interest groups will try to undermine the reform process in order to maintain the status quo. What eventually will evolve in the Hong Kong health care reform of 1999–2000 will be scrutinized carefully in Taiwan, Singapore, throughout Southeast Asia, and of course in Beijing.

Many resources have been used in preparing this examination of the Hong Kong system, including the *Hsiao Report*, primarily for the extensive data that were available to the Harvard team during the year they conducted their research. The annual report of the HA, which is published for public consumption, is also of great importance and interest. In addition, private correspondence with key players in the health care reform process have been most helpful in evaluating the health care system at a time when this region is going through rapid changes.

Historical Perspective

In 1842, at the end of the now-famous Opium War, the island of Hong Kong was ceded to Great Britain outright; the Kowloon peninsula, along with the New Territories, likewise came under British rule on an extended lease of over 150 years. All this changed in a highly publicized ceremony on July 1, 1997, when Prince Charles, representing Queen Elizabeth II, returned the island of Hong Kong, Kowloon, and the New Territories to China; these lands are designated by the current Chinese government as an SAR.

Before that historic event, international and local experts were predicting major changes in Hong Kong and saying that the changes would come quickly. Surprisingly, little changed at the beginning, and the subtle political rumblings were only discernable by the most astute and observant scholars. However, the recent economic downturn throughout Asia has certainly affected the real estate market, the stock market, economic growth (being negative for the first time in fifty years), and the mood of the people. Other changes include the relative absence of British influence and the increased use of Mandarin as the official language, as well as the language used on the street.

The health care system has undergone little change compared to its political and economic counterparts. Perhaps the well-entrenched laissez-faire philosophy is responsible for this; minimal government intervention or regulation allows the free-market system to structure itself and organize. System change has been successful primarily because of the unprecedented economic boom over the past five decades, allowing the low tax rate to continue (a 15 percent tax for all wage earners, with no tax on capital gains or unearned income) and continuing the policy of linking the increase in public expenditure on the health care system with GDP growth. Recently, in response to an increasing demand for government health services, a more definitive position on the health care system has been articulated for Hong Kong. This response by the government includes the building of more government hospitals, thus increasing the bed-to-population ratio and providing a safety net for all Hong Kong residents for their health care needs at nominal charges.

In 1989–1990, in a major reform process, the Medical and Health Department was divided into two major divisions: the Department of Health (DOH) and the HA, both answerable to the secretary of health and welfare.

The DOH has a myriad of functions, including the promotion and education regarding public health issues, management of public primary care clinics, licensing, and food and drug safety. All employees in the DOH, including physicians, are civil servants.

The HA, which has grown considerably in size and budget, manages the forty-four public or government hospitals and forty-eight specialty outpatient clinics; the majority of employees of these facilities are not civil servants. The HA is autonomous and has its own powerful board of directors.

Meanwhile, the private sector has thrived over the past five decades, serving the ever-expanding middle and upper-middle classes. Total private health expenditures in 1996–1997 were HK$26 billion (about US$3.4 billion), as compared to the public sector expenditure of US$4.0 billion. The majority of private expenditures are financed by patients' out-of-pocket payments, which they make on a fee-for-service basis.

The private sector primary care physicians remain the primary providers of care for over 80 percent of the residents in Hong Kong. However, because of the rising costs of private hospitals and increasing specialist fees, more patients are opting for the public hospital care. The HA provides close to 90 percent of all inpatient care.

Current Dilemmas

Hong Kong is in the unenviable position of having a growing and aging population. In 1977 the total population of Hong Kong was 4.58 million and is projected to top 8.2 million by 2016. Although the total population is projected to nearly double, the population over the age of sixty-five is projected to triple in the same time frame, with 5.7 percent of the population in 1977 over sixty-five and projected to rise to 13.3 percent by 2016. The government is keenly aware of the reality of rising expenses in health care, and yet it must exercise restraint in keeping the health care budget at a fixed percent of GDP in order to maintain other public services at the same level.

Government expenditures on health care are channeled through the DOH and the HA, with the latter taking the lion's share of the budget (over 70 percent). The Hospital Authority's *Annual Plan, 1997–1998* illustrates the enormous task and financial responsibility of taking care of such a large number of patients. At the end of 1996, HA had 25,500 hospital beds, which represented 4.05 public hospital beds per 1,000 population. There were 47,247 full-time staff, with a budget of HK$22 billions. In addition, the volume of secondary and tertiary care was increasing steadily on a yearly basis. There was a 6.2 percent increase in the number of patients discharged in 1996–1997 over the previous twelve months. Surgical outpatient and emergency room visits are also up 11.6 and 7.9 percent, respectively (Hospital Authority, 1996, 1997).

Ever since the formation of the HA nearly a decade ago, there has been a gradual shift of inpatient services from the private to the public sector. First, under the capable leadership of Dr. Yeoh, the HA has progressed considerably in providing a high level of care at affordable costs (HK$68, or US$9, for a hospital day, inclusive of all costs). A centralized infrastructure is well established, with a capable and cost-conscious administrative staff. Internationally renowned physicians and surgeons fill the academic posts in some of the flagship hospitals. Private rooms (for a slightly higher fee) with modern amenities are attracting more middle-class residents to the public sector, particularly for more expensive and complicated tertiary care. Over the years, the annual budget for the HA has increased considerably, but because of economic expansion, the budget has remained a relatively constant percentage of GDP.

Since 1998, as the economy has slowed and the GDP has shown negative growth for the first time in modern history, the HA has been struggling with increasing demands in the face of a shrinking budget. This is made worse by the immense cost differential between the public and private sectors in the secondary and tertiary care arena. Naturally, just on the cost issue alone, the middle class is shifting into the HA system, with a decline in the patient census in private hospitals over the past eighteen months. Even the upper middle class is reconsidering health care options. Although statistics are not available, there is the general perception that the truly well-to-do residents are having their major tertiary health problems taken care of in the United Kingdom and in the United States.

In 1998 the HA, with legislative approval, commissioned Dr. Hsiao and his associates from Harvard University to assess the present health care problems in Hong Kong in both the public and private sectors. The *Hsiao Report* took nearly a year to complete and was made available to public perusal in April of 1999. It has been received with mixed reactions among the local health experts, considered by some to be long on citing problems and short on offering solutions.

On the strengths or achievements of the current system, the *Hsiao Report* states:

Our assessment of the Hong Kong health care system shows that Hong Kong has a relatively equitable system, in terms of access and utilization, resource distribution, and financing. Because of the 1990 reform of the public hospital system through the establishment of the HA, Hong Kong has also benefited from improvements in certain aspects of quality and productive efficiency in specific areas. Evidence indicates that the cost-effectiveness of the Hong Kong health system is similar to its neighboring Asian nations and compares favorably to European advanced economies.

On weaknesses, the *Hsiao Report* continues:

Our assessment of Hong Kong's health care system shows that the system suffers from three inter-related weaknesses—highly variable quality of care, inefficient allocation of public funds, and questionable financial and organizational sustainability of the system. These results point to the need to seriously rethink and redevelop an overall coherent health care policy and health care financing/delivery system that will meet the needs of the population of Hong Kong.

Based on the *Hsiao Report,* the private health insurance companies are waiting in the wings, watching with interest how the government will eventually implement the changes recommended and what role, if any, private insurance may have in the new system. At this time, private insurers have only a small stake in the health care industry. Health insurance policies are usually inexpensive, bought primarily by employers for their employees, and with coverage mainly for office visits and minor tests or medical services. United Healthcare has an office in Hong Kong, and American International Group (AIG) is strong in the general insurance market; managed care companies such as those in the United States have had little impact. Private sector physicians and surgeons, as well as the private hospitals, are openly opposed to the introduction of American-type managed care models. Dr. Kai Ming So, president of the Hong Kong Medical Association, speaking for the majority of his colleagues in the private sector, has stated repeatedly in newspapers and on television his position that managed care and the capitation system will be unacceptable at this time. At the same time, he and many of his colleagues in both sectors acknowledge that change is inevitable. They say they hope the change will be gradual and acceptable to all concerned.

Options for Future Reforms

In 1997, even before Hsiao and his colleagues were commissioned, the HA quietly discussed several options that could bring about changes in health care financing. The mission statement then and now has remained the same: "It is the policy of the government that no one should be prevented, through lack of means, from obtaining adequate medical treatment" (Hospital Authority, 1996). The proposals put forth by the *Hsiao Report* have provided further fuel for discussion.

One simple option, which the government will naturally consider, is to do nothing. But the option of maintaining the present status quo is unacceptable, even to the most conservative. The rising cost of medical care and the aging population will place an increasing financial burden on the government budget, leading to reduction of spending on other public services with the risk of adversely affecting the standard of living of all Hong Kong residents.

Another simple option is to limit the government budget for health care. However, there is serious concern that the quality of services will deteriorate. Well-to-do patients will shift back to the private sector and will encourage the entry of for-profit insurance companies into Hong Kong. They in turn will drive down the high cost of health care in the private sector by the introduction of cost-containment systems. Indemnity insurance coverage will be significantly more expensive, thus excluding those who are not affluent enough to afford the high premiums. The overall result will be inequity and lack of access.

Currently, user fees account for only 3 percent of the cost of the government health care expenses. As the public perceives the government health system to be so inexpensive, there is the obvious overuse of facilities and services. Adding a small copayment for every clinic visit could affect utilization. Care must be taken to avoid setting copays at such levels as to burden the poor and low-income families unfairly by raising economic barriers to access. The concept of means testing is slowly gaining acceptance. However, it is clear that means testing alone would not be a panacea.

Another option being considered is to redesign the basic infrastructure of the health department. From an administrative standpoint, the division of responsibility between the HA and the DOH, initially an innovative concept, may prove inefficient as the new millennium approaches. Currently, the public primary care clinics are under the supervision of the DOH; hospitals are managed by the separate HA. The lack of shared incentives and management makes it difficult to promote the concept of a seamless continuum of care. The growing elderly population and their need for comprehensive coordinated care will only augment this problem in the years ahead.

The medical savings account concept is not new. This savings account can be used to purchase long-term care insurance offered by private companies at the time of retirement or disability. As proposed by the *Hsiao Report*, this will be a mandatory contribution to an individual savings account. This will not be a short-term fix, as it needs time to build up a substantial savings account for future use. Because the government is not providing long-term care and the cost for elderly care is escalating, this concept should appeal to the younger age groups, even though it will affect their disposable income for the moment.

Another model is for the government to set up a not-for-profit insurance plan that would be administered by a separate regulatory agency headed by the secretary of health and welfare. In such a plan, there would be only one premium level for Hong Kong residents. For the poor and unemployed or the retired with little unearned income, there would be no premium; they would use existing public clinics and hospitals as before except they would make a small copayment for a clinic visit. The level of the premium for everyone else to buy in would be set at a level affordable by the average wage earner. This reasonable and affordable premium could essentially allow all Hong Kong residents to have health care coverage, even for costly, catastrophic illnesses.

Need for Improved Information Technology

In a region as diverse as Hong Kong, with overlapping authorities within the government agencies and with patients crossing back and forth between the public and private medical facilities, any reform process must take into consideration the need to upgrade information technology, particularly through the Internet. Innovative companies have created systems that can store almost a limitless amount of data, with easy retrieval and flexibility as well as the capability to network with health care providers, laboratory, hospitals, and clinics instantaneously. The programs are also immensely efficient in checking eligibility, processing claims, updating demographics, and approving of medical and surgical services. In addition, the new millennium will likely see a paperless medical record-keeping system, including the elimination of the conventional X-ray and CT-scan films. Moreover, medical knowledge can be shared simultaneously via the website, as consultants can discuss complex cases on-line. When the new facilities are built to accommodate the health care reform process, visionary designers and engineers will play a major role in adding all these new technology capabilities to the system in order to be ready for the fast-paced advances in the technological arena.

Conclusion

The health care system currently in place in Hong Kong must and will change sooner rather than later, as the government has made all the strategic steps through the timely use of the best consultants locally and internationally. For the first time, the appointed secretary of health and welfare is a physician; Dr. Yeoh has the extensive training, the vision, and the energy to move ahead with the reform process with deliberation and caution. It is an exciting moment, and a new era is about to begin.

References

Hospital Authority. *Annual Report, 1995–1996*. Hong Kong: Hospital Authority, 1996.
Hospital Authority. *Annual Plan, 1997–1998*. Hong Kong: Hospital Authority, 1997.
Hospital Authority. *Hsiao Report*. Apr. 13, 1999. [http://www.info.gov.hk/hwb/english/consult/hcs/hcs.htm].

CHAPTER TWENTY-EIGHT

INDIA

Neelam Sekhri

India spends almost 6 percent of its GDP on health. However, unlike most developing and developed countries, nearly 80 percent of health care services are financed by the private sector (World Bank, 1997). Private health spending as a share of national income in India is among the highest of any nation in the world, financed largely through out-of-pocket expenditures (Berman and Khan, 1993). Voluntary insurance is available to a very small percentage of the population and covers limited hospital services with numerous exclusions. Fewer than 2 million people out of India's population of 1 billion currently have insurance coverage. (This refers to voluntary insurance rather than mandatory schemes such as Employees' State Insurance.)

Although health care spending has increased slightly over the past decade, funds have not been efficiently allocated. Urban residents and hospitals receive the majority of public funds to pay for the high costs generated by inefficient use of equipment and pharmaceuticals. As health care costs increase, quality health care becomes less and less accessible to more Indian residents. This particularly affects the access of the middle class and poor to appropriate health services. Whereas the rich can afford to purchase high-priced private care, the middle class and poor are often unable to obtain health care services of reliable quality.

Financing and Flow of Funds

Both as a percentage of GNP and in real terms, India's expenditures on health care are similar to those of many lower- and lower-middle-income countries (World Bank, 1997). Overall, India spends 5.6 percent of its GNP on health services. This amounts to only US$17 per capita in nominal terms; however, when purchasing power parity is considered, annual expenditures are US$69 per capita (World Bank, 1997).

What distinguishes India from other lower-middle-income countries and from the Asian region is that public spending on health care is low, with only 22 percent of health expenditures publicly funded (see Figure 28.1). Households finance almost 80 percent of expenditures privately, primarily through out-of-pocket payments. Of the 75 percent of health care dollars spent by individuals, 48 percent goes to purchase primary care services; 27 percent is spent on inpatient care (Naylor, Prabhat, Woods, and Shariff, 1999).

An important feature of the health care system in India is the strong role played by the state governments in the financing and provision of health care. Consequently, there are significant variations among states in

- The health status of the population
- The relative importance of public sector finance and delivery

FIGURE 28.1. HOW INDIA'S HEALTH CARE SYSTEM IS FUNDED.

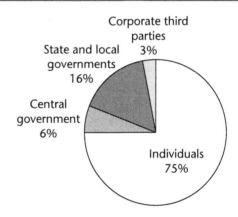

Source: Adapted courtesy World Bank.

- The quality of publicly provided services
- The degree of regulation of the private sector
- The political and legal climate for foreign investors and the protections afforded to them

Overall, populations in the southern states of Kerala and Tamil Nadu and in the wealthier states such as Punjab and Maharastra enjoy better health and better health services than in other states. Kerala, a relatively poor state, is an exception to this; its residents have by far the best health and public health services in India. For example, the infant mortality rate in Kerala is 17 per 1,000 live births, whereas in the much wealthier state of Harayana, the infant mortality rate is 69 per 1,000 live births (Measham and others, forthcoming). Kerala's statistics highlight that good public policy and stable government are at least as important to health as the absolute amount of resources spent on health care services (see Figure 28.2).

Components of the Health Care System

India's health care system is pluralistic, with large public and publicly mandated systems of care, state-owned enterprise systems, hospitals and clinics run by NGOs, and a large and unregulated array of private providers (see Figure 28.3).

FIGURE 28.2. HOW INDIA'S HEALTH CARE MONIES ARE SPENT.

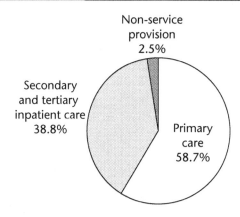

Non-service provision 2.5%

Secondary and tertiary inpatient care 38.8%

Primary care 58.7%

Source: Adapted courtesy World Bank.

FIGURE 28.3. INDIA'S HEALTH CARE SYSTEM.

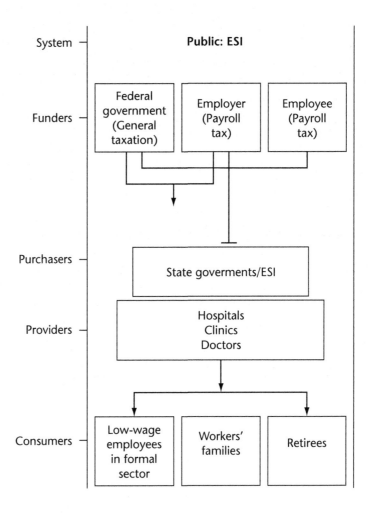

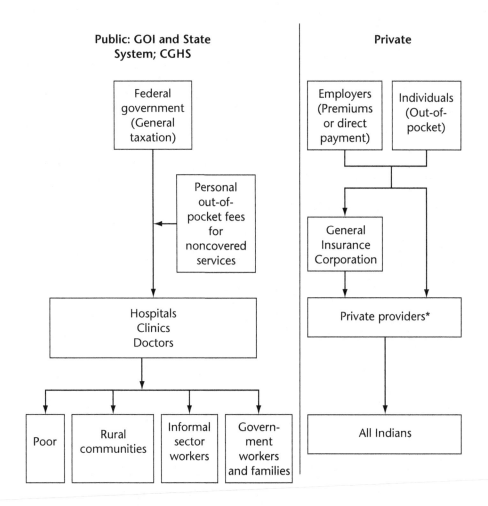

*Several *parastatals* and large corporations operate their own health care systems; these are not depicted.

The central government sponsors two major, publicly mandated programs to which the states contribute financially. These programs are the Employees' State Insurance Scheme (ESIS) and the Central Government Health Scheme (CGHS). These systems function as both insurers and providers of care with their own ambulatory facilities and hospitals. The government of India (GOI) and the states also operate a public system of hospitals and clinics, which serves as the provider of last resort for rural and urban Indians.

Voluntary health insurance is very limited and is offered only through the nationalized General Insurance Corporation (GIC). Employers often augment this limited coverage with direct payments to employees, allowing them to use private providers for care. Some large employers, such as Tata, operate their own health care systems for employees and their dependents. Despite these schemes, most Indians pay out-of-pocket on a fee-for-service basis for health care services.

The following sections describe each of the major public and private systems in greater detail.

Public Purchasers and Providers

Employees' State Insurance Scheme

ESIS was established in 1948 as a self-supporting social security program for the organized labor sector. This insurance scheme is operated through an autonomous body and is mandatory for employees earning less than 6,500 rupees per month (US$162). ESIS covers over 28 million workers, their families, and retirees and is largely funded through mandatory employer (4.75 percent of wages) and employee (2.25 percent of wages) contributions (Naylor, Prabhat, Woods, and Shariff, 1999).

ESIS operates an extensive network of 124 hospitals, with 18,527 beds in twenty-two states and territories, and contracts with hospitals outside the system for subspecialty services. The program also provides a variety of cash, death, and disability benefits to employees and dependents. Although ESIS is a central government program, provision and management of facilities is largely through the states, with ESIS acting as a purchaser of care.

As is typical of the public systems in India, ESIS facilities suffer from a poor quality of care and service. As a result, many of those covered under ESIS choose to go outside the system and pay for services by fee-for-service providers. Ellis (1996, cited in Naylor, Prabhat, Woods, and Shariff, 1999) states that "detailed patient surveys conducted in Gujarat found that more than half of all survey respondents covered by ESIS did not seek care from ESIS facilities for treatment."

Central Government Health Scheme

The CGHS covers central government employees, dependents, retirees, and a variety of special groups such as employees of the defense industry, senior government officials, and high court judges and employees (Naylor, Prabhat, Woods, and Shariff, 1999). The scheme currently has over 4 million beneficiaries who receive care through a combination of CGHS-operated ambulatory facilities, public hospitals, and referrals to private hospitals. As a purchaser of health services for its employees, the GOI provides significant subsidies to CGHS. Given the population to which it caters, benefits are generous, allowing more luxurious accommodations at public and private facilities. Despite this, beneficiaries complain of poorly operated clinics and long waiting times to receive reimbursement for private services. Again, many go to private providers for their care and pay out of pocket.

Government of India and State Systems

The national government and the state governments operate very extensive urban and rural systems of hospitals, primary health centers, and clinics. The states provide the majority (75 percent) of funding for rural and urban curative care and manage hospital and clinic facilities. Rural networks focus on ambulatory and basic inpatient services; urban centers concentrate on more complex tertiary and specialty care.

With the exception of certain high-technology academic centers that are operated by the GOI, the public system is often considered the system of last resort. Rural facilities are poorly staffed and suffer from supply and drug shortages, impersonal service, and long waiting times (Naylor, Prabhat, Woods, and Shariff, 1999). Primary health centers are not easily accessible. Wyatt and Bhat (1997, cited in Naylor, Prabhat, Woods, and Shariff, 1999) indicate that greater than half the population must travel over 5 kilometers to access a primary health center. As a result, those in rural areas either seek care in urban clinics and hospitals or go to private, often unlicensed, providers for their care.

In urban areas the poor typically rely on public facilities for hospital care and visit private providers for ambulatory care. Those who can afford it use private hospitals and nursing homes. (Nursing homes are small, inpatient facilities that provide a limited range of services such as maternity care.)

State-Owned Enterprise Delivery Systems

The Indian Railways and other state-owned enterprises operate their own extensive health systems. The Indian Railways is particularly interesting because as the largest publicly owned enterprise in the world (Naylor, Prabhat, Woods, and Shariff, 1999), it has a health care system that serves over 10 million beneficiaries.

Its infrastructure of ambulatory and diagnostic facilities, secondary hospitals, and tertiary hospitals is one of the most sophisticated in India.

Private Purchasers and Providers

Insurance

Currently, only the General Insurance Corporation (GIC) a quasi-governmental agency, is allowed to sell health insurance in India. The general insurance industry was nationalized in 1971, and the GIC was formed a year later. GIC works through four subsidiary companies, which are located in different geographical regions, but operate on an all-India basis and sell insurance policies in competition with each other. Despite the creation of this internal market, little innovation has occurred in the development of insurance products. The few health insurance policies that exist contain numerous exclusions and deductibles and require beneficiaries to pay out of pocket for services with subsequent reimbursement by GIC. Beneficiaries complain of very slow and restrictive reimbursement practices. Most private hospitals do not bill GIC directly; they expect the individual to pay cash at the time of service. This causes an unmanageable financial burden on policyholders and, as a result, only the highest-risk individuals voluntarily purchase individual coverage. Most GIC policies are purchased by employers who provide health insurance as a managerial and executive benefit.

In late 1999, after years of lobbying, a bill passed the Indian Parliament that will permit foreign private companies to enter the Indian health insurance market in defined joint venture arrangements with local firms. This is seen as the first step toward the eventual privatization of the entire insurance industry.

Given the restricted insurance environment, it is not surprising that India has one of the lowest levels of insurance density (per capita spending on insurance) as well as insurance penetration in the world.[1] The insurable population of India is officially defined as all males between twenty and sixty years of age. Of a potential of 241.6 million insurable lives, only 2 million lives are covered by voluntary health insurance. The definition of the insurable population excludes a substantial population of working women who can also afford to buy insurance products.

Providers

The majority of health services in India are purchased through direct out-of-pocket expenditures on a fee-for-service basis. In the case of the urban and rural poor, out-of-pocket payments buy primarily ambulatory medical services by qualified as well as unqualified physicians and folk healers; they also buy pharmaceuticals. Inpatient care for the poor is provided through the public hospital system and through a vast network of small private hospitals (five to thirty beds) called nursing homes.

India's growing middle class, however, which is estimated at between 425 and 700 million (Naylor, Prabhat, Woods, and Shariff, 1999), requires a very different mix of services from India's poor. The middle class expects a level of quality and service that the public sector is often unable to provide.

As in most emerging economies, India is undergoing a health transition. The burden of disease is shifting from predominantly diseases of poverty (communicable, neonatal, and maternal illnesses) to an increasing incidence of the diseases of affluence, urbanization, and aging (for example, cardiovascular diseases, cancers, and injuries). This transition changes the emphasis to interventions that demand greater management of disease across the primary, secondary, and tertiary levels of care. It also requires the use of expensive technologies and pharmaceuticals, and places greater emphasis on prevention, early diagnosis, and intervention.

In response to these changes, India's private health sector is growing rapidly, with large multihospital groups establishing a national presence. Although they function as fee-for-service hospitals with a focus on filling beds, these groups could create the basis for integrated delivery systems with salaried specialists and integration of ambulatory and inpatient services at a single site of care.

The growth of these "corporate" hospital chains has led to tension with the Ministries of Health. The government believes that many of these private, for-profit systems, which cater to the upper-middle class and rich, have not honored their commitment to provide care to the underserved in exchange for receiving substantial governmental subsidies. As a result, many of the subsidies previously provided by the government have been withdrawn, causing the private sector to scramble for new sources of capital.

The repeal of government subsidies for private hospitals makes the economics of operating these systems more risky than in the past. However, the unavailability of high-quality private beds in urban areas and the great demand generated by the middle class have resulted in private hospitals having long waiting lists for beds. Employers often pay thousands of rupees just to reserve access to a bed when it is needed for their senior employees.

In addition to the newly emerging investor-owned systems, the highest-quality private hospital facilities have traditionally been provided by NGOs—religious and charitable foundations. These facilities, however, are often filled to capacity, and private bed shortages are frequent in urban areas.

Regulation and Market Opportunities

Since 1991, there has been a considerable shift in the foreign investment and technology transfer policy of the Indian government. The major changes in this policy are as follows:

- Automatic approval for foreign equity holding up to 51 percent in a large group of industries and automatic approval of foreign equity up to 74 percent in nine groups of core industries.
- The creation of the Foreign Investment Promotion Board (FIPB), which is the apex body for approving foreign investments in India. The board was created to expedite the approval process for foreign investors.

India has also accepted the norms of intellectual property rights under the World Trade Organization (WTO), affording protection to both process and product patents. As a member of the WTO, India has made a commitment to promote free trade. After four decades of controls on the import of consumer goods, India has finally agreed to liberalize the import of consumer goods.

Because of this liberalization, the market is already experiencing a surge in private capital investment in health care. The internationally renowned group of pundits, McKenzie & Co., states that "health care is India's next big business opportunity" (Dhawan, 1999, p. 20) A significant group of Indian private investors, including Fortis Healthcare, Wockhardt, and Apollo Hospitals, is planning to invest over $500 million in new hospitals in India, Malaysia, Sri Lanka, and other neighboring countries. Experts estimate that India's health care industry will grow 13 percent per year for the next six years.

The boom is not only affecting the hospital industry but is causing an expansion of the entire health care sector. Medical equipment manufacturers like Siemens and GE have entered the market in a major way; PPOs are being developed and medical software has become big business, with a single Indian firm, Himachal Futuristic, making $150 million in 1998 through medical software sales. Diagnostic clinics are springing up, and private investment in clinical research is increasing (Dhawan, 1999).

This, however, is just the precursor to the surge that will occur when insurance is privatized. *Business World's* Radha Dhawan (1999) says it well: "While hospitals may be akin to vital organs like the heart . . . insurance will function as the circulatory system that keeps the money flowing" (p. 20). Many major international insurers have already entered India and formed joint ventures in anticipation of the passage of the insurance bill. Cigna has entered this market with plans to develop new products and introduce smart card technology targeting 100 million enrollees in fifteen major cities by the year 2010. Aetna estimates that once insurance is available, 6 percent of household income will be spent on health care, as opposed to the current 2 percent (Dhawan, 1999).

Regulations to implement the insurance bill that allows private and foreign investment in health insurance are currently being implemented. This will undoubtedly have profound effects on the purchase and provision of health care services in India during the next decade. Not all these effects will be positive, however, and the Ministries of Health are concerned that private insurance will cover only the wealthiest (and healthiest) individuals and leave the largest, most needy populations without coverage, exacerbating the burden on the public system. The government also fears the cost escalation spiral that indemnity insurance often unleashes. This fear is not unfounded, given the entrance of large U.S. insurers. As a result of these concerns and protests by labor organizations, the version of the bill that has passed the lower house includes numerous social obligations that companies must meet and inserts safeguards to prevent skimming by insurance companies. Foreign ownership in insurance will be limited to 26 percent, and requirements to provide coverage for the poor and disadvantaged will be included. Despite these restrictions, foreign investors are publicly calling the legislation a watershed bill that will not discourage foreign entry into the market.

Some government officials view managed care models as much friendlier to their agenda of providing high-quality, broad-based coverage. Although there is limited awareness of alternative health care financing and organization models in many government circles, international donors support these ideas. A meeting of state and national health secretaries, convened by the World Bank in Goa in 1997, highlighted the opportunity for public and private sector collaboration in the development of health models and managed care pilots. The World Bank has funded several state health care reform projects and is beginning a major national analytical study on health care and policy reform.

Several firms are anticipating this direction with preferred provider organizations (PPOs) and third party administrators (TPAs) beginning to form in a number of cities. These Indian-run organizations are likely to form partnerships with insurers and hospitals and become risk-bearing entities like HMOs when the insurance legislation passes.

Conclusion

Given India's financial growth, burgeoning middle class, changing disease patterns, and supportive political climate, opportunities for private investment in health care will continue to expand. McKenzie & Co. estimates that the insurance business will increase five-fold to over $4 billion by 2005 (Dhawan, 1999). However, as in many countries with long-standing socialist traditions, regulatory control over market forces is likely to remain strong. This is particularly true for the social sectors where the government is naturally wary of profit-making motives, and trade union interests are defensive of the status quo.

Despite the sometimes-cautious approach taken by the government, India has an urgent need to promote and develop private health care services of high quality, as well as health insurance products that can serve the needs of all segments of the Indian population. There can be little doubt that the next decade will see rapid development of the private health care market, with an important role for foreign investment and partnerships.

Because international firms consider India as offering an investment opportunity, several lessons can be learned from the experience of high-technology companies that have created small Silicon Valleys in southern India. The technology industry has spurred a new class of professionals in India, providing access to one of the most underutilized, educated labor markets in the world. Its focus has been on creating opportunities for the best and brightest to remain in India, thereby helping to build India's long-term human resources capacity. This investment in India has not been without its challenges, and the success of technology companies has depended on considering a long-term investment horizon. It is clear that with the continued growth of technology, the availability of a skilled labor force, and increased foreign investment in a number of major industries, India is emerging as one of the most exciting health care markets of the twenty-first century.

Note

1. In an unpublished paper, Modhi Charu states that India measures its insurance penetration as a percentage of the number of lives covered by life insurance of the insurable population. The term *insurable population* includes all males between the ages of twenty and sixty. Recent statistics show that 48 million males out of an insurable base of 217 million males were covered, yielding a penetration of 22 percent.

References

Berman, P., and Khan, M. E. *Paying for India's Health Care*. Thousand Oaks, Calif.: Sage, 1993.
Dhawan, R. "The Fever Is Rising." *Business World*, Oct. 18, 1999.

Measham, A., and others. "The Performance of India and Indian States in Reducing Infant Mortality and Fertility, 1975–1990." Article submitted for publication; forthcoming.

Naylor, C., Prabhat, J. D., Woods, J., and Shariff, A. *A Fine Balance: Some Options for Private and Public Health Care in Urban India.* Washington, D.C.: World Bank, 1999.

World Bank. *Sector Strategy Paper: Health, Nutrition and Population.* Washington, D.C.: World Bank, 1997.

CHAPTER TWENTY-NINE

JAPAN

Aki Yoshikawa

The greatest strength of Japan's health care system, aside from its low cost, is guaranteed access to comprehensive medical care provided for virtually every member of the population. A national survey by the Koseisho (Ministry of Health and Welfare) showed that only 0.2 percent of the respondents cited problems of access and 0.4 percent cited economic problems. The guaranteed access and the lack of economic burden may explain the fact that the per capita number of physician visits is higher than in other nations (Utsunomiya and Yoshikawa, 1993).

The Japanese Universal Health Insurance System

Japan's universal health insurance system, which covers its entire population, is segmented according to workplace. The type of employer determines the insurance society to which one belongs and the required financial contributions. The three basic groups are (1) employee health insurance for employees of firms and other public sector organizations and their dependents; (2) national health insurance, or *Kokuho* (short for *Kokumin Kenko Hoken*), for the self-employed, retirees, and their dependents; and (3) the *Roken* system, a special pooling fund for the elderly.

Employee Health Insurance

Employee health insurance is a system for employees and their dependents and can be broken down into three main categories:

1. *Seikan:* Government-managed health insurance covers the employees of small and medium-sized companies and their dependents.
2. *Kenpo:* Society-managed health insurance covers those employed by larger firms and their dependents. Companies such as Toshiba, Honda, and Sony maintain their own *kenpo* societies. There are about 1,800 *kenpo* associations.
3. *Kyosai:* Public employees' insurance covers both national and local employees and private school teachers, staff, and their dependents.

For an employee health insurance system such as *kenpo,* the employer is withholding an employee's monthly premium. An employer's mandated contributions provide funds to its *kenpo* association.

The amount of copayments varies between 10 and 30 percent, depending on the type of the insurance. For example, copayment obligations are greater for *Kokuho* members than for those insured under employee insurance such as *kenpo,* *Seikan,* and *Kyosai.*

The Pooling Fund for Geriatric Care

The health and medical services system for the elderly (*Roken* system) is a pooling fund through which the Koseisho has attempted to distribute across all Japanese the burden of paying for geriatric care. Established in 1983, the pooling fund covers all those over seventy years and bedridden people who are over sixty-five. The fund pools contributions from all insurance schemes such as *kenpo* and *Kyosai.*

Under the current system, elderly patients are charged fixed amounts of 1,200 yen (approximately US$11.50) per day for hospital care and 530 yen (just over US$5) per outpatient visits. Seventy percent of medical costs for elderly people, excluding the portion paid by the people themselves, are covered by contributions from health insurance societies for company employees and national health insurance schemes run by municipalities for non-wage earners. The government pays the remaining 30 percent.

The *Roken* system is a macro-level cost-shifting mechanism. It was created when the employer-based *kenpo* associations were fiscally strong and when the elderly population was small enough to be supported by a good-sized working population.

As will be discussed next, with the increasing proportion of elderly persons seeking assistance from *Roken* relative to the number of workers paying into the pooling fund, Japan's ability to sustain this financing system is now facing imminent collapse.

Nursing Care Insurance

The new nursing care insurance scheme *(kaigo hoken)*, designed to assist senior citizens, was implemented in April 2000. Under the plan, the elderly are classified into six categories, based on care needs, with each category of user assigned maximum coverage under the public nursing system. Ceilings are established for the use of two services (care and bathing assistance, which are provided by visiting home helpers), as well as for short stays at nursing care facilities. (Because all elderly people are covered by health insurance today, the new law will force some to be covered under the new nursing care insurance.)

Under the system, 10 percent of the cost of nursing care services will be paid by the recipients themselves; half of the remaining 90 percent will be publicly financed, and the other half will come from mandatory contributions by people aged forty or older. Even though the elderly will only have to pay 10 percent of care expenses within the limits of the categories, they will be asked to pay the full amount for services that exceed their limits. (A typical elderly person in the category of those needing the most intensive care can receive in one week some thirteen hours of home nursing care, about two hours of home medical care, and one rehabilitation session at home.)

Catastrophic Coverage

The High-Cost Medical Care Benefits Law of 1973 was amended in 1984 to introduce a cap on monthly copayments. The measure established the monthly ceiling on copayments, most recently set at 63,600 yen, or about US$600, per month. With this ceiling, the actual daily copayment rate for an inpatient suffering from a major catastrophic illness approaches zero over time.

Fee Schedule

Under the Japanese system, all medical facilities are reimbursed for medical services according to the official uniform fee schedule *(shinryo hoshu)*. The fee schedule, based on the so-called point system, lists the amount of reimbursement that medical facilities will receive for individual procedures and pharmaceuticals. The fee schedule is a very detailed form of pricing control, listing more than 3,000 medical procedures for physicians alone.

This fee schedule has proved to be a useful resource for the nation's health care policymakers because it gives them the power to influence and alter the behavior of health care providers and facilities. Manipulation of the fee schedule has been serving as one of the primary mechanisms by which the Koseisho regulates the supply of medical services, utilization rates, and aggregate health care expenditures. Lower health care expenditures have not been realized accidentally; systemic manipulation of the fee schedule has been a cost-containment tool.

Anachronistic Reimbursement Procedures

All costs incurred by medical facilities are reimbursed on a fee-for-service basis. When patients receive medical services, they are responsible only for the copayment at the point of services. Upon providing medical services to a patient, a hospital prepares a reimbursement claim. The claim, called *receputo*, is prepared and submitted monthly in order to receive the reimbursement. The *receputo* itemizes each procedure, including the dispensing of drugs, for which a predetermined number of points are assigned according to the fee schedule.

Prepared and submitted in paper form, the *receputo* is overwhelmingly detailed and complicated. Each contains a variety of demographic, diagnostic, and procedural data. There are line items for each billable item, and some *receputo* are tens of pages in length.

Most hospitals and clinics use specialized computing machines commonly known as *rececom* (abbreviation for *receputo computer*) in preparing these *receputo* claims. The *rececom* is a rather primitive stand-alone machine fostered under the unique fee-schedule-based financing environment. Currently, the *rececom* has little useful analytical applications for hospital management.

The task of preparing *receputo* is extremely labor-intensive work. Many workers input detailed fee schedule points to the *rececom* machines, and the billing department *(iji-ka)* in a hospital resembles a garment factory sweatshop.

After receiving the original paper *receputo* from clearing houses, an insurance organization such as Toyota *kenpo* then calculates the total payment and sends the amount with the original *receputo* back to the clearinghouses; hospitals receive payments from the clearinghouses. The process between the submission of a *receputo* by a hospital and the reimbursement payment takes approximately two months. It is an irony that in Japan, the country famed for its technology, all reimbursement claims are submitted on paper and processed manually.

Official Pharmaceutical Prices

In addition to the official fee schedule, there is a separate reimbursement schedule for pharmaceuticals. The Koseisho sets official medicine prices every two years, based on a weighted average of market prices plus a fixed profit margin for hospitals and clinics. (Drug expenses are predicted to total 6.47 trillion yen in fiscal 2000, or about 23 percent of all medical spending.) The existence of *yakka saeki,* the so-called doctor's margin—the difference between the official reimbursement rates for pharmaceuticals and the actual purchasing prices the drug companies charge physicians—is a classic example of distortions generated by price control. It is common knowledge that doctors augment their earnings from regulated medical services by freely prescribing drugs. With the existence of *yakka saeki,* predictably, Japanese physicians often sell higher-priced drugs.

National Medical Expenditures

Spending for Japanese health care reached 28 trillion yen in 1997. It was approximately $231 billion (at the exchange rate of 121 yen to the dollar). In the same year, the medical expenditures in the United States, where its population is roughly twice that of Japan, was estimated to be $1.035 trillion.[1] Per capita medical expenditures were 230,4000 yen (or US$1,900) in Japan, compared with $3,645 in the United States. Health care expenditures as a percentage of GDP are 7.3 percent, compared with 14.0 percent in the United States.

Hospitals and *Byoin*

In Japan, the definition of the term *hospital* is a medical facility with twenty or more beds; facilities with fewer than twenty beds are classified as clinics. In comparison with other industrialized countries, the number of hospitals and beds in Japan is extremely high. For example, whereas the United States had 6,201 hospitals with 1,062,000 beds in 1997, Japan had 9,413 hospitals with 1,660,784 beds. For each 1,000 population, there were 13.2 beds in Japan, compared with 4.0 in the United States.

This difference is even greater when one considers that Japan's population is half that of the United States. Some of the disparity between these countries may be attributable to differences in what is considered a hospital and a hospital bed in the different countries. For example, some of Japan's hospital beds are used for long-term geriatric care, making an accurate comparison difficult. The hospitals, known as *byoin,* may also function differently than hospitals in other nations.

Private ownership dominates the hospital system and represents approximately 70 percent of total hospital beds. The so-called *iryo-hojin* hospitals, a form of private hospital, are the most prevalent in Japan. *Iryo-hojin* is a special legal status for a nonprofit entity in the medical care sector. It is illegal to operate health care facilities on a for-profit basis in Japan. An *iryo-hojin* is prohibited from distributing profits to anyone outside the hospital (such as shareholders).

Even though the prohibition on distributing profits may make *iryo-hojin* private hospitals superficially seem like not-for-profit hospitals, an *iryo-hojin* hospital is essentially a private entity—an entrepreneurial business owned by a doctor (or doctors) operating under more or less the same financial incentives as for-profit enterprises. Japanese law merely prohibits the distribution of profits to non-insider shareholders.

Under the country's uniform fee schedule, there are few incentives to refer a patient to other medical facilities, and this has engendered an environment in which hospitals of various sizes and ownership types compete for the same pool of patients without a clear division of specialization.

Long Stays in Hospitals

The average length of stay (ALOS) in hospitals, which was 32.8 days in 1997, is far longer than that found elsewhere. Under fee-for-service medicine, there is a strong incentive for a hospital to keep hospital beds occupied. Instead of discharging a patient quickly, the hospital can earn the daily hospital reimbursement fees by delaying discharge.

The extremely long ALOS is also due to hospitals often being used as geriatric nursing facilities. However, this alone cannot fully explain the country's long ALOS because it is considerably greater in Japan for any specific disease categories, including normal pregnancy.

High-Technology Purchases

Under Japanese fee-for-service medicine, with its uniform fee schedule, hospitals cannot engage in price competition. Under such market conditions, hospitals tend to engage in non-price competition in order to attract patients. With legal restrictions on advertisement, a hospital's options are limited; many may be purchasing high-technology medical equipment to signal a level of medical sophistication that will attract more patients. There is an interesting relationship between the level of competition among hospitals in a market and incentive to acquire high-tech medical equipment (for further information, see Vogt and others, 1995).

The two imaging technologies—computed tomography (CT) scanning and magnetic resonance imaging (MRI)—have become symbols of high-technology, high-cost medicine and have shown very high diffusion rates in Japan. The diffusion of CT, as well as MRI, in Japan has been extensive. Even though Japan's fee schedule was instituted as part of an extremely effective cost-control system, such price control has had unintended consequences and has led to aggressive non-price competition among hospitals.

It is interesting to note that, despite the use of high-technology medical devices, the rate of surgical procedures per capita is low. Estimated numbers of annual surgeries is 4.8 million, and the estimated annual surgical rate is 27 per 1,000 population.

Changing Dynamics

Today the health care system is facing some important changes (see Figure 29.1). Following are some of the major changes Japan is facing, as well as their implications and challenges.

A Rapidly Aging Society

Currently, the ratio of the elderly (sixty-five years and over) to the productive population (fifteen to sixty-four) in Japan is approximately 1 to 5. By 2025 it is projected to fall to about 1 to 2, which means that five younger people now financially support each elderly person, whereas in 2025 each Japanese person over sixty-five will have the support of only two people of working age. It is also important to note that the proportion of elderly in the Japanese population will increase at a far faster rate than in any other industrialized nations, a point illustrated in Table 29.1.

The number of senior citizens who will need care is expected to double to 5.2 million by 2025. The rapid aging will place substantial burdens on the health care delivery and financing systems in Japan. An essential question is whether Japan can prepare quickly enough to accommodate such rapid aging.

The Failing Health Care Financing

In fiscal year 1998, *Kokuho* posted a deficit of 102 billion yen, an increase of about 250 percent from the previous year. *Seikan* experienced a similar dismal performance. Traditionally it was *kenpo* that cross-subsidized the financial losses of *Kokuho* and *Seikan*. Various *kenpo* associations have maintained the surplus pre-

FIGURE 29.1. CHANGING DYNAMICS IN JAPAN'S HEALTH CARE.

Major Change Drivers	Challenges and Opportunities

Rapidly aging society	Improved management and operational effectiveness
	    – Reduces costs
	    – Enhances quality
	New and changing health service needs
	    – Skilled nursing facilities
	    – Home health care

Failing health care financing system	Risk: from "reimbursement" to "insurance"
End of the fee-for-service	New information requirements New approaches to better utilize information

Deregulation of the hospital and health insurance markets	Changing industry structure
	    – Provider integration and consolidation
	    – New entrants

Information technology	New choice, more competition

mium with their young and healthy employers. As described earlier, this macrolevel cross-subsidization has been the foundation of the Japan's health care financing mechanism.

One of the most serious problems Japan is facing today is the fact that many of *kenpo* associations are now suffering financial losses. The rapidly aging society and its shrinking economy can partially explain that performance. *Kenpo* associations have to pay 40 percent of the premiums they collect to cover care of the elderly. Although each *kenpo* association traditionally made its "contribution" to the pooling fund for the geriatric care, some *kenpo* have started to resist. Today more than three-quarters of *kenpo* associations are in the red, and their predicament poses

TABLE 29.1. RAPID AGING IN JAPAN.

Country	Percentage of the Population over Age 65 in 2025	Years It Will Take to Go from 10% to 20% over Age 65
Japan	27.3	22
Switzerland	23.4	54
Germany	23.2	62
Italy	22.8	48
Sweden	22.4	66
Finland	22.2	45
Netherlands	21.3	52
Canada	21.2	39
France	20.8	95
United States	19.8	—
United Kingdom	19.4	—

a serious threat not only to corporate management but also to the foundation of Japan's health care financing mechanism.

In order to improve the financial condition, the Koseisho introduced several measures; however, they are merely cosmetic in their nature and cannot solve the fundamental problem Japan is facing. At first the government introduced a measure to increase copayment. The current cap on copayments is uniformly set at 63,600 yen a month, and the Koseisho is planning to increase the monthly cap on payments to 121,800 yen. In addition to doubling the cap amount, the Koseisho is also planning to introduce a copayment to the elderly. The Koseisho also proposes having patients aged seventy or over shoulder 10 percent of their medical costs instead of fixed amounts under the current system. According to a set of five proposals presented to a panel advising the Health Minister, elderly patients to be hospitalized would pay 10 percent of the costs, with a maximum monthly payment 40,800 yen, up 3,600 yen from the present ceiling. The Koseisho has also proposed setting a monthly ceiling for elderly outpatient care at 3,000 to 5,000 yen.

An important observation, which can assist in explaining *kenpo*'s performance, is that *kenpo* associations have become essentially bureaucratic and inefficient organizations that merely provide jobs for retiring corporate executives and bureaucrats. Under Japan's fee-for-service medicine with the uniformed fee schedule, there is little entrepreneurial leadership *kenpo* executives can play. If in fact they save the medical expenses, the government as a "contribution" will take their surplus premiums away to the geriatric pooling fund. Entrepreneurial efforts by various *kenpo* associations have not been rewarded; they have been often punished by bureaucratic control. Over forty years of tight bureaucratic control, *kenpo* associations lost their entrepreneurial instincts and the cost-minimizing incentive.

Faced with criticisms made by many corporate leaders, the Koseisho announced that its plan allows more autonomy to *kenpo* associations. A government panel recommended that insurance organizations such as *kenpo* develop a more efficient auditing and utilization review capacity to screen hospital bills to ensure they are getting value for money. The panel also wants *kenpo* associations to provide more information on hospitals for their members. Some view this as an initial attempt to transform a *kenpo* to a U.S.-type HMO. To the author, the idea of transforming bureaucratic and rigid *kenpo* with little entrepreneurial incentives into efficient HMOs is unrealistic. Deregulating the health insurance market entirely and permitting life insurance and other companies to enter the market to replace the inefficient *kenpo* is a quicker more direct way to accelerate reform.

The Imminent End of the Fee-for-Service Medicine

Even though health economists often cannot agree on a simple issue, one thing they do agree on is that the fee-for-service medicine is not the most effective tool for containing national health care costs.

Even if the government can set the unit price, it cannot control utilization. The government of Japan has attempted to set artificially low unit prices in order to control the total medical expenditures. However, this created a wide gap between the fee schedule reimbursement amount and the actual cost of providing a specific service. With such an increasing disparity between the official fee and the actual cost, it becomes less justifiable for the government to maintain the micro-level price control.

An advisory panel to the Koseisho recommended an introduction of a DRG-type prospective payment. Under the current fee-for-service payment scheme, medical institutions can generate higher revenues by increasing prescription drug volume and the number of medical examinations. The proposed system would pay fixed amounts for treating patients suffering from certain symptoms, regardless of how they are treated.

The transition from the fee-for-service to a DRG-type system will trigger a major structural change in Japan's hospital industry. Today Japan has more hospitals and more beds than the United States, and the ALOS at Japanese hospitals are several times longer than at American hospitals. With a DRG-type prospective payment system, the ALOS in Japan will drop drastically; consequently, there will be an excess of hospital beds. Many smaller private hospitals will be driven out of the hospital market in Japan. This is why many Japanese hospital owners are opposing an introduction of a DRG-type system.

Deregulating the Hospital Industry

Various regulatory reforms have been discussed in Japan, including the possible opening of the hospital industry to private corporations. Such a proposal faces immediate and direct opposition from the Japan Medical Association (JMA).

However, even though no private for-profit enterprise is permitted to enter the market, the new nursing insurance-related long-term care market is open for private enterprises. The Koseisho seeks to resolve a possible shortage of nursing care service providers by using private sector initiatives. Various private firms are actively seeking new business opportunities in the new long-term care market. This may be viewed as a subtle but important prelude toward the opening of the hospital market.

What will be the timing and the extent of such a deregulation in the hospital market? We must remember that the existing laws protect physicians' interests. Any regulatory changes affecting such interests will be opposed and delayed by the powerful JMA.

New Information Technology

Policymakers may not be the source of reform measures to change the health care system in Japan. The new information technology will undermine many of today's existing laws and restrictions and may trigger a profound and fundamental reorganization.

Even though JMA could defeat the government, it may not be able to stop the impact of the Internet. Today a growing number of homepages post details about doctors and medical staff, pictures of hospital rooms, approaches to treatment, and results. Even though Japanese law regulates much of the information that can be used to publicize hospitals and clinics, it is difficult to put restrictions on Website content.

The Price of Yesterday's Glory

Recognizing a serious threat to its health care financing system, the Koseisho planned to propose several major reform measures such as a DRG-type prospective payment method. Many of these fundamental reforms of Japan's health-insurance system scheduled for April 2000 have been either postponed or aborted due to the strong opposition from JMA. As major reforms are deferred, government spending is rising. In the proposed fiscal 2000 draft budget, social security is estimated to be 16.76 trillion yen, up 4.0 percent from a year earlier, accounting for 35 percent of the general account. Growth will outpace the overall increase in the general account, and the government will depend on borrowing for nearly 40 percent of the revenue to finance the bloated budget. Total bond issues in the new fiscal year will amount to 85.8 trillion yen, surpassing general account spending of 85 trillion yen for the first time.

The question is whether Japan can reform its once highly acclaimed health care system quickly enough to avoid a crisis. Ironically, the great success of its universal health insurance system in the past is the reason people are not willing to change the system today. As long as the financial resources are abundant (as in the past, with its young and healthy population and strong economic growth), fee-for-service medicine remains the choice of both patients and physicians. The Japanese liked the system, and introducing health care reform will not be popular. Because it will not be economically feasible to maintain the existing Japanese fee-for-service medicine for long, is it politically feasible to change the system?

Note

1. When Japanese health care expenditures are compared to those of other OECD countries, four items excluded from the official Japanese data become particularly important: (1) various costs associated with government hospitals, including construction costs and financial subsidies; (2) research and development funding for medical research; (3) welfare-related expenses such as nursing home costs; and (4) medical expenses not covered by the universal health insurance system.

References

Utsunomiya, J., and Yoshikawa, A. "Health Status and Patients in Japan." In D. I. Okimoto and A. Yoshikawa (eds.), *Japan's Health System: Efficiency and Effectiveness in Universal Care.* New York: Faulkner & Gray, 1993.

Vogt, W. B., and others. "The Role of Diagnostic Technology in Competition Among Japanese Hospitals." *International Journal of Technology Management: Series on Management of Technology in Health Care,* 1995, *1.*

PART SIX

NORTH AMERICA

Until 1973, the United States and Canada had similar models of health care financing and service delivery, with comparable health expenditures. Then Canada introduced universal public hospital and medical insurance, after which the systems differed significantly. In this last section, contributors look at the two systems of the neighboring giants.

In Chapter Thirty, T. W. Noseworthy traces the evolution of Canada's health care system to its present-day construct, size, and scope. In operation for nearly thirty years, Canada's Medicare system covers virtually all hospital and doctor services. Fiscal restraints and shifts in services are forcing the reconsideration of Medicare operations and funding. Noseworthy describes directional changes and their implications for service provision and restructuring, as Canada moves into the new millennium.

Concluding the book, in Chapter Thirty-One, Neelam Sekhri analyzes the U.S. health care system—a system that remains unique among wealthy industrialized countries in the extent of its reliance on the private sector for financing, purchasing, and delivery of services. The U.S. system is renowned worldwide for its advanced medical technology, excellent clinical quality, and consumer choice, yet nearly 47 million people have no insurance and little access to these medical resources. And although the United States devotes 14.5 percent of its GDP to health care—a higher percentage than any other country in the world—

it compares unfavorably to other developed countries on most measures of health status. The country is now at a crossroads in how it manages the conflicting priorities of equitable access and affordability, according to Sekhri. The chapter ends with a recounting of recent reform efforts in both public and private sectors.

CHAPTER THIRTY

CANADA

T. W. Noseworthy

At the millennium, Canada's Medicare system has been operating for almost thirty years. What was originally designed as a single-payer, publicly funded system actually operates as a hybrid model of public-private funding, with mostly private delivery. Canadian Medicare covers virtually all hospitals' and doctors' services. However, fiscal restraint and an ambulatory shift in services are forcing reconsideration of how Medicare operates and is funded.

This chapter traces the evolution of Canada's health care system to its present-day construct, size, and scope. A description of the system as it exists today is used as a basis for describing directional changes and their implications for service provision and restructuring.

Evolution of Canada's Health Care System

Until 1973, when Canada introduced universal public hospital and medical insurance, the United States and Canada had similar models of health care financing and service delivery, with comparable health expenditures. Patients paid physicians directly on a fee-for-service basis. Similarly, hospitals were paid directly on a per diem basis. This traditional health care market model existed in the United States prior to the 1980s but changed with the introduction of Medicare,

Medicaid, the DRG system, and managed care. Prior to the introduction of Canadian Medicare, the extent of hospital and medical insurance was markedly limited.

Hospital and Physician Services

The Canadian government passed the landmark Hospital Insurance and Diagnostic Services Act in 1961, providing for comprehensive hospital coverage, and the Medical Care Act in 1966. These acts laid the framework for federal transfers and financial support to the provinces and formed the legislative basis for virtually complete coverage and government financing of hospital and physicians' services and for "medically necessary" services by 1971. All provinces agreed to participate with the federal government by 1973. The initial understanding was that there would be equal cost sharing by federal and provincial governments. The reality became apparent by 1977 that the federal government commitment for cost sharing would or could not be maintained. The federal contribution has subsequently decreased to 30 percent of the publicly funded share, or approximately 20 percent of total health care costs, leaving the provinces to shoulder more financial responsibility.

By the early 1980s, physicians in some provinces became progressively unhappy with the annually negotiated fee schedules used to determine fee-for-service reimbursement. Some began to extra-bill patients directly for discretionary fees. Correspondingly, some hospitals planned or implemented user fees for patients. The federal government believed that these actions constituted a threat to universal accessibility by introducing financial barriers to care. At that time and since then, the federal government has penalized provinces that permit extra-billing and user fees for medically necessary services provided by hospitals and doctors. Surprisingly enough, there never has been and likely will never be a universally accepted definition of "medically necessary services" in Canada. Furthermore, the federal government has never financially penalized provinces under the Canada Health Act for other than direct charges at the point of care.

Fundamental Principles: Canada Health Act (1984)

In 1984, the federal government promulgated five principles constituted within the Canada Health Act: universality, accessibility, comprehensiveness, portability, and public administration (Table 30.1). The *Canada Health Act* and agreements pursuant to it set forth an understanding that the federal government would transfer both funds and taxation powers to the provinces and would not deliver direct services other than for aboriginal peoples, military, and selected personnel.

TABLE 30.1. CANADIAN HEALTH CARE EXPENDITURES.

Total health expenditures:	$79.9 billion
Public:	$55.6 billion (69.6%)
Private:	$24.3 billion (30.4%)
Health expenditures per capita:	$2,609 (9.1% of GDP)
Use of funds	
Hospitals:	$26.8 billion (33.5%)
Other institutions:	$8.0 billion (10.0%)
Physicians:	$11.4 billion (14.2%)
Other professionals:	$9.7 billion (12.1%)
Drugs:	$11.2 billion (14.0%)
Capital:	$2.1 billion (2.6%)
Other:	$10.8 billion (13.5%)

Source: Canadian Institute for Health Information.

Provinces, correspondingly, would be responsible for funding and organizing health service delivery and would recognize reciprocity of Canadians visiting from but residing in other provinces.

Although each province funds and administers its own programs, actual provision of care is and always has been a mixture of public and private delivery. This, in effect, represents the organizational construct to date (see Figure 30.1).

Single-Payer, Publicly Funded System

Medicare at the millennium is a series of interlocking pieces, including ten provinces, the territories and the federal government, with a financial model, which is single-payer and publicly funded. This is to say that the majority of hospital and doctors' services are universally insured, with no direct charges at the point of delivery. This is funded from the national and provincial tax bases. Public funding has traditionally accounted for approximately 75 percent of total expenditures on health care in Canada. Growth in private spending has significantly outpaced growth in public spending, however, resulting in the public share declining to 70 percent by 1998. The sectors of care that have expanded with restructuring and with reducing acute care, many of which are now in the community, operate within a hybrid of public, private, and other financing arrangements.

By the early 1990s, most provinces were spending at least 30 percent of revenues on health care that, in combination with reduced federal transfers, caused what might be referred to as an "affordability crisis" for Canadian Medicare. This triggered substantial federal and provincial expenditure reductions. These reductions had their greatest impact on the acute care sector.

FIGURE 30.1. CANADIAN HEALTH CARE SYSTEM.

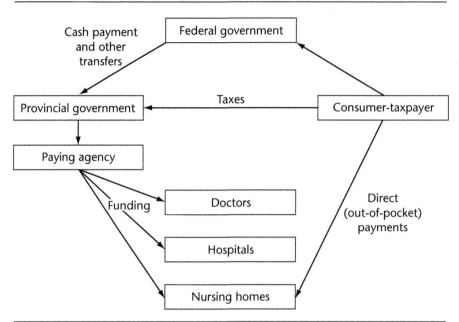

Source: Noseworthy and Jacobs, 1996. Copyright © 1996, Futura Publishing. Reprinted with permission.

Public-Private Financing and Delivery

Canada has a system characterized by public funding and private delivery, yet with many and large exceptions. The terms *public* and *private*, when referencing delivery, are ambiguous and confusing in Canada. Physicians, for instance, are largely community-based private practitioners and retain hospital privileges, which define their participation in and use of the hospital system. Virtually all fee-for-service income is derived from direct payment by provincial health insurance programs. On behalf of the physician membership, provincial medical associations negotiate directly with their governments for the total funding envelope. Provincial medical associations determine allocation across and within specialties. Notwithstanding a growing interest in alternate reimbursement systems for physicians, it remains the case that Canadian physicians are, for the most part, private practitioners. Yet with virtually all reimbursement coming from the public funds of provincial insurance programs and in light of the regulations prohibiting extra-billing for services, one might reasonably argue that Canadian physicians are "public practitioners," particularly those who derive a large portion of their income from hospital and inpatient services.

Hospitals and Community-Based Care

Hospital services in Canada are a mixture of public and privately financed institutions, varying across provinces. Most private facilities are aligned to a religious or denominational orientation. In all cases, there is a strong government regulatory presence, and provincial governments generally provide the vast majority of annual revenue. Table 30.2 characterizes the services in the Canadian system, in terms of both financing and delivery.

Economic Organization

Taxpayers of both federal and provincial governments finance the public component of Canada's health care system. By 1998, Canada was spending $79.7 billion on health care, or 9.1 percent share of GDP, amounting to $2,609 per capita.

In accordance with the Canada Health Act, provinces receive fund transfers from the federal government through what is known as the Canadian Health and Social Transfer (CHST). The balance of federal support for provincial health care is provided by taxation "points" provided by the federal government. This in effect is an agreement whereby the federal government reduces its taxation power in favor of provinces garnering their own tax room and implementing their own taxation plans. Between 1992 and 1993 and from 1998 to 1999, the CHST was reduced from $18.5 to $12.5 billion, in cash. It is apparent that federal leverage over Medicare was diminished with reduced cash transfers.

In the face of widespread pressure and with improved economic conditions in February 1999, the federal government reinstituted $3.5 billion for health care funding as an immediate, one-time supplement to the CHST. Current budgets forecast an increase in federal cash expenditure to $15 billion by 2002.

In the early 1960s, hospitals were funded based on historically derived global operating budgets. Following the example developed by Medicare in the United States, case mix funding systems, with adjustments determined by DRG-like weights, were introduced in many Canadian provinces in the early 1990s. Over the past ten years, several provinces have moved toward some form of population-based funding model, with reimbursement determined by case mix and severity and adjusted by such other variables as gender, age, and other surrogate measures for morbidity or socioeconomic status.

TABLE 30.2. PUBLIC-PRIVATE FUNDING AND DELIVERY.

Service Type	Financing	Delivery
Hospital services	100% public for medically necessary services (no user charges permitted); private payment for upgraded accommodation or non–medically necessary services provided in hospitals.	Mixed public-private; varies across provinces. Government generally exerts a strong regulatory presence.
Physician services	100% public for medically necessary services (no extra billing permitted); private payment for non–medically necessary services.	Private; physicians are independent and self-regulating; some models of primary care delivery (for example, CLSCs in Quebec) are more akin to government agencies.
Services provided in private clinics	Privately funded for services not defined as medically necessary. Some clinics charge a facility fee to patients for medically necessary services over and above the funding provided by the provincial health insurance plan.	Privately owned and operated; limited regulations.
Dental and optometry care	Mostly private (insurance or out-of-pocket); some provincial plans provide coverage for children and seniors.	Private and self-regulating (dentists and optometrists).
Prescription drugs	Mixed public-private; provincial plans pay for approximately 40% of all prescription drugs dispensed outside hospitals. Coverage is typically limited to seniors and welfare recipients. Drugs dispensed in hospitals are covered in hospital budgets. Balance is funded by a combination of private insurance plans and out-of-pocket.	Private; delivery includes prescription by physician and dispensing by pharmacist or hospital.
Nonprescription drugs	Mostly private (out-of-pocket).	Private; over the counter.
Services of other professionals	Mostly private (insurance or out-of-pocket).	Private (for example, psychologists, physiotherapists, chiropractors, midwives, private duty nurses).
Alternative medicines	Mostly private; some limited coverage provided by provincial plans; remainder is paid for through private insurance plans or out-of-pocket.	Private (for example, naturopaths, homeopaths, practitioners of oriental medicine, traditional (aboriginal healers).

Service Type	Financing	Delivery
Long-term care (residential)	Mixed public-private; public portion covers insured health care services; private portion covers room and board.	Mixed public-private.
Home care	Partial public coverage provided in most jurisdictions; informal caregivers play an important role.	Mixed public-private.
Ambulance services	Partial public coverage in some provinces; special programs for residents of remote areas.	Mostly private operators.
Public health programs	Public.	Public.
Services to status Indians and Inuit	Public.	Mixed public-private (federal government employees deliver some services directly).

Source: "The Public and Private Financing of Canada's Health System," National Forum on Health, 1995. Copyright © 1995, National Forum on Health. Reprinted with permission.

Cost, Size, Growth

As in the United States, health care is a major industry in Canada and one of the largest employers. Not surprisingly, it is also the largest public expenditure, from which is derived a great deal of public scrutiny and concern. Hospitals remain the single largest cost component, despite a rapid decline in beds and utilization (see Table 30.2).

In terms of international comparisons of health expenditures, regardless of the measurement used, Canadian expenditures until recently ranked second only to the United States. Restructuring and expenditure reductions of the 1990s and improvements in the Canadian economy have changed this. At the millennium, Canada's total expenditures as a proportion of GDP appear far more comparable to Europe than to the United States.

Despite financial restraint, certain sectors have had increasing costs, most notably pharmaceuticals. The cost of pharmaceuticals has doubled over twenty years, to approximately $360 per capita by 1998. Accordingly, current pharmaceutical costs in Canada approximate the cost of all physician services. Unlike most of Medicare, which is 70 percent publicly funded, pharmaceuticals are limited to 30 percent public and 70 percent private funding. Not surprisingly, given the cost of pharmaceuticals and the lack of Medicare coverage for out-of-hospital medications, 88 percent of Canadians hold some form of insurance for pharmaceuticals, often through employer drug benefit programs or government-operated programs with significant copayments and deductibles. Cost containment and access to medically necessary pharmaceuticals in Canada are gaining attention as substantial health policy issues. Although now there is broad-based interest in expanding public funding for medically necessary pharmaceuticals, there are no federal-provincial agreements for doing so; there is much concern about the affordability of such an expansion of Medicare.

Health Workforce

Health care is a very labor-intensive industry. This is particularly true for hospitals. Directly and indirectly, health care employs 7 percent of the labor force in Canada. During the 1960s, roughly 70 percent of hospital costs were directed toward wages and benefits. This increased to 75 percent by the early 1990s, with nursing wages being the largest component (30 percent of hospital expenditures). Economywide inflation, greater-than-average wage rates in the 1970s and 1980s, unionization of most health care workers, and increased educational qualifications, among other factors, have contributed to the rising cost of labor and the health workforce. Under these conditions, reductions in health care expenditures clearly have a direct impact on income and employment. Not surprisingly, labor unrest has followed federal-provincial reductions in the early 1990s. Nurses and physicians in many Canadian provinces have best exemplified this in 1998 and 1999 by a volley of strikes and withdrawals of service.

In 1995 there were thirty-one categories of health professionals in Canada. Up to that time, the rate of growth in physician and nursing numbers increased at a greater rate than the growth of the population. For physicians in the twelve years from 1981 to 1993, the doctor-to-population ratio decreased from 1:538 to 1:460. However, reduced undergraduate and postgraduate enrollments that were introduced into Canada's medical schools in the early 1990s now raise ever-increasing concern that there is a developing physician shortage in Canada.

In terms of the output of Canada's sixteen medical schools, approximately 50 percent of graduates choose family medicine (primary care), as distinct from an approximately equal number that enter specialty training in accredited programs of the Royal College of Physicians and Surgeons of Canada. This reflects the general distribution of primary care and other specialists among practicing physicians.

Restructuring markedly affected nursing training and numbers in Canada in the 1990s. Many hospital-based training programs for nurses closed, and education was concentrated in universities and postsecondary institutions. Canada is currently experiencing what is widely believed to be a serious nursing shortage, and both federal and provincial governments are responding with wage and benefit increases, along with special funding and programs to stabilize and sustain an adequate supply of nurses.

Restructuring in the 1990s

Fiscal restraint in the late 1980s and early 1990s triggered unavoidable change in Canadian health care. Yet winds of change preceded financial perturbations, brought on in part by a series of provincial royal commissions and task forces during the 1980s. Many health reforms later, and yet to be introduced, are recommended in this work. One consistent theme appeared: that the system as a whole was fundamentally sound and adequately funded but could be improved.

Affordability Crisis

It remains debatable whether substantial changes would have occurred in Canadian health care had these not been precipitated by major expenditure reductions by federal and provincial governments. By 1992, most Canadian provinces had experienced the economic downturn and were deficit budgeting. The same held true for the federal government. Hospitals represented 42 percent—the largest component of total health costs—then at 10.2 percent of GDP. Given the declining federal portion of public funding, widespread deficit financing by provinces, and the increasing cost of health care annually in excess of consumer price index, all but one Canadian province brought in strict expenditure reductions, with examples of precipitous decreases such as approximately 20 percent over three years, as in Alberta.

Provincial governments, especially those in Alberta and Ontario, were accorded large election majorities to reduce the costs of public spending and programs, most notably on health care. This precipitated major lay-offs, wage reductions, and controls for the health workforce, most particularly directed to acute care. Not surprisingly, a financial lever in the form of an affordability crisis triggered substantial restructuring.

Governance and Management of Services

In reaction to the realities of fiscal restraint, nine of ten provinces restructured through the 1990s, becoming fundamentally different forms of governance and management; the intent was to develop integrated delivery systems. Individual hospital and institutional boards and management were dissolved and replaced by cross-sectoral regional health authorities and districts, each with broad financial and programmatic controls. In most cases, regional health authorities were, and continue to be, direct service providers; they assumed the control and operation of public facilities. Accordingly, there is no clearly delineated purchaser-provider split of services in the Canadian system, as has been the case in the United Kingdom and elsewhere.

In the face of widespread reform largely at the provincial level, the federal government with the election of Prime Minister Jean Chretien in 1993, set out to review the Canadian health care system with a long-term view to its future. In doing so, they established the National Forum on Health.

National Forum on Health

In October 1994, the newly elected government activated a pre-election commitment and established the National Forum on Health, chaired by the prime minister; the twenty-four volunteer members had wide-ranging knowledge of the health system. The mandate of the forum was to involve and inform Canadians and advise the federal government on innovative ways to improve the health of Canadians and ensure that the Canadian health care system would be equipped for the challenges of the future.

In February of 1997, after Canada-wide consultation with stakeholders and the public in seventy-one discussion groups in thirty-four communities, the National Forum on Health released its recommendations to governments and the people of Canada. Priorities for action called for maintaining the single-payer, publicly funded model but building on it with necessary changes in primary care, pharmaceuticals, and home care. The forum focused attention on transforming current knowledge about health into action, through awareness and action on the broader determinants of health. Further, the forum called for federal leadership in establishing a culture of evidence-based decision making in health and developing a national health information system that would be a fundamental cornerstone in such a transformation. Critical elements of the national system, of course, would be provincial health infostructures.

Federal Investment

Provincial health infostructures were necessary for other reasons. Establishment of regional health authorities, and the necessary requirement for cross-sectoral, multi-institutional information and reporting, meant that health information requirements had to be met as a critical feature of developing an integrated delivery system. This has led to early actions and high expectations by provincial governments and at the local level.

At the federal level in 1997, the minister of health established the Advisory Council on Health Infostructure. The twenty-four-member body, with representation from a wide range of stakeholders in the health sector, provided strategic advice on the development of a national strategy.

The council promulgated a vision for Canada Health Infoway that reads as follows:

> Canada Health Infoway empowers individuals and communities to make informed choices about their own health, the health of others and Canada's health system. In an environment of strengthened privacy protection, it builds on federal, provincial and territorial infostructures to improve the quality and accessibility of health care and to enable integrated health services delivery. It provides the information and services that are the foundation for accountability, continuous improvement in health care and better understanding of the determinants of Canadians' health.

In February 1999, the council released its final report: "Canada Health Infoway: Paths to Better Health." In the same month, the federal government budget allocated $328 million in expenditures to be directed at a broad range of strategic and infostructural initiatives and projects aimed at developing a national health information network and at strengthening provincial health infostructures.

Federal-Provincial-Territorial Collaboration

The Canadian Institute for Health Information (CIHI) was formed in 1994 by the amalgamation in whole or part of four pre-existing organizations involved with health information. CIHI is supported by federal and provincial health ministries and acts as a national health information repository and dissemination agency, collecting, analyzing, and distributing hospital separation and other relevant health care information on over 80 percent of Canadian utilization. In all, $95 million was allocated in this recent federal budget for CIHI to integrate data management and information exchange systems in order to give Canadians access to timely and accurate information on health matters. CIHI is a national resource for Canada; together with the development of provincial infostructures and national initiatives, CIHI is becoming a critical component of Canada Health Infoway.

Arising out of the advisory council's recommendations, the federal-provincial-territorial Advisory Committee on Health Infostructure has been established as a standing committee reporting to the deputy ministers of health.

Provincial Initiatives

There has been enthusiasm for the development of provincial health information networks, with each provincial government at some stage in the development of an integrated system aimed in the first instance at supporting health care. One rapidly developing provincial example—Alberta Wellnet—has ambitious plans to have a provincewide telehealth network with over fifty videoconferencing sites in operation by the end of 1999. A provincewide pharmaceutical information network and several projects and applications associated with registries, screening, and integrated cancer care are developing. Wellnet's approach of facilitating common opportunities for Alberta's nineteen regional and provincial health authorities and physicians is capitalizing on common strategies, standards, and procurement methods. This is seen as central to fostering a collective approach, achieving economies, and promoting the interoperability of systems.

Public-Private Sector Collaboration

Integrated health information systems are a notable example of a growing tendency toward public-private sector collaboration in health care. There are, and will continue to be, innumerable opportunities for private sector alliances and business relationships with the publicly funded system, particularly in diverse areas of technology development.

The scope of arrangements is potentially great but likely to provoke a great deal of public scrutiny from those who fear that private sector involvement in health care is contributing to Medicare's demise. Realistically, the public, private, and social sectors in Canada will each have to be major players in sustaining the health care system.

Directional Change and Policy Implications

There is a view in Canada today that if Medicare were being built from scratch, it would be structured much differently and might be less expensive. There would be less reliance on hospitals and doctors, and there would be a broader range of community-based services, delivered within primary care models by multidisciplinary teams with strong emphasis on health promotion, disease prevention, and injury control. Canada is in transition in attempting to achieve this. In the meantime, the ambulatory shift in the focus of care has cost Canadians directly and has contributed to what might be referred to as "passive privatization." In short, a growing component of care is being financed from private insurance and directly by the public. This now accounts for 30 percent of total health expenditure in Canada, second only to the United States among G7 countries.

It is well recognized that community-based services are key to preventing, delaying, or substituting for long-term institutional care and acute care hospitalization. Accordingly, the National Forum on Health and many others have argued that home care should be included as an integral part of publicly funded health services. At present, however, there is a patchwork of home care and community-based services across provinces, with variable degrees of public and private financing and delivery.

As the ambulatory shift in services from institutions broadens, the impact in Canada is likely to be increased investment in home care, particularly services for the frail elderly. There is no doubt that a great deal of program development and reengineering is needed for community-based services to be successful and cost-effective.

Accessibility and Comprehensiveness

With the ambulatory and cost shifts brought on by restructuring, constrained funding, and other factors, the pressure for more privately delivered services will undoubtedly increase; without substantial federal and provincial commitments, the proportion of public-to-private financing is likely to decrease. At some point, risk-averse Canadians may purchase insurance or wish to buy services directly. To a very limited extent this happens now. This scenario will, nonetheless, prompt the introduction of financial barriers to access, as is happening with prescription pharmaceuticals. Alternatively, it will encourage limits to the principle of comprehensiveness and what is covered. A current example, is that most provinces do not insure MRI, and the federal government has not challenged this on the grounds that it is a medically necessary service.

In the end, the federal and provincial governments and regional health authorities will be forced to use the breadth of supply- and demand-side management of health services to make them affordable. Furthermore, through whatever arrangement is negotiated, all governments committed to Medicare will need to share in funding it if they wish to deal with the leaks in the system that occur under universal and comprehensive coverage or to avoid financial barriers at the point of access.

Private Investment

Given the structure of Medicare to this point, the scope of private investment in health care is limited but probably will expand in terms of delivery and service provision, if not in the financing of services. Most dental, optical, and abortion services are not covered by Medicare; neither are out-of-hospital pharmaceuticals and a broad range of home and community-based services. These are the principal elements that account for the 30 percent of privately funded health care.

On supply side management, most hospitals and regional health authorities have consolidated nonclinical services such as food production and delivery, laundry, and some clinical laboratory services; varying degrees of the regional management of programs have been achieved. In most of these cases, private sector investment and involvement has helped to capitalize the changes, or the private sector has assumed operations. "Contracting out" has had a threatening and provocative effect on unions.

Will managed care be implemented in Canada? This question requires a careful definition of the term *managed care*. That matter aside, the regionalization of governance and management of services and the implementation of population-based funding formulas, together with the development of primary care models of delivery and alternate funding arrangements for doctors, makes the distinction between many features of the Canadian and American systems less apparent. The fundamental difference is, and likely will continue to be, who pays and how. In Canada, at present, legislation prohibits private insurance for services covered by Medicare. Nonprofit organizations like Blue Cross may act as intermediaries in processing and paying Medicare benefits, or may offer additional insurance for services not covered by Medicare. The market for private insurance may change if different directions are taken with regard to funding or to the delivery of services, or if the comprehensiveness of services included in Medicare is constrained.

Public Accountability

Regardless of how health care systems are funded or delivered, they exist to serve the needs of the public. Accordingly, purchasers and providers of care, as well as policymakers and administrators in Canada, have accountability to the public. The trend to greater consumer participation in health care decisions, together with the exploding use of the Internet, will rebalance the current asymmetry in health information availability and access between providers and patients. Canadians want to know more about their health, the health of others, and the health of the system itself. Public accountability means that they should be enabled to do this.

Accordingly, the key to accountability is providing user friendly, understandable information about health and health care. The Advisory Council on Health Infostructure recommended using Canada Health Infoway as a means of developing report cards. Council recommended that federal and provincial governments should work together to develop performance measures and to provide a fair evaluation of the health system to ensure accountability. The range and nature of indicators will, no doubt, foster a great deal of debate and analysis.

Reference

Noseworthy, T. W., and Jacobs, P. "The Health Care Industry: An Overview." In W. J. Sibbald and T. A. Massaro (eds.), *The Business of Critical Care: A Textbook for Clinicians Who Manage Special Care Units.* Armonk, N.Y.: Futura, 1996.

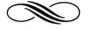

CHAPTER THIRTY-ONE

UNITED STATES OF AMERICA

Neelam Sekhri

The U.S. health care system is unique among wealthy industrialized countries in the extent of its reliance on the private sector for financing, purchasing, and delivering health care services. Public expenditures, through federal, state, and local governments, total 45 percent of overall health spending—primarily for purchasing health services for specific populations such as the elderly, disabled, and poor. The large majority of U.S. residents receive health insurance benefits through their employers and access services delivered by the private sector. Although the United States has established a system that is renowned worldwide for its advanced medical technology, excellent clinical quality, and consumer choice, the country still lacks a national policy of universal coverage for all of its population. Almost 44 million people are not covered by any continuous public or private health insurance scheme and have limited access to the United States' vast medical resources (Kronick and Gilmer, 1999).

At 13.5 percent, the United States devotes a higher percentage of its GDP to health care than any other country in the world. This percentage has remained essentially flat since 1992 and is attributable to the strong U.S. econ-

This chapter is adapted from Neelam Sekhri, Octavio Gómez-Dantés, and Tracy MacDonald, *Cross-Border Health Insurance: An Overview* (Oakland: California HealthCare Foundation, 1999). Copyright 1999, California HealthCare Foundation.

omy, the Balanced Budget Act of 1997, and the dramatic shift away from indemnity insurance into managed care plans. Although annual per capita health expenditures of US$4,094 in 1998 are still well above other OECD countries, they are growing more slowly than in the past (Health Care Financing Administration, 2000a).

Components of the Health Care System

Figure 31.1 shows an overview of the U.S. health care system; the funders and purchasers of health care are distinct from the providers of care. Different levels of purchasers further complicate the system. For example, employers may directly purchase health services from providers or may go through health insurers who in turn purchase services from providers. Similarly, managed care organizations may serve as insurers (pooling the risk) as well as providers of care, or they may only serve as insurers and purchase services from providers.

The major public funders of health care services are the federal government (for the Medicare program for the elderly) and the state and federal governments (for Medicaid programs for the poor and disabled). The federal and state governments also directly purchase health care for their own employees and dependents, for the armed forces, for veterans, and for certain special populations such as Native Americans.

Private funders are primarily employers who purchase health insurance benefits for their employees. Employees often share in the cost of these benefits. Individuals can also purchase health care services separately, either through purchasing private health insurance or directly paying providers on a fee-for-service basis.

The provision of health services in the United States is predominantly through private providers, including hospitals, integrated health care organizations (which link physicians, hospitals, and other providers), and physicians.

Financing and the Flow of Funds

As shown in Figure 31.2, despite the significant contribution of employers to health care, federal and state governments cover almost half the nation's bill for health care services.

Surprisingly, the heavy reliance on the private sector for financing health services has not resulted in significant individual out-of-pocket expenses for most

FIGURE 31.1. THE U.S. HEALTH CARE SYSTEM.

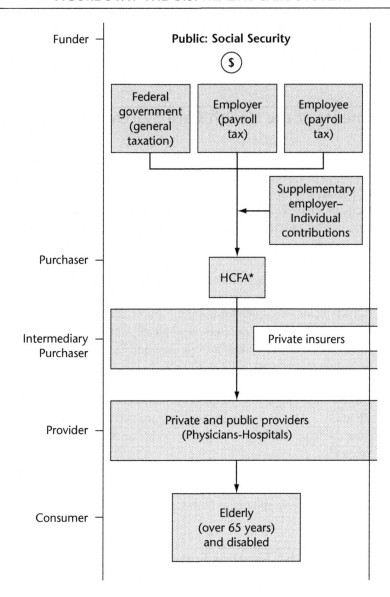

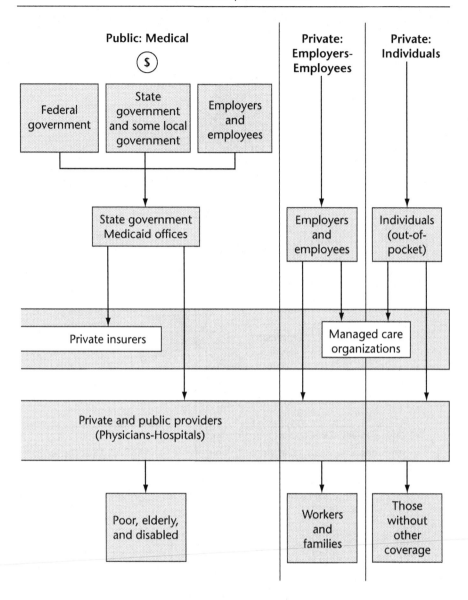

Source: Health Care Financing Administration.

FIGURE 31.2. FOLLOWING THE U.S. HEALTH CARE DOLLAR.

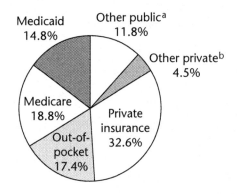

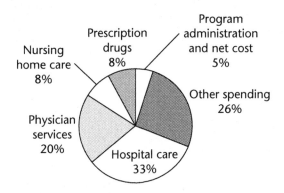

Source: Health Care Financing Administration.

[a]Includes programs such as workers' compensation, public health activity, Department of Defense, Department of Veterans Affairs, Indian Health Services, and state and local hospital and school health.

[b]Includes industrial in-plant, privately funded construction, and nonpatient revenues, including philanthropy.

Americans. Individual contributions account for only 17 percent of total health expenditures in the United States (Health Care Financing Administration, 2000b).

Public Sector Financing

Thirty percent of total expenditures for health originate with the federal government. The major categories of federal spending are

- The Medicare program for the elderly and disabled
- Shared funding with the states for Medicaid programs covering the poor
- Purchase of health services for federal employees
- Specific purchasing and delivery programs for veterans, Native Americans, military personnel, and other special populations

All states spend a significant portion of their annual budgets on health, primarily for Medicaid programs, which they finance jointly with the federal government. States also play a major role in regulating health facilities, health professionals, and health insurance.

County, district, and city governments expend resources on clinics and hospitals that they own and operate. Federal and state governments, while not insignificant, heavily subsidize these expenditures through various cost-sharing mechanisms.

Private Sector Financing

Employers are the major funders of health services for those under sixty-five years of age. Nearly all large government, public, and private employers, most medium-size private employers, and a minority of small private employers contribute to the cost of their employees' health care premiums (Astra USA, 1998).

Employers buy private health insurance as a tax-deductible business expense and provide it to employees and often their dependents as a tax-free benefit. Because health benefits represent a major cost of doing business for U.S. firms, many have taken an active role in trying to reduce or stabilize these costs in recent years. Strategies include (1) establishing business coalitions that exert power for reduced premiums with insurers and health plans, (2) eliminating or sharing the cost of coverage for dependents and family members, and (3) self-insuring for medical costs.

Individuals spend an average of US$711 out of pocket per year on health care services. These expenditures represent payments for services not covered by insurance, copayments, or deductibles, or through health insurance premiums.

Purchasing of Health Services

U.S. residents are covered by a variety of public and private health insurance programs. The major types are described next.

Medicare

In 1965 the U.S. government enacted legislation creating the Medicare health insurance program for the elderly and permanently disabled. Fourteen percent of the population currently receives coverage through the Medicare program (Hoechst Marion Roussel, 1997).

Workers contribute to Medicare through a payroll tax that funds hospital care and some skilled nursing care. Outpatient services are funded through revenues from premiums paid by Medicare beneficiaries and through general taxation. Beneficiaries can also purchase supplemental coverage from private insurers for outpatient prescription drugs, optometry, and other specialized services. Long-term care is not covered.

In fiscal year 1998, Medicare's costs totaled US$216 billion—about 20 percent of national health expenditures (Health Care Financing Administration, 2000a). To reduce the growth rate of these expenditures, the federal government has been actively encouraging Medicare beneficiaries to receive their health care services through managed care organizations (MCOs). The Medicare program contracts with these MCOs to provide coverage and health services on a per capita basis.

At this writing, Congress, the Clinton administration, and lobbyists for the pharmaceutical industry and for the elderly are debating whether and how to extend Medicare benefits to cover outpatient prescription drugs for the elderly. The administration initially favored an approach that would have established the federal government as a major purchaser of prescription drugs for Medicare beneficiaries. The pharmaceutical industry resisted this concept and contended it could lead to federal price controls on drugs. A compromise introduced by Congress and supported by the administration, the pharmaceutical industry, and advocates for the elderly would have Medicare beneficiaries purchasing prepaid outpatient prescription drug benefits from their choice of private insurers, with the federal government subsidizing their premiums. Advocates of major structural reforms of the Medicare program, however, are resisting this proposed compromise on the basis that any freestanding reform may raise barriers to future structural reforms.

Medicaid

Medicaid is a jointly funded federal and state health care coverage program that covers 36 million low-income individuals, including women, children, and the poor who are elderly, disabled, or blind. The program also covers those who are eligible to receive certain types of federal assistance (Urban Institute, 1997). Although children represent the largest category of Medicaid beneficiaries, spending is disproportionately directed toward the aged, blind, and disabled.

The number of children covered by Medicaid, already large at one-fifth of all children in the nation and one-third of all babies born in the United States, is growing significantly. Between 1985 and 1995 the number of Medicaid beneficiaries under age twenty-one nearly doubled, increasing from 9.8 million to 18.7 million. This growth is primarily due to mandatory and voluntary expansions of the program to cover children living in higher-income families (Urban Institute, 1997).

Federal regulations require that state Medicaid programs cover a minimum set of services, including hospitalization, physician care, and nursing home services. States then have the option of covering additional services, including prescription drugs, hospice care, and personal care services.

The disproportionately high spending for the disabled and elderly has resulted in a cost for each eligible beneficiary in 1995 of US$3,700 (Urban Institute, 1997). Due to escalating health costs, an increasing number of states have begun to shift all or a portion of Medicaid recipients into managed care programs.

Private Health Insurance

Nearly two-thirds of the non-elderly population in the United States is covered by private health insurance. Most of this coverage is employment-based, and 89 percent of these employees receive their coverage through managed care plans (Best Week Insurance News & Analysis, 1998).

Employers often "self-insure" for the health care costs of their workers. Rather than purchase health insurance from an established insurance company, firms that self-insure create a fund for medical costs and pay these expenses as they are incurred.

At this writing, Congress, the administration, and various interest groups are debating whether and how to protect "managed care patients' rights" when managed care plans deny coverage for services that arguably may be medically necessary. This debate has led to an unusual alliance. The politically conservative American Medical Association (AMA) is aligned with liberal Democrats and plaintiffs' lawyers in supporting the farthest-reaching proposal that would enable aggrieved managed care patients to sue their managed care plan for both denial of coverage and medical malpractice.

The AMA had earlier made another policy decision in its efforts to stem the growth of managed care plans in which physicians' professional prerogatives may be overridden by managed care plan administrators. At its 1999 annual meeting, the AMA amended its long-standing policy against physicians unionizing. It now supports and facilitates physicians who organize collective bargaining units and negotiate with managed care plans.

The Uninsured

Forty-four million Americans—nearly 18 percent of the population—had no health insurance coverage of any kind in 1996, and this number appears to be growing, especially among certain segments of the population such as children and immigrants (Kronick and Gilmer, 1999). A majority of those without regular health insurance coverage are employed persons and their dependents, whose employers do not provide health insurance as a benefit of employment. These individuals often cannot afford to purchase insurance and do not qualify for publicly funded programs.

The uninsured often defer preventive or primary care services, relying instead on episodic urgent or emergency care. The costs of this care are absorbed directly by providers and indirectly borne by other purchasers, including state health departments, taxpayers, and health insurers. As the pressures for cost containment grow, however, such cross-subsidies for the uninsured are being threatened.

Indemnity Insurance and Managed Care

Under traditional indemnity insurance, the money follows the patient. Patients select health care providers and visit them as they choose. Providers then bill the insurer or government agency and are reimbursed on a fee-for-service or per case basis, with little or no constraint on patient utilization.

This form of insurance is rapidly disappearing. Currently, managed care covers 89 percent of workers with employer-sponsored benefits (Best Week Insurance News & Analysis, 1998). In 1996, 12.8 million Medicaid beneficiaries and Medicare beneficiaries were enrolled in managed care programs (Urban Institute, 1997).

Managed care describes a continuum of arrangements in which purchasers contract with selected providers to deliver a defined set of services at an agreed-upon, per capita or per service price. Managed care plans have been successful in controlling costs and improving quality by

- Giving providers and patients incentives to use services cost-effectively
- Promoting delivery systems that monitor and coordinate care through the entire range of services (primary care through tertiary services)
- Providing access to preventive and primary care services and encouraging the provision of care in the most appropriate setting (such as outpatient clinics)

In practice, managed care encompasses a wide range of arrangements, some of which resemble a traditional private practice (such as PPOs) and others, like many HMOs, that are tightly managed, integrated systems.

Real and potential benefits of managed care include its emphasis on prevention and wellness, integration of services, promotion of primary care providers, and focus on population-based measures of quality. Real and potential disadvantages of managed care include restricted access to care, incentives for providers to skimp on patient care, and, ironically, an underinvestment in preventive care.

Health Care Providers

The delivery of health care services in the United States is predominantly private and occurs in a variety of settings and by various provider groups.

Hospitals

U.S. hospitals are primarily (70 percent) community-based, nonprofit institutions. Government-owned hospitals are usually operated by counties and states and provide care for low-income and uninsured (usually urban) populations (Health Care Financing Administration, 2000a). Those with insurance receive most of their hospital care in private facilities.

Since 1992 both the number of hospital admissions and of hospital bed days have decreased significantly. As the demand for hospital care has shifted to ambulatory and home health settings, occupancy rates have plunged, leaving some hospitals in precarious financial positions.

A recent study by the American Hospital System Institute concluded that if the entire population were enrolled in managed care plans with lengths-of-stay at HMO rates, and all hospitals averaged 67 percent occupancy, there would be 447,545 excess hospital beds (48 percent of the current capacity) (Astra USA, 1998).

Physicians

Most physicians in the United States, both primary care practitioners and specialists, are in some form of private practice. Thirty-nine percent operate solo practices, and 61 percent are in group practices of two or more physicians, based on 1995 data (American Medical Association, 1996). The majority of nonfederal physicians contract with one or more managed care organizations, and an increasing number receive all their compensation from managed care plans.

Average net income for nonfederal physicians increased by nearly 66 percent from 1985 to 1994 but has remained relatively flat for the past several years. During the same period, the supply of physicians has exceeded population growth by 18 percent. In a joint statement, the AMA, the National Medical Association, and representatives of U.S. medical schools announced that "the United States is on the verge of a serious oversupply of physicians" and recommended a 20 percent decrease in the number of physicians being trained (Astra USA, 1998).

The United States has a higher ratio of specialists to primary care physicians than either of its North American neighbors. With the rapid spread of managed care, however, demand for primary care providers (PCPs) has grown dramatically. PCPs are becoming coordinators of clinical care for their patients and managing referrals to specialists. Today PCPs account for almost 40 percent of the U.S. physician supply (Health Care Financing Administration, 2000a). One study estimated that if 40–65 percent of the population were enrolled in plans that capitated physicians and demand for physician services were at the rate for HMOs, the supply of specialists would outstrip the demand by 60 percent by the year 2000 (Weiner, 1994).

Other Providers

Outpatient services are provided through private physician offices and a growing number of primary care and specialty care clinics, rural health centers, ambulatory surgery centers, and family planning clinics. Some of these are freestanding; some are chain-operated. Hospitals, managed care plans, or various levels of government own others. Like hospitals, clinics may be public or private, for-profit, or not-for-profit.

As the U.S. population ages and as illnesses can increasingly be managed without acute hospitalization, a significant industry has developed around home health care, skilled nursing facilities, and long-term care.

Pharmaceuticals

Expenditures for drugs as a percentage of total health expenditures have been declining for the past thirty years in the United States (Astra USA, 1998). This decline, however, is due primarily to controls on physicians' choices of drugs and to discounted purchasing rather than to declines in the retail price of drugs. Drug prices have been escalating at rates of up to 15 percent annually.

Since 1992 the annual rate of growth for pharmaceuticals has ranged from a low of 7.0 percent in 1994 to a high of 12.3 percent in 1998 (Hilman and others, 1999). Spending for prescription drugs accounted for 8 percent of personal health spending in 1998 and was responsible for 20 percent of the increase in health spending for that year (Levit and others, 2000).

Most private insurers provide drug coverage, at least for inpatient drugs. Managed care plans have extended outpatient drug coverage to the general population and to the elderly. They are increasingly adopting formularies, however, that limit the group of drugs covered or provide full coverage for generic drugs and impose higher copayments for brand-name drugs. Managed care companies have also created pharmaceutical benefits management systems based on clinical practice guidelines for the management of chronic diseases. In addition, large managed care plans negotiate highly discounted purchasing contracts, having a significant effect on the pharmaceutical industry.

Health Status

Despite spending more on health care than any other nation in the world, the United States compares unfavorably to other developed countries on most measures of health status, including life expectancy at birth, infant mortality, immunization levels, and rates of avoidable death. Like most wealthy, industrialized countries, the main causes of death in the U.S. population are cardiovascular diseases, cancer, cerebrovascular diseases, and accidents.

The strong reliance on private sector financing and provision has made it difficult for the United States to set health status targets as a nation. A recent breakthrough in this area is an initiative called "Healthy People 2010," which is a cooperative effort by the public and private sectors to set goals for national health promotion and disease prevention for the year 2010. The broad objectives of this initiative are to increase the span of healthy life for all Americans, reduce disparities in health status, and achieve universal access to preventive health care services.

Health Care Regulation

Strong regulation of health care services exists in the United States and is largely the responsibility of state governments and independent accreditation organizations. The federal government regulates the interstate trade of medical supplies and the licensing of pharmaceuticals and medical devices.

Hospital licensure is a state responsibility. In addition, to receive Medicare funding, hospitals must achieve accreditation through the Joint Commission on Accreditation of Healthcare Organizations (JCAHO). This private, nonprofit organization surveys hospitals and health care systems and certifies those that meet its standards.

States are responsible for licensing physicians, sanctioning them for malpractice, and reporting sanctions to the federal government. They also regulate other health professions and occupations, including registered nurses, physical therapists, and ancillary staff such as respiratory therapists and medical assistants. There have been few efforts over the past decades to establish workforce targets for most health professionals; hence, shortages and surpluses of nurses and other health care personnel have occurred at various times.

States are also responsible for regulating the health insurance industry and managed care organizations. Regulating bodies and standards often differ significantly among states. For example, the Department of Corporations in California is responsible for licensing HMOs, whereas the State Insurance Commissioner oversees the operation of traditional indemnity insurers. In some states, all MCOs are licensed by the Department of Insurance; in others, separate agencies are established for MCOs. Regulations require compliance with stringent financial standards, and managed care organizations must demonstrate appropriate access to services and meet patient satisfaction standards.

Although the federal government continues debating whether to enact some form of a managed care patients' bill of rights, many states have extended their regulation of managed care plans to include various measures for increasing consumer protection.

Regulation of the Quality of Care

Measuring and regulating the quality of services is an important issue facing the U.S. health care system. The measurement of quality has historically emphasized the technical aspects of care delivery through licensure and certification activities. In recent years, however, there has been a movement toward research on health care outcomes. Many managed care organizations are leading quality outcomes research and the creation of clinical practice guidelines to identify and promote best practices in caring for patients with specific conditions.

The National Committee for Quality Assurance (NCQA) conducts a voluntary accreditation program for managed care plans. In collaboration with employers and managed care organizations, NCQA has developed a set of indicators of performance, or "report cards," called the Health Plan Employer Data and Information Set (HEDIS). HEDIS includes measures on preventive care, access to screening services, and patient satisfaction indicators.

Augmenting HEDIS, managed care plans are increasingly issuing their own performance-focused report cards, typically focusing on gross indicators of performance such as levels of immunization among children and the prevalence and frequency of cancer screening.

The measurement of quality and quality improvement is a dynamic field, and there is a great need to improve indicators and systems for measuring outcomes and adjusting for risk factors such as comorbidity, severity of illness, and demography in quality comparisons.

Challenges

Major challenges face the U.S. health care system today. Like most countries, the United States is grappling with escalating health care costs. At the same time, the nation has been unable to guarantee access to health care for all residents and must address these inequities.

The key challenges for the U.S. health system include the following:

• *Ensuring equitable access to health care for everyone.* The large number of people who are uninsured and who have inadequate access to health care continues to be an embarrassment for the wealthiest nation on earth. New ways to address this issue must be explored, although there are widely divergent opinions on how this problem can be solved. Some combination of market-based reforms and expansions of public programs are the most likely solutions. Current reform efforts are beginning to address equity issues for children. Medicaid reforms may result in greater access for Medicaid recipients through MCOs and expansion of eligibility.

• *Developing strategies to control escalating costs.* Although managed care has had a significant impact on rising costs, the "managed care backlash" is now a key political issue that necessitates new models that build on managed care principles but are more responsive to patients and providers. At the same time, the U.S. population is aging. This demographic shift poses challenges to the health care system, as more and more people live longer with chronic conditions, placing an additional financial burden on the federal government.

• *Measuring quality and ensuring value for the health care dollar.* As mentioned earlier, research on clinical effectiveness and the creation and adoption of best practices are areas that will require major effort in the next several years.

Plans and Proposals for Reform

In 1994 President Clinton proposed an elaborate health reform scheme that would have expanded insurance coverage to millions of U.S. residents primarily through private sector efforts. The proposal, which many believe was too complex and far-reaching, failed to pass in Congress and was never enacted. Incremental reforms of the health care system, however, are occurring in the public sector as well as in the private health care market. These reforms address some of the challenges confronting U.S. health care and are described next.

Increased Access Through Extension of Coverage

In the Balanced Budget Act (BBA) of 1997, the U.S. Congress established a goal to reduce the number of uninsured children in the United States from 10 million to 2 million by the year 2002. The State Child Health Insurance Program (SCHIP) was passed to expand access to health care services for children through less restrictive Medicaid eligibility, enhanced outreach, subsidy of private coverage, and the creation of new health insurance programs for children. Twenty-four billion federal dollars over the next five years have been allocated for this effort (Urban Institute, 1997).

Because of SCHIP, states have new authority and greater flexibility in restructuring their Medicaid programs and in developing programs for uninsured children. States can target children who are not receiving welfare and whose parents are employed in low-wage jobs that do not offer health insurance coverage.

Insurance reforms, which guarantee greater portability of health insurance coverage when individuals leave their employment and place restrictions on exclusions to care, have been enacted. These reforms also expand coverage to those with preexisting conditions and chronic illnesses.

A step in the other direction (reducing access to health care) was taken in the form of the Personal Responsibility and Work Opportunity Reconciliation Act of 1996 (PRWORA). This act makes major changes in the eligibility of legally admitted immigrants for health insurance under the Medicaid program. Prior to 1996, legal immigrants were eligible for the full range of Medicaid benefits, whereas undocumented (illegal) immigrants were eligible only for emergency benefits. Under the new welfare reform law, with certain exceptions, noncitizen immigrants who arrive in the United States after August 1996 will be barred from Medicaid, although they may still be covered for emergency services.

Cost Containment

In 1997 the Medicare program initiated its most significant reform since the inception of the program in 1965 through the creation of Medicare Part C. This reform is aimed at encouraging Medicare beneficiaries to enroll in managed care arrangements and will allow direct contracting between provider organizations and the Medicare program, eliminating the role of the insurer or managed care organization. In addition, the types of managed care options available to beneficiaries will be significantly increased.

Many state Medicaid agencies have launched extensive reforms in recent years to enroll Medicaid beneficiaries in MCOs. For Medicaid recipients, this represents an opportunity for increased access to private providers who, historically, have hesitated to see Medicaid patients due to poor fee-for-service reimbursement. In 1996, Medicaid enrollment in HMOs increased 30.6 percent to 12.8 million enrollees nationwide. California, Tennessee, and Florida led these increases (Hoechst Marion Roussel, 1997).

Private Sector Reforms

Notwithstanding the reforms just described, the most dramatic changes in the U.S. health care system are occurring not because of government legislation but due to forces at work in the private health care market. The most significant features of these market-driven reforms are described in the sections that follow.

Disease Management

Managing disease through the continuum of care has been an exciting area of development in U.S. health care. Shifting from fee-for-service, in which providers are paid for sickness, to capitation, in which they are paid to keep people well, has generated innovative practices and launched dozens of enterprises focused on better managing the quality and costs of the chronically ill. These companies have accumulated valuable evidence on the most effective treatment protocols, how to involve patients and families in the care of chronic illnesses, how to promote compliance with drug and treatment regimens, and the most appropriate settings for each level of care. It can be argued that many of the programs that have been developed lead the world in providing high-quality, comprehensive care for difficult chronic syndromes at reasonable cost.

Quality Measurement

Managed care firms have used several techniques that represent progress toward improving the quality of health care. These include using guidelines based on clinical best practices, developing quality report cards that provide information about providers and health plan performance, and using evidence-based medicine that incorporates the latest clinical findings and cost-effectiveness data. Although the data-gathering and comparison methodologies still need refinement, they have served as a catalyst for insurers and providers to develop population health management and measurement programs.

Alignment of Incentives

There has been a great deal of experimentation on how best to pay providers and structure incentives for cost-effectiveness, productivity, and quality. A significant amount of information has been gathered on different ways to blend capitation and fee-for-service payments for providers. Of particular global interest are structures that contain costs by limiting the unnecessary or inappropriate use of the health care system. For example, a recent study of the impact of financial incentives on the use and cost of prescription drugs found that the introduction of a $10 copay was "almost as effective at controlling drug spending as is switching physician payment from fee-for-service to a capitated risk payment" (Hilman and others, 1999).

Conclusion

The United States is once again at a crossroads in how it manages the conflicting priorities of equitable access and affordability. Although managed care has been the single most significant contributor to cost containment, strong public and provider reaction against some managed care excesses have slowed the growth of the most tightly managed models of care such as HMOs (Health Care Advisory Board, 1995).

There is growing evidence that the original managed care practices, which place a heavy emphasis on control of specialist referrals and strict restrictions on provider practice, have achieved the maximum savings of which they are capable. Large HMOs have experienced significant financial losses in recent years, and managed care premiums are rising after many years of flat or declining rates.

Some analysts cite the trend toward investor-owned HMOs and managed care plans as one reason for this industry's current financial problems. When the federal government amended its national health policy to include the promotion of HMOs by adopting the HMO Act of 1973, only about two dozen health plans met its criteria for an HMO; the majority were nonprofit organizations. Today the majority of HMOs and managed care plans are for-profit, investor-owned organizations. Their critics contend that managements are too vulnerable to making financial decisions based on pressures to maximize short-term financial returns.

Whatever the next generation of managed care holds, many managed care practices are attracting international interest. OECD and middle-income countries wish to benefit from the experience of both the United States and other countries in such areas as quality measurement and improvement, disease management, and incentive structures. These experiences are relevant and applicable across a wide range of European Community, Eastern European, and Latin American health care systems. It is clear that market-based reforms will continue to provide learning opportunities for health care systems globally.

References

American Medical Association. *Physician Marketplace Statistics, 1995.* Chicago: American Medical Association, Center for Health Policy Research, 1996.

Astra USA. *Compass Report on Health Care.* Vol. 1: *The Direction and Alignment of Health Care Systems.* Westborough, Mass.: Astra USA, 1998.

Best Week Insurance News and Analysis. *Four Year Trends Show Drop in HMO Net Income Despite Steady Rises in Enrollments, Revenues.* Nov. 9, 1998. [www.bestweek.com].

Health Care Advisory Board. *Emerging from Shadow: Resurgence to Prosperity Under Managed Care.* Washington, D.C.: Advisory Board Co., 1995.

Health Care Financing Administration. "Highlights of National Health Expenditures, 1998." [http://www.hcfa.gov/stats/nhe oact/hilites.htm]. Jan. 10, 2000a.

Health Care Financing Administration, Office of the Actuary: National Health Statistics Group. "Personal Healthcare Expenditures Aggregate and Per Capita Amounts and Percent Distribution, by Source of Funds: Selected Calendar Years, 1960–98." [www.hcfa.org]. 2000b.

Hilman, R., and others. "Financial Incentives and Drug Spending in 'Managed Care.'" *Health Affairs,* 1999, *18*(2), 189–199.

Hoechst Marion Roussel. *Managed Care Digest Series, 1997: HMO-PPO/Medicare-Medicaid Digest.* Kansas City, Mo.: Hoechst Marion Roussel, 1997.

Kronick, R., and Gilmer, T. "Explaining the Decline in Health Insurance Coverage, 1979–1995." *Health Affairs,* 1999, *18*(2), 30–47.

Levit, K., and others. "Health Spending in 1998: Signals of Change." *Health Affairs,* 2000, *19*(1).

Urban Institute. *Medicaid: National and State Estimates.* Washington, D.C., Urban Institute, 1997.

Weiner, J. "Forecasting the Effects of Health Reform on U.S. Physician Workforce Requirement." *Journal of the American Medical Association,* 1994, *272*(3), 222–230.

INDEX

A

ABRAMGE (Brazilian Group Medicine Association), 222, 223, 224, 225

ABRASPE (Brazilian Association of Company Services), 223

ACC (Accident Compensation Corporation) [New Zealand], 310

Accident Insurance Act of 1998 (New Zealand), 309–310

Accidental Logics (Tuohy), 7

Accreditation. *See* Global health care accreditation

Act to Strengthen Solidarity in SHI (Germany), 146, 150

Acute medical care (The Netherlands), 130–131

Adams, O. B., 34

Advertising regulations, 68

Advisory Council on Health Infostructure (Canada), 377, 380

Aetna International, 43–44

Aetna U.S. Healthcare, 47

Agenda for Leadership in Programs for Healthcare Accreditation (ALPHA), 85, 86

AHMOPI (Philippines), 290

AID (U.S. Agency for International Development) Quality Assurance Project, 83

AID Quality Assurance Project II, 89

AIG (American International Group) [Hong Kong], 335

AIH (*Autorização da Internação Hospitalar*) system (Brazil), 220

Alma Alta Declaration (New Zealand), 304

Altenstetter, C., 23, 139

Alternative medicine: Chinese health care system and, 327; Malaysian health care system and, 276

AMA (American Medical Association), 389–390, 392

AMA (Australian Medical Association), 301

AMA's CPT codes, 47

Amelung, V. E., 150

American Association of Health Plans (AAHP), 74

American Hospital Institute study, 391

American Medical Association (AMA), 73

Anderson, G. F., 1, 24, 307

Anglo American Corporation, 58–59

Annual Plan, 1997–1998 (Hospital Authority), 334

Anti-kickback laws, 70

Argentine health care system: background of, 230–231; described, 229–230; future developments of, 235–236; initiative for change of, 233–235; investments/opportunities of, 235; *Mandatarias* of, 234–235; medical providers of, 233; structure and organization of, 231–233; work-related accident coverage separation from, 235

Assurance-maladie. See French health care system

Australia, 84–85

Australian health care system: cost containment of, 298–299; historical context of, 295–297; hospitals of, 300; Medicare programs of, 297; opportunities of,

401